D0768698

DATE DUE

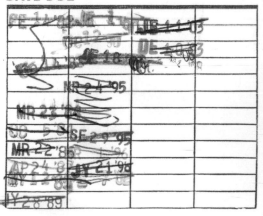

MANTRAS
Words of Power

MANTRAS
Words of Power

Swami Sivananda Radha

Timeless Books

(*publishers of timeless wisdom*)

ISBN 0-931454-05-0

Library of Congress Cataloging in Publication Data

Sivananda Radha, Swami, 1911-
    Mantras: Words of Power
    Bibliography: p.
    Includes Index
    1. Mantras   2. Yoga   I. Title
    BL1226.3.S57   294.5'43   80-10293

Book Design by Richard A. Reeves.

Published by

Box 60
Porthill, ID 83853

in association with
Yasodhara Ashram Society
Box 9, Kootenay Bay
B.C. V0B 1X0 Canada

Printed and Bound in Canada

Dedicated. . .

To Swami Sivananda Saraswati of Rishikesh, India
and all the Gurus before him who have
prepared the Path.

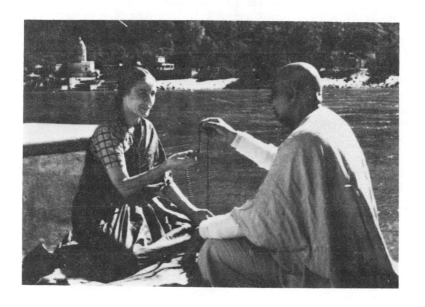

*Know that by prostration, by question and service,
the wise who have realised the Truth will instruct
thee in that knowledge.*

• from the *Bhagavad Gita* •

vi

Acknowledgements

The publication of this book is an effort of many years preparation and involves the patience, time and energy of a "team," a group of individuals who have both knowingly and unknowingly made their contributions.

My gratitude initially goes to those who were my teachers at Sivananda Ashram in India: Swami Nada Brahmananda, my music guru who instructed me in Mantra chanting; Swami Venkatesananda who, when I went through arduous training and despaired, would quietly play on his veena and lift my spirits by the power of the Mantra; Professor Shastri who gave me the theory and history of Mantras; and to Swami Saradananda who took the photographs.

There have been many others who have given encouragement and financial assistance. In the actual production of the book, the high calibre of the editors, designers and printers is evidence of their dedication to the Work. To all of them I express my deep gratitude.

preceding page:

Swami Radha receiving her mala from Swami Sivananda
on the day of her Mantra initiation in India in 1955.

CONTENTS

Mantras: Words of Power

Mantras

Mantras: Guru & Disciple
Excerpts from the Writings of Swami Sivananda Saraswati

Cover and title page illustrations:
The Archer, a Thai sculpture, is one of the pieces of Oriental art from the author's collection. It depicts the moment of the aspirant having released the arrow (the tool or practice, in this case the Mantra) to meet the target which will be the goal decided upon at various levels until the final target of Liberation is hit.

List of Illustrations

MANTRAS
Words of Power

Chapter One

What is Mantra?

A mantra is a combination of sacred syllables which forms a nucleus of spiritual energy. This serves as a magnet to attract or a lens to focus spiritual vibrations. According to the Upanishads, the ancient scriptures of India, the original abode of the Mantra was the Parma Akasha or primaeval ether, the eternal and immutable substratum of the universe, out of which, in the uttering of the primal sound Vach, the universe itself was created. (This same account is found in the Gospel of St. John, "In the beginning was the Word.") The Mantras existed within this ether and were there directly perceived by the ancient Rishis, or seers, who translated them into an audible pattern of words, rhythm and melody.

The root *man* in the word *Mantra* means in Sanskrit "to think"; *tra* comes from *trai*, meaning "to protect or free from the bondage of *samsara* or the phenomenal world." Therefore *Mantra* means, "the thought that liberates and protects." But there are many levels of meaning in a Mantra which must be experienced to be truly understood. An intellectual explanation encompasses only a very small part of its meaning.

The chanting or recitation of mantras activates and accelerates the creative spiritual force, promoting harmony in all parts of the human being. The devotee is gradually converted into a living center of spiritual vibration which is attuned to some other center of vibration vastly more powerful. This energy can be appropriated and directed for the benefit of the one who uses it and that of others.

Every Mantra has six aspects: a *Rishi* or seer, a *raga* or melody, a *Devata* or presiding deity, a *Bija* or seed sound, *Sakti* or power and *Kilaka* or pillar.

The *Rishis*, through their intuitive perception, opened themselves to the revelation of the Mantras and were able to recognize their own effectiveness as channels for the flow of grace, knowledge and power from the Divine. These ancient seers understood that their powers were intended to be used in the service of others, as a guide to mankind.

The Mantras were transmitted from generation to generation, from Guru to disciple, and in this process the power of the Mantras was greatly increased. The repetition billions of times by countless devotees over the centuries has brought about a vast reservoir of power which augments the inherent spiritual potency of the Mantras.

The raga is comparable to a western melody line — a sound, or sequence of single sounds, without harmony. When chanting a Mantra it is extremely important that the raga and its key should not be changed, because the rate of vibrations on which the sound is based is an integral part. All Indian music is based on the understanding that there are two aspects to every sound: the audible expression; and the subtle sound-essence which carries the meaning and which arises from the eternal Spirit. This essence is called *Shabda* or *Vach*. When the spoken word is perfectly sounded within and without, contact is made with this power which manifests as an image.

There is a certain power in a word even on a human level — one's own name has a special significance, and the way in which it is pronounced can convey numerous messages. Different tones cause different vibrations affecting the bodily, as well as the emotional, response.

The practice of Mantra Yoga for a long period of time makes one aware of sounds actually creating images, and of certain images having an inherent sound.

In his book "Japa Yoga" Swami Sivananda Sarasvati says that sounds are vibration which give rise to definite forms. The repeated chanting of the name of the Lord gradually builds up the form or special manifestation of the deity worshipped (the *Devata*) and acts as a focus to concentrate this influence, which then penetrates and becomes the center of consciousness of the worshipper.

The *Devata* is the presiding deity of the Mantra, the informing power, a very personal aspect of God. It is the wisdom that comes from a higher source and is like a single beam of sunlight, one beam that is singled out and given a name so that the disciple can develop a personal relationship and worship an aspect of God that he or she can understand. In the beginning, God is too awesome for the human mind to grasp and only later can the Divine Energy be perceived in its pure form.

Each Mantra has a *Bija* or seed. This is the essence of the Mantra and gives it special power — self-generating power. Just as within a seed is hidden a tree, so the energy in the Mantra is the seed from which will grow a beautiful spiritual being.

The *Kilaka*, or pillar, is at first the driving force, the persistence and will-power that the disciple needs to pursue the Mantra. But when the power of the Mantra begins to take on a self-generating "flywheel motion," the kilaka becomes a very fine thread joining the disciple to the Mantra, to the power of the Mantra, to the Guru and to the Deity, until all become one.

The power, the consciousness within the Mantra, is *Sakti*, Divine Mother, the Goddess of the Spoken Word. The male aspect of God is energy in a state of equilibrium; the female aspect is dynamic energy which manifest as creation. There is only one Energy in all created things; in the Mantra that energy is present in pure form. The potency of the Mantra is released through repetition until the individual finally comes to his or her *Devata* (the particular aspect of the Divine associated with the Mantra) and a spiritual experience may take place.

"Mananat Trayate Iti Mantrah" means that by constant recollection or thinking of the Mantra one is protected from the impact of Maya, the illusory world. Through repetition of these words of power, the goal of Mantra Yoga is achieved — that is (as with all Yogas) unity of individual consciousness with Cosmic Consciousness.

Mantra is not prayer. Prayer consists of words of supplication chosen by the spiritual aspirant, while Mantra is a precise combination of words and sounds — the embodiment of a particular form of consciousness or Sakti.

Mantra is the song of a star. . .
and it will transport you to that star.

Chapter Two

Mantra and Japa Yoga

Mantra Yoga is one of the manifold Yogas, of which there are about 40, all intertwined like threads of a cloth. The four principal ones are: Bhakti Yoga, the Yoga of love and devotion; Karma Yoga, the Yoga of action, of selfless service; Jnana Yoga, the Yoga of knowledge and wisdom; and Raja Yoga, called the "Kingly Yoga," a combination of several Yogas based on the Yoga Sutras of Patanjali. One type of spiritual practice is sufficient to attain God realization, but since there is an interaction of the body forces, the Yogas cannot be totally separated. Also because of physical problems, such as restlessness, poor blood circulation, it is recommended that several different Yogas be included in a balanced practice.

The chanting of a Mantra is called Mantra Yoga. When the Mantra is spoken aloud, this is known as Vaikhari Japa; when whispered or hummed it is Upamsu Japa; when repetition is mental it is Manasika Japa; written Mantra is called Likhita Japa.

The use of Mantra in any of these forms is effective in securing single-pointedness of mind. The most subtle, Manasika Japa, although it is very powerful, may be difficult for those who are just beginning a Mantra practice. Alternating it with vocal repetition helps to keep the mind from wandering. Likhita can be done in any script, in any language, but should be consistent for the chosen length of time. This repetitive writing brings peace, poise and strength within, and may also be used to alternate with the other forms of Japa.

Chanting a Mantra with devotion and concentration attunes the individual through divine melody and has a harmonious influence over the whole body and mind. It is most important to use the correct raga (melody) always, since precise rules govern the interrelation and sequences of sound. Each raga, which is a particular combination of sound, is claimed to reflect the laws of the universe and to be in perfect harmony with it at the time it is sounded. Since sound results from the union of breath and intellect of the human being, the one who chants will be brought to harmony also.

Through constant repetition of the Mantra one becomes like a magnet attracting the spiritual power of the Mantra to oneself and becoming aware of the Self. This repetition gradually awakens the higher faculties in a person and raises the consciousness towards the level of the Mantric resonance. According to Vedic teaching, "A Mantra has the power of releasing the Cosmic and Supra-cosmic Consciousness," and it bestows freedom, ultimate illumination and immortality. Not only does the singer benefit, but also those who listen and attune themselves to the spirit of the singing. This serves not only as an aid to meditation but is, in fact, a form of meditation in itself.

Chanting produces a whole series of psychological and spiritual effects. The concentration brings a deep sense of peace and joy, as often arises with other forms of meditation. The Mantra serves the same function as the "koan" in Zen or the mandala of Tibetan Buddhism: it functions as a device for focusing the ordinarily dispersed powers of the mind to a sharp point that is capable of penetrating through the sifting sands of thoughts to the deeper layers of mind beneath.

When a Mantra has been received from a Guru, the power of that Mantra increases after the initiation. As the initiate practices, the

Mantra becomes a self-generating force, uniting the individual with this power. Through your own efforts you are drawn towards the chain of Gurus who have found Realization through the use of the Mantra. In due time, you must become a link in that chain.

By reciting the Mantra you carry its force and power, and this will be a blessing for all those you meet. At times the Mantric Power may take over so that it will not even be necessary to speak. As a person, as a mind, you do not need to get involved. This is a much more valuable communication which can take place on the soul level.

The practice of this form of Yoga is as effective today as in former times, and is still taught and practiced by the Gurus and spiritual teachers of India. In fact, it is said that Mantra Shastra is the easiest means by which the aspirant may reach Self-realization in the present era. Mantras are used at every significant step of the religious life in the Indian spiritual tradition. In the Guru/disciple relationship, both are under an obligation throughout their lives to chant the Mantra which has been given to the disciple. It constitutes a permanent spiritual link between them.

Mantra is an accumulation of power that is activated by the one who practises it, drawing this power to oneself and merging in it through surrender. Through the use of Mantra, one becomes conscious of the self, beginning with a small "s" and expanding the awareness that will eventually lead to becoming aware of the Self with a capital "S". This results eventually in achieving unity of the lower and the Higher Self. Mantra leads the Spirit, lost in trivialities and worldly pursuits, back to pure Essence.

Om Krishna Guru Om Krishna Guru Om Krishna Guru Om Krishna Guru Om Krishna Guru Om Krishna Guru Om Krishna Guru Om Krishna Guru Om Krishna Guru Om Krishna Guru Om Krishna Guru Om Krishna Guru Om Krishna Guru Om Krishna Guru Om Krishna Guru Om Krishna Guru Om Krishna Guru Om Krishna Guru Om Krishna

Chapter Three

Mantra Practice

When you begin to recite and practice Mantra you need to clarify to yourself what you want to achieve. What are your ideals? You can rightfully pin your hopes on the Mantra to help bring these ideals into manifestation in your life in the purest form possible. But to what extent and how soon this will come to pass depends on you. Obviously, the more you put into it the more you will achieve. The pearl exacts its price.

As you chant, observe the mind. You may be shocked at how easily the mind can be side-tracked and how quickly you get bored. You may even begin to doubt your sincerity in desiring God or desiring to become single-pointed, as you watch the mind finding 95,000 excuses. Perhaps you will tell yourself that doing a charitable act would be a more worthwhile way to spend the time. But you are missing the point when you start thinking this way. You will be of far more help to others when you have gained some spiritual power.

The choice of the Mantra is extremely important because the greatest success lies with the Mantra to which you can best surrender. There is a specific Mantra for each person — their Ishta Mantra. This does not mean that no two people will have the same Mantra. However, in Nada Yoga, the Yoga of sound, there is a particular sound, a particular vibration to which your body will best respond. The Mantra that is designated for you corresponds to your spiritual nature.

There are many ways in which a Mantra may be chosen. You can chant a Mantra to which you simply feel drawn and naturally attracted. Or, if you are fortunate enough to find a true Guru, your Guru may choose the Mantra to which you are best suited.

Having chosen or been given your Mantra, stay with it until you have had some experience of its power. Resist the temptation to change to another one, thinking perhaps you made the wrong choice, or because you are bored or because the high notes are too difficult for you to reach. Begin with one Mantra and lay a good foundation. Only at a much later stage of your development can you use two or three Mantras simultaneously.

In the practice of Japa Yoga, a mala is used to assist in counting the repetitions of the name of a Divine aspect such as Siva or Divine Mother. A mala is a string of 108 beads, usually made of sandalwood, tulsi, or rudraksha seeds. The number 108 is a holy number. 1 means one line, symbolizing God, the Supreme Energy, the power from which all other lines, circles or movements come. 0 is completeness, a circle representing God's creation as complete and perfect. 8 is the sign of eternity — creation goes on eternally, so this brings in the time element. Time can be stretched or compressed. This understanding comes only through practice.

The mind is constantly moving, using energy unproductively because the "mental background noises" mostly concern past or future events. Life is a chain of cause and effect. The beads of the mala are also an endless chain and the endless thoughts are now given with each bead a specified, significant meaning relating to the particular Mantra. There is a special bead called Mount Meru where the mala is tied together. When the fingers reach Mount Meru, the mala should be turned and the movement continued the other way. This bead symbolizes God-realization and each time you reach it you have a reminder that you do not have to continue the chain of cause and effect. Another reminder is given in holding the mala at heart level, signifying the devotional aspect of this practice, the attempt to transcend the lower levels of being.

The use of a mala gives the body some activity and thereby releases nervous energy or restlessness. The beads are moved between the third (ring) finger and the thumb, never the first (index) finger and thumb, as the Mantra is repeated with each bead. Through use of the beads they take on some of the energy of the user and they become spiritualized. The mala is made from the tulsi tree and is a little rough at first, but the beads become smooth from the practice. The mala should be worn around the neck with Mount Meru in front. Wearing the mala reminds you of your purpose in life, to realize God, the Self, because you feel it when you move in all your daily activities. Place it under your pillow or on your altar at night. Especially for the busy Western person the practice of the mala has therapeutic value because of its benefit of concentrating the mind, directing the emotions and focusing the body, all of which leads to the spiritual realm.

To get the greatest benefit from your Mantra practice, set a definite period of time aside each day and make a written commitment to yourself to continue the practice for a sufficient length of time that you can feel its effects. Three months is a good beginning. Begin small and build up — this develops enthusiasm and perseverance to handle greater things. Do not be over-ambitious, letting the ego convince you that you will be able to sustain a long period of chanting immediately. A little seedling needs the greatest care and attention. Handle your spiritual growth with at least as much care as you would a plant.

The recommended time for Mantra practice is four o'clock in the morning because at that hour there are few troubling vibrations in the air. However, this may be difficult unless you are living in an Ashram or by yourself. When you set your time for practice, remember that you should not chant for at least an hour and a half after meals. As you become accustomed to the idea, increase the time of practice. You will become very conscious of time, how you spend it and how, perhaps, you waste it. Make a practice of writing down everything that you do. See where you waste time and learn to be efficient so that you can find the time you want for spiritual practice.

Before beginning to chant take a bath, or at least wash your hands, face and feet. As you wash, think that the impurities of your mind are being washed away. Put on fresh clothes and think that your soul is being clothed with a new garment of a Divine nature. These thoughts will help to uplift you. Put into your mind a clear, commanding thought that your full attention will be given to chanting for a specific period of time. Free the mind of all other things by going through any worries or duties, firmly promising yourself that you will deal with them when your period of chanting is over but they are not to intrude on the time you have set aside to be holy.

Choose a quiet spot where you will not be disturbed and use it each time, facing north or east. Sit in a comfortable chair or on the floor with a cushion. If a cushion is used for support of the back, be sure that it is placed below the waist to straighten the spine, not to fill in the curve at the waist. There is a subtle power in the thought of straightening the spine, suggesting straightforwardness, thinking straight, moving with uprightness and strength.

Put down a pure wool blanket or a pure silk cloth at the place you have chosen. A deerskin or tigerskin are traditionally used for this purpose, to conserve energy and keep out the vibrations of the earth. We want to create a very different magnetism that will release us from the magnetism of the earth, from our needs and instincts, that will carry us to great heights of consciousness and awareness. A cloth of natural fibre covering the body fulfils the same function and helps to retain the spiritual vibrations you generate.

Sit on the floor with the left leg over the right, or in one of the traditional Yogic asanas such as *siddhasana* (the perfect pose), *padmasana* (the lotus), *vajrasan* (kneeling pose), or *sukhasan* (easy pose); or in a chair with your back straight. The spine must be straight so that the electrical current which is created or stimulated through the chanting can flow freely. A crooked spine is like a broken wire; sometimes the connection is made and sometimes it is not. From the Yogic point of view this pranic circuit of the body should be closed by crossing the ankles to maintain the beneficial effects of the Mantra. Rest the hands in your lap, with the palms up, thus suggesting surrender and receptivity to divine insights.

Before beginning to chant make sure that not only the large muscles of your body are relaxed, and the neck and shoulders, but also the muscles of the tongue, jaw, forehead and eyes. Focus the eyes gently on the space between your eyebrows.

As you chant, pull the abdominal muscles in, thus forcing the air out of the lungs. Let the chest widen by itself as the air comes in, not by lifting the shoulders. Use all the breath, all your energy. Put yourself completely into your chanting. It is important to breathe through your nose. The right kind of deep breathing will naturally begin to take place when you chant; there is no danger, as there is with some breathing exercises. Watch your breath and keep expelling it evenly.

Learn to sit motionless for increased periods of time and check the position of the body at the end of the time to be sure that your head, shoulders and back are straight, but relaxed, with the vertebrae one on top of the other.

To summarize: sit erect, relaxed, in a quiet place, on a piece of cloth of natural fibre, left leg crossed over right, hands in lap, palms up. Deal with objections and obstacles before you start to chant, then give yourself a clear commanding thought of what you are about to do. Focus attention on the space between the eyebrows. Then begin to chant, drawing in the abdominal muscles to expel the air and, as you breathe in, feel the chest widening. Set the length of time for chanting and stick to it. Work at keeping the mind interested and concentrated. Afterwards write down observations that easily come to mind. As time goes on you will find it revealing to read them over.

At the beginning and end of your practice, offer a prayer of thanksgiving to those who have chanted the Mantra. In this way you attract those who have found God-realization by the use of the Mantra. If you say, "Help, help, please come and help me," they will come to support you. By accepting that this is possible, you help yourself to have the experience. Do not let your intellect decide what can or cannot be. Hold judgement suspended and see what happens.

The melody of the Mantra must never be changed. The combination of sounds is based on the perception of the Rishis who translated the etheric vibrations into those particular combinations for the purpose of creating a magnetic effect in the human being.

If you have difficulty in reaching the high notes, do not let the ego get in the way and discourage you from continuing. The voice needs training, and with time, patience and practice you will get there. That is one of the little miracles along the way, as you find your voice becoming clearer, smoother and more able to reach notes you never thought possible. Not being able to reach the high notes should be seen symbolically. As the voice needs training, the mind and consciousness also need to be trained with the same diligence to reach heights you never dreamed of.

Really put yourself into the chanting. If you allow it to become mechanical, or if you let yourself think it is monotonous, or if you let your interest drop, it will take a longer time to be effective. As with learning a language; the more you give yourself to it, the faster you will become fluent. When you study and practice Mantra you will learn the language of the Divine, the Most High.

After your Mantra practice remain quiet and receptive, surrendering your will to the Divine. Allow the still, small voice to speak. Come out of your practice gently and slowly. Don't get up and rush into something new. Try to keep the sensitivity, peace and quiet for as long as possible. Time is needed following spiritual practice for the effects to be absorbed.

Chapter Four

Worship:
Cultivating the Imagination

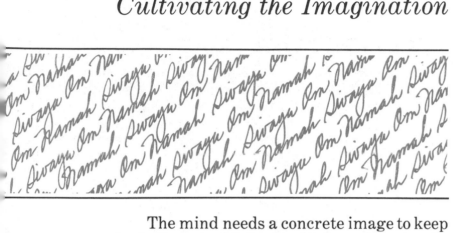

The mind needs a concrete image to keep it single-pointed during Mantra practice. In Bhakti Yoga, the Yoga of Love and devotion, the devotee concentrates on the picture of the Deity connected with the Mantra. This Deity, the *Ishta Devata*, creates a great longing in the devotee. There is a link of love and mercy, an extended help from the power of the deity, which the picture represents. This happens because of the complete surrender of the body, of the mind and of the ego at the feet of the Deity. The image stands for the Most High, everything that is holy, perfect, beautiful to the mind of the devotee, and there is a response of those qualities within the individual.

We can only understand and see God as we create Him in our mind, and we begin by creating God in our own image. You can paint an image, take one from a book, or you can use a picture of your spiritual teacher. This can be most helpful, since you already know what he or she looks like. Any image of the Divine that you charge with the power of your mind, your prayer, your love brings the image to life. In this way you cultivate your imagination while practicing the Mantra.

There is great wisdom in entering into a personal relationship with a particular aspect of God. As a method of overcoming the temptation to be side-tracked and to pacify the rebellious mind you can intersperse the recitation of Mantra with brief periods of worship, using flowers, making garlands, caring for an altar, thus bringing into your consciousness that aspect of the Divine.

For example, if your chosen deity is Lord Siva, the aspect of the Divine as the destroyer of all obstacles, you can grow white flowers and place them on an altar for Him. Designate and keep some spot in your home as a holy place. By the law of thought asociation the white flowers will put you in touch with the snowy peaks of the Himalayas, the abode of Lord Siva. If you chant Hari Om, invoking the aspect of the Lord as Vishnu, the preserving one, for Him you could use blue flowers. Roses or other colourful flowers may be used as an offering to Divine Mother when you use Ave Maria as your Mantra.

These images of worship can also be invoked in the mind's eye, and so increase the power of positive imagination. Desire is born out of imagination. In worship we put God into our mind so He becomes part of our desire, and we raise the scheming for the fulfillment of desire to a higher level.

The eyes may be kept closed, focused on the space between the eyebrows. If the mind cannot be stilled when you are chanting, open your eyes and chant straight to heaven, invoking the name of God with a deep feeling of expectancy that Someone is really listening. Use the power of your imagination and, looking into the sky, imagine an enormous ear. Sing into this ear and see what happens. Or take an image of God and establish it firmly in your mind. Then try to reproduce it in the sky and feel a deep longing to be near God. Imagine Christ on the Cross, or in a fishing boat calming the storm; or Krishna, with his beautiful Indian jewelry, his peacock feather, his flute, his ankle-bells and his blue skin, which shows that he is God and not another human being, that He stands for the divine principle.

Another method of cultivating imagination is to imagine that you are placing a flower before the image of God; this gesture will help you to realize that only after you have done the preliminary work with your imagination can you recognize God in the flower or see the Light Force in it.

Place a flower, real or imagined, before an image of Christ, the Virgin Mother, Siva, Buddha, or whomever you wish. Then say, "God, here is a flower. I have not made the flower. I have no power to create a flower. I have really nothing, not a single thing I can call my own. But I take this little part of your creation and I give it back to you, charged with my love, my emotion and my devotion. Please accept my offering."

You could put flowers on your altar, burn a candle and say, "God, I wish you to accept the flowers as a symbol of my devotion; may the candle be a symbol of my false desires, may they be burned in the Light of Wisdom as this candle burns before my eyes."

Put a little vessel of water on the altar and leave it there for three months without renewing the water. Every day drink just one sip and wonder as you experience that the water stays fresh as you raise the vibrations of your mind because of your chanting and prayers. Let each sip of water be symbolic of the Mantras and prayers that will wash away the debris of the mind. You may find that water will remain fresh without being covered throughout the whole time of your spiritual practice. Do not be ashamed to perform such acts of worship. You have a right to expect a great deal, but you have to open the doors for these things to happen.

After some time is spent in cultivating the imagination through a variety of forms of worship, the mind may achieve a level of concentration in which it will willingly resort to more subtle images of the Divine, such as breath or Light.

Om Krishna Guru Om Krishna Guru Om Krishna Guru Om Krishna Guru Om Krishna Guru Om Krishna Guru Om Krishna Guru Om Krishna Guru Om Krishna Guru Om Krishna Guru Om

Chapter Five

Benefits of Using a Mantra

The repetition of a Mantra is a means of improving the powers of concentration. There are Indian spiritual masters who maintain that the meaning and the content of the Mantra do not necessarily have to be understood by the aspirant in order to bring about the desired effect, that the practice of Mantra alone is sufficient to achieve the spiritual awakening which is its purpose. Certainly, the use of the Mantra purifies the subconscious and even if it is repeated mechanically some purification will take place. However, each Mantra is devotional by nature and has the Divine as its form and essence. With concentration on the meaning, the attainment of the ultimate goal is surer and quicker.

One of the results that comes quickly with the practice of Mantra is control of the breath which is the means by which we can develop the ability to control the emotions. In chanting we can give all our emotions to the Mantra, to the deity of the Mantra, and ask that deity to help us gain control. In this way we find a safe release for negative feelings. Rather than throwing them on someone else, we offer them back to their source. Continued chanting will lead to greater awareness and the replacing of negative feelings with positive affirmations.

Mantra practice stills turbulent emotions and thereby stills the turbulent mind. In yogic terms there is a difference between emotions and feelings, since a purified emotion becomes a true feeling. Mantra Yoga gives an opportunity to know the emotions, what they are, where they come from and what their proper place is in our lives. Through Mantra Yoga we can learn to deal with the emotions properly, to control and refine them and to encourage the harmonious development of all aspects of the human potential.

When emotions are purified they develop into love, which is an important step in the awakening of further levels of consciousness. Feelings which have been purified bring us into the presence of the Divine and from the Divine we feel a sense of protection. The Mantra is like a shield against all that is negative and disturbing. It is not a magic pill, rather it is like a steady stream of water which gradually wears down the hardest stone.

Although you may have experienced fears, worries, loneliness, and had limited encounters with love and joy, do not despair. Even if your feelings are easily hurt, in that oversensitivity you have a wonderful, if as yet undeveloped, tool. As these negative emotions evolve into more refined feelings, you will find that your concepts of love and joy also change, and that such sensitivity is exactly what is needed to enter new dimensions of understanding on the path to Self-realization.

The voice can become an instrument for expressing and controlling the emotions. All stray thoughts and emotions should be offered with the chant, as though the singer were "telling all" to the Lord who is called upon. As thoughts crowd in, the intensity of chanting can be increased in a determination to surrender all to the Divine.

Your voice can be caressing, gentle, intense, full of longing or surrender. At other times it may be strong and powerful as you put into it all your anger and disappointment, your requests and demands. Honestly express to God what you feel, even your anger and impatience toward Him for not bringing you sooner to Him. In chanting out the emotions, from the ugliest to the most exalted, in giving them back to the One who gave them to you in the first place, you learn to accept both parts of yourself, the good and the bad, and to transcend the pairs of opposites, from which we are trying to free ourselves. On the spiritual path, by channeling the emotions toward God, we find that He accepts our struggle and aids and sustains us in our search for Him.

Emotions in themselves are not bad, but when running wild they can be extremely damaging. Even love, when not shared, not given freely and generously, becomes self-love which turns destructively back on the individual. When emotions are directed, they are a source of strength for great achievements. Through the power of emotions men and women have overcome their limitations and attained a higher purpose in life. Emotions channeled through a Mantra towards the Divine can take you close to God.

As the Mantra is chanted, moods will in time be brought under control and awareness in the here and now will grow. Attention, and therefore energy, will be withdrawn from the old thought patterns that, like tapes on a tape recorder, play over and over. The mental background noises keep us tied to the past and future, to fearful imaginings and senseless fantasies, which cause our self-created sufferings. The energy will now be channeled to the Most High, to a positive affirmation of one's innermost Self.

Do not let the intellectual mind distract you from attempting the practice of Mantra and Japa. No amount of words or book knowledge can give you the experience. You have to practice yourself for their effect to be understood. The benefits depend on the individual, on where you start off, where you stand now, what your past lives have been, and the intensity and degree of longing in your desire. When you chant a Mantra your whole being changes for the better. Build up the habit of repeating the Mantra at all times. The work you do will become easier and more joyful because the Mantra is continuously in the back of your mind. If you repeat it while doing Hatha Yoga you will be able to penetrate the deeper levels of the asanas. Holding an asana, chant mentally, becoming absorbed in what you are doing. Gradually you will become aware of the pranic flow in the body, the deeper aspects of the asana and finally you will experience its mystical meaning.

If you have found your teacher, chant his or her name as an offering, an act of love. Channel the emotions by giving admiration and gratitude for the inspiration you have received. This offering and recognition of the divine spirit within the Guru will aid in developing humility and overcoming the ego. Learning to surrender to the Mantra and to the energy of the Mantra puts in motion the process of purification of the self, facing up to and eliminating selfishness, self-glorification, self-justification and self-gratification.

When chanting a Mantra the emotions express themselves in the breath and the voice. Every time the breath is uneven it means the emotions are involved and we are out of balance. As long as the emotions are running high, this imbalance exists, but gradually they subside and we begin to experience the equilibrium that is our goal. Then, as quietness descends, we can tune into the great rhythm of the Cosmos and become one with that rhythm. Chanting helps us to achieve this stillness by bringing the breath and the emotions under control. In these moments of complete stillness of the mind, indescribable bliss is experienced. By repeated practice it becomes possible to hold onto the contact made with your innermost being.

Through the use of Mantra a greater sensitivity, a refinement of the senses, comes about which may eventually bring you to the point where you can see with the inner eye and hear with the inner ear. When the inner ear is developed, the music of the spheres may be heard, music of such exquisite beauty as no instrument, no human voice, is able to produce. The Cosmic AUM might be heard. The impact and effects of such experiences will bring an intense desire to change for the better.

Through the practice of Mantra and Japa Yoga you will find yourself in direct confrontation with the lower self, the ego or "body-mind." You will become aware of those personality aspects that have been in control and have ruled your life. Now the Higher Self begins to take possession.

Chapter Six

How to Use the Mantra

One of the greatest problems in concentrating the human mind stems from the "mental background noises." These are an accumulation of influences from the world around us, memories and impressions that are triggered by the law of thought association. It is difficult to be completely quiet because we seem to be forever in the company of all these imprints which the mind has stored and turns out at random. When you first attempt to develop single-pointedness, you will become aware of this inability to keep the mind still. To deal with this, you can trick the mind into concentrating by a variety of techniques which vary the monotony without essentially changing the focus, by allowing the mind to be active within the framework of the Mantra.

Think of all the detail of chanting, how the sound is produced, the breathing, the effect of the sound on the body. Speed up the tempo of your chanting, including a greater number of repetitions within the span of one breath. Slow down the tempo, extending a name or syllable, stress the first syllable, or the last. (This is dealt with more specifically in the section on individual Mantras). Vary the voice from very loud, swelling the sound, to very soft and gentle. This kind of variety keeps the mind interested while still involving it fully and helps to keep the repetitions from becoming mechanical.

You may notice that your voice becomes smoother as you chant, that you can sing as you never could before. Delight in these improvements and put into your mind positive thoughts that you want to reach God by means of your voice, that you wish to be an instrument of God's love, and that the Mantra you chant will be of help to those in need. In this way you are master of the situation rather than becoming the slave of intellectual doubts and false pride. Watch the flow of your breath and its relation to emotions to understand the difference between expressing them and indulging in them. Indulgence indicates that you have become the victim of undisciplined emotions.

When chanting we often get in touch with emotions we did not know we had and tears that have been held back from childhood will come flooding out. You must use discrimination to recognize when these become tears of self-pity and deny yourself that indulgence. Sometimes the tears will be part regret and part joy — that the soul is at last on its way back home, regret that so many lifetimes have been wasted. Symbolically collect your tears, whatever their origin, and offer them to the Divine. Or wash the feet of Divine Mother with your tears.

Realize also that we cannot control the emotions through sheer will-power and when they are too strong, give them back to God, ask Him for help as a child asks its mother. At that moment, when you cry out from the depths of your being, you are most sincere and you are single-pointed in your anger, disappointment, or anguish. In doing this, you will experience true humility, perhaps for the first time. You can be either God's child or God's servant. If you are the kind of person to whom pleasing others is important, be God's servant. Then He is your Master; please Him. Offer yourself as an instrument through which He can love others. As you try to become more pleasing to God, you will find that His love comes to you through people, who are His creation. If God can love you, everybody can love you.

Combine formal Mantra practice with daily reflection and the keeping of a spiritual diary. This will help you to cultivate awareness and make the necessary changes in daily life to remove all aspects of egoism. The diary will also provide a record of mental reactions to the practice and the obstacles encountered, as well as the changes you observe within yourself and any experiences you may have. It is only by keeping a close watch on your practice over the entire period that a full understanding, not only of the Mantra, but also of the functioning of the mind will be achieved. Knowing the impasses the mind encounters and also how it can overcome them can be very helpful in any situation in life.

Try this experiment: chant your Mantra and watch your dreams. Do this for a definite length of time — you are working with the laboratory of your mind, and you must allow a reasonable period of effort to give it a fair trial. You cannot become a saint in a weekend. It takes nine months for a baby to be born and many more years to grow into an adult; the beginner on the spiritual path is like a spiritual baby.

Chanting is an individual matter and each person has a right to his or her own understanding. There can be no hard and fast rules. If you seek God, it is like a love affair between you and God. As you approach the Most High you grow and your understanding grows. You approach Truth differently, gaining new perspective and insights.

The power of the Mantra becomes most effective when practiced regularly and for a sufficient period of time — that is, until you get results. How long you chant at one time or how frequently is your decision.

When you begin chanting you will find that a wave of enthusiasm carries you through the first period. Unfortunately, this soon passes as the mind wants a change, something new. Mantra practice is upsetting to the mind, forcing it out of its normal habits into a very narrow path, making it single-pointed through discipline, and cutting the attachments to which it has clung. Like a child with new toys, the mind has a tendency to flit from one thing to another without discrimination. But the true reward will come only by perseverance and practice; only then will its secret be discovered, its mystery and power revealed.

Awareness is essential; mere dreaming during the chanting will not "light the fire that consumes." With application, with the purifying of the emotions and the mind more single-pointed, stillness will ensue and a sense of the "ever-present Presence" may be felt.

Record the changing reactions of the mind in your spiritual diary. After the first wave of enthusiasm there comes rebellion and opposition. The first critical point is at the end of two weeks, then three months, then two years. If you know the pattern ahead of time, you can take precautions.

The mind is like an elephant. You cannot force an elephant to move rigidly along a fixed line, but you keep the reins in your hand and allow him to sway a little from side to side. You don't let him go sightseeing and forget his destination. Similarly, you can give the mind a little leeway but do not let it go entirely its own way.

When the practice of Mantra goes on for several hours at a stretch, mental chanting as well as the various forms of Japa can be alternated in order to maintain concentration. Mental repetition is considered by some Yogis the most powerful form but for many people the audible chanting which helps to express emotions is more successful while the mind is still very active. At a much later stage the mental repetition will be found more potent. Sometimes it is a good idea to recite the Mantra mentally when you are in the presence of others. This will restrain the urge to show off. When the awareness of this desire arises, say "thank you," because such awareness will increase when gratitude is felt. As the Mantra is put into the subconscious, the mind is purified to an extent of which we would be incapable without this aid. So the power of the Mantra is a great protection from fear. Slowly the ego is overpowered by the Higher Self. It is like pouring milk into black coffee until, little by little, it becomes pure milk.

Another variation is Likhita Japa, in which the Mantra is written down in lines like sentences, or in shapes and forms, as in the diagram of a lotus, or a cross, or in any design that will help to reinforce your devotions. One uniform system of writing will help concentration. If you work in an office, it is an excellent way of using any free time for your spiritual development, rather than wasting it in socializing. Writing the Mantra may also be alternated with other forms of Japa to maintain the focus on the Mantra, while providing variation to keep the mind interested. Keep all sheets of paper or notebooks in which you have written the Mantra, because these things have a very subtle effect on the subconscious. Keep them near your bed or on your altar.

You may find that different forms of Japa are effective at different times. Whatever form you are using, take the first few minutes of

An example of Likhita Japa using the Mantra
Om Namah Sivaya in floral form.

your practice to get the mind in order, to focus the feelings and emotions on what you are doing. Then direct all your efforts to the glorification of God, expressing your feelings of gratitude for having received knowledge of this practice and being able to help yourself. This attitude may not always be possible for you. If it is not, acknowledge your negativity and offer it to the Divine. Remember that being involved with God, even in anger, is better than being lukewarm and indifferent.

Later, when the practice is established, you will find that inspiration, the answers to your prayers, will come when you have finally surrendered, when you have chanted or repeated the Mantra to the point that the mind is exhausted. It is like the scientist in the laboratory who has tried and tried and when he finally lets go of his reasoning, inspiration comes.

If, after a year or two of practice, there emerges by itself a different way of practicing Mantra Yoga, it should not be suppressed. This may be guidance from a higher level. But make sure it is not the ego that wants to have its own way. First do your practice the way you have been taught and see what the results are. Then allow yourself to try and see if the same results can be reached in a different way. If changes are made too soon, based on assumption rather than experience, the results cannot be obtained. Dig one deep well rather than many shallow ones. Only when, through expanding awareness, you realize that one lesson is completed, are you ready to move on to another.

If you are completely serious in your efforts, extended Mantra chanting brings steadily deepening God-communion and release from emotional imbalance, bringing the self into harmony with the Self.

Chapter Seven

Practice and Understanding of Individual Mantras

The mind is creative; as soon as you give it some material it weaves with it a pattern all its own. This can be easily mistaken during chanting as coming from some higher divine source. The advantage of not knowing what the Mantra means is that the mind has nothing to work on. Then, when the Mantra does reveal itself to you, there will be no doubt of its meaning. Although an intellectual explanation encompasses only a small part of its significance, knowing the meaning, while understanding the creativity of the mind, may hasten the revelation.

The Cosmic sound *AUM*, or its condensed form *OM*, is the origin of all other sounds and is itself a Mantra. It is called the *Pranava* or sacred syllable, and symbolizes Brahman or the essential spiritual reality. The Mantra AUM gives birth to rays of Light, bringing illumination to the mind.

All sounds are blended into the beautiful Cosmic AUM, which can reverberate in the hearts of men and women. Mantra is speech most profound, sound at its purest, and when that supreme sound of Om becomes sovereign, it takes you past the little selfish ego, so that you are clothed in new cloth of thought and sound. You will be lifted beyond all other existence and when you speak, you will hear the sound of the Self, your innermost Being.

The flute of Lord Krishna is also symbolic for the Pranava. By the sound of His flute, Krishna created the world, and with its sound, He calls His devotees back to their heavenly home. Like the flute, the devotee must be empty, with egoism and self-importance removed. In that perfect and complete surrender, the mortal aspect, the self-will, becomes merged with the Divine and blends in joy and harmony, producing a sound of great inspiration, the Cosmic sound of AUM. Swami Sivananda has said that in this kind of self-surrender, which comes from the very core of one's heart, spiritual practice or Sadhana is not necessary, because one has truly become the Lord's property, the flute of Lord Krishna.

AUM must be chanted in three parts, with equal time given to each part; *Ah* is chanted in the region of the navel, *OO* in the sternum and *MM* in the throat.

Here is an example of a meditation you can use, and which can help you develop your own, to gain understanding and insights into this Mantra. When you chant Ah, place the sound at the navel or solar plexus. Visualize a lotus representing life itself. See a fluctuation of light energy on its petals. Imagine a change in colour from bright red to that of rain clouds. Allow these fluctuations to move, almost as if they have a life of their own. Think of them as symbolic for changing moods. Now see the tips of the lotus petals become faint pink, then let the lotus gradually become a shimmering white. Think of this as the Divine Light of insights, understanding and love dispersing the rain clouds of ignorance.

As the Light expands, let the next lotus, the Heart Centre, come into focus.

Chant OO and place the sound at the area of the sternum. See the petals as red at the centre of this lotus, pink in the middle and with the tips becoming clear white. As you chant, think of how refined the emotions can become when cultivated by such practices as this.

When the last letter, the M, is chanted with closed lips, you will become aware of your physical response and vibration of the many, many cells of your body. When you chant, listen with great attention and contemplate the innate power of sound and its ability to manifest. This will lead to hearing the Cosmic AUM which is not a physical experience, but one that is heard by the inner ear, always the right. M becomes symbolic for surrender and for the response of the body as it reverberates to Pranavanada, the sound of the Most High.

The chanting of AUM will purify the mind, destroy all evil, all egoism. *AUM* represents the trinity of the physical, mental and spiritual bodies; waking consciousness, dream consciousness and dreamless sleep; and also individual, universal and transcendental consciousness.

Listening to the sound of Lord Krishna's flute, all consciousness is submerged in the Divine. Listening to the reverberations of the *OM* within, the devotee becomes Divine. In the chanting of *OM* one empties oneself and is filled with an essence that is beyond description.

Krishna Invocation

The name of Krishna may be invoked and used as a Mantra. The *Krishna Invocation* contains an allegorical story with the sequence of notes resembling the crying of a child for its father or mother. The devotee is a child of God, and just as the child calls out for its parent, the devotee cries for God in the manifestation of Lord Krishna. Krishna may also be seen as the Cosmic Lover, or as the Oversoul, with the singer as the soul in search of the Lord.

This Mantra begins at a low tone and works up gradually, like the child who does not get an immediate response, until there is the realization that attention cannot be commanded of either the parent or of God. Then there is resignation as the voice drops. But soon the demands start again with strength and energy, feelings and emotions. Just as the human mother or father knows and responds only to the real cry for help, so God pays little attention to us as long as we are caught up with our wordly games and toys, the cars, houses, position, achievements.

The devotee must learn that Lord Krishna cannot be commanded, and will not produce a vision or spiritual experience at the individual's convenience. When there is surrender to the fact that God comes in His own time, and when the flood of uncontrolled emotions is cleared away, only then, in that silence there may come a response. This Mantra is a devotional fire that consumes the emotional dross, brings the heart to pure longing, the mind to stillness, and the soul to peace.

Om Krishna Guru

Om Krishna Guru is especially helpful if you are seeking a teacher. Its practice can bring you to your Guru.

The Mantra begins with Om, the Supreme, beyond all names and forms, the Supreme Energy, the essence of all Energy. Krishna is this Energy manifested in shape and form for the convenience of the human mind. The impersonal power thus becomes personalized. Siva, Krishna, even Jesus, are all creations of the human mind, manifestations of the Supreme Energy. If you want to love God, you can only love that power when it manifests as creation. Loving God means loving people, loving plants, loving animals, loving all that you think of as God's creation. This may be difficult, but we can begin by having reverence for life in all its forms.

Lord Krishna is always shown standing when He plays the flute, His body making a cross. This means that He is lenient with human frailties, but it also symbolizes the control of the three gunas of this world. Very often He is shown standing on a Lotus or with one flowering near Him. The Lotus is untainted by the muddy water in which it grows; the inner Light of every human being is untainted; the universe is untainted. The dark blue colour of Krishna signifies the unknown; although He is in human form, the Divine can never be known in its entirety.

Guru is the spiritual teacher, the one who dispels our ignorance and brings us to the Light.

Radhe Govinda

Radhe Govinda is a charming representation of emotions and the spiritual search, and the relationship of the individual soul to the Oversoul. Govinda means "the one who tended the cows" and is another name for Lord Krishna, just as Jesus is sometimes called the Good Shepherd, the Christ, the Nazarene. Radha is His mortal companion, who through her unceasing love for God became the symbol of the soul in search of her Lord, the Overself.

When love has become Cosmic, it no longer has a "because" attached to it. The human relationship can have these divine qualities when the love for God obliterates self-centeredness. The story of this Mantra, like the Krishna Invocation, displays an understanding of human nature and an acceptance of it as the vehicle through which we reach the Divine.

Radha calls for Krishna and they play a game of hide-and-seek. Krishna withdraws, Radha searches. He returns, but keeps disappearing and reappearing. Radha becomes bored and drops the search; she is distracted and petulant. Now it is Krishna's turn to take the initiative and win over Radha. This is to reveal and to illustrate the sublime truth that God loves his devotee at least as much as the devotee loves Him.

The chanting of the Radhe Govinda Mantra should be infused with the most intense feelings of love; it should be sung with God-centered aspiration: to find God within, which deepens that love; to find God in all mankind, which broadens that love.

Ave Maria

Ave Maria, although not as short as some of the Indian ones, will produce similar results when used as a Mantra. In Hindu mythology and religious thought the female principle is seen as the creative power through which the universe is manifested. In Christian terms, the Ave Maria, the Hail Mary, is worshipping the mother, the love aspect of the Divine. This brings out the noblest feelings in the human being. In Hindu teachings, the seeker can approach the ultimate spirit of God, which is beyond all manifestation, only through the mother principle of the manifested universe. The devotee who wants to enter the house of the Lord has first to go to Divine Mother for the keys — love and devotion — before entry can be attained.

The Ave Maria creates a deep feeling of love for the Divine. It will bring you in contact with Divine Mother Herself. Dedicate the chanting to those whom you wish to bless.

Hari Om

Hari Om is the healing Mantra. Hari is a name for Vishnu, the preserving aspect of the Supreme Spirit. Krishna is also an aspect of the preserving or sustaining force, and so Hari may be thought of as the healing aspect of Lord Krishna. God assumes many aspects in order to provide us with the means of tackling our dificulties in a variety of ways, according to individual characterstics and temperament.

In Sanskrit, *Hari* means "to take away." Vishnu takes away the consequences of offences, errors and follies, when there is repentence. These are the impurities that bring about grief and sickness. If they are removed, health and strength are conserved for spiritual endeavours.

Om or *AUM* is the Hindu trinity, which here means creation, preservation, and destruction: the generation within us of that which is pure, sacred and noble; the sustaining and strengthening of these qualities; and dissolving all that is impure and negative.

This Mantra calls on Vishnu (or Lord Krishna) to preserve the human body and the mind in the best state of health for the purpose of finding Self-realization, attaining to the Om, the very Cosmic concept that absorbs all aspects in One, finally becoming formless.

The Hari Om Mantra is most powerful from midnight until three o'clock in the morning. At this time the vibrations are calm and mental activity is less. This is the time at which you are most likely to have a spiritual experience.

Since the science of sound and breath control applies to any religion, Christians can chant "Jesus Christ" to the tune of *Hari Om*, while Jews can use "Adonai" or "Elohim." A Buddhist might choose one of the names of Lord Buddha; or you can chant to Divine Mother, or use any one of Her 108 names such as Radha, Lakshmi or Saraswati. When a spontaneous feeling of gratitude wells up towards your teacher or Guru, this may be expressed by using that name as a way of blessing and giving thanks for all that has been received. You can go from one to another of these names, in order to give greater variety to the chanting, without changing the notes and the key in which the Mantra is sung.

Through the various ways in which it can be chanted, Hari Om is effective in efforts to make the mind single-pointed. To control the restlessness of the mind and overcome feelings of doubt, changes may be made by stressing syllables or sounds differently, while keeping the melody the same. Here are some possibilities:

a. Soft voice, normal breath comes slowly under control.

b. Sing full sequence of Mantra in one breath, so the concentration is again gathered, like light through a magnifying glass, to become single-pointed, and returned to the Mantra. Continue chanting for as long as you can keep the concentration single-pointed. If the mind begins to behave like a monkey, jumping here and there, then it is time to make a change once more.

c. Chant two sequences in one breath. This will again help to bring concentration back to the Mantra. When it begins to wane it is time to attempt three Mantras in one breath.

d. When thoughts crowd in and you cannot keep them out by any effort of will, try another change. Express your distress by emphasizing the "ee" in *Hari Om.*

e. Another variation is to stress the Om, extending the sound as long as possible.

f. Stress the "ha," with emphasis on the breath and tension of the muscles in the region of the solar plexus. Link this with the mind and throw out everything that is negative.

Om Namah Sivaya

In this Mantra the devotee appeals to God in His aspect as destroyer of all ignorance and illusion that stands in the way of the divine Union. We need assistance in our efforts to overcome the ego. Self-centeredness cannot be mastered by sheer will-power; we must surrender and ask for divine help. Om Namah Sivaya is a call upon God to eliminate our negative qualities, to dissolve our difficulties and to destroy the obstacles to higher spiritual life. Siva is called "The Compassionate One," removing obstacles like selfishness and jealousy that impede our development. Lord Siva's destruction is really a blessing.

We must be prepared to have our concepts, our preconceived ideas, even our relationships destroyed. What we believe to be true and unshakeable today may be meaningless tomorrow. Some of our obstacles may be things to which we are very strongly attached. In seeking higher values, we have to ask, "Am I willing to pay the price?" The Most High is a pearl of great price. Attachment, whether to possessions, to name and fame, or to another individual, stands between the devotee and God.

Sometimes blessings come in disguise. An illness gives us time to be holy, time to think and to reflect on the purpose and direction of our life. Destruction on any level means turmoil and this is especially true on the spiritual level. But the old must be destroyed to make way for the new and in chanting this Mantra the devotee is asking Siva to perform this kind of destruction.

However, a mistake can be made in concentrating on the destructive aspect without invoking a feeling of gratitude that help is being given to overcome the obstacles. This involves two important human emotions: humility, to recognize that one needs help, and gratitude that, whenever it is sincerely asked for, this help is given. Imagine yourself driving along a road that has many potholes. Then someone appears ahead of you and begins filling in the holes. You would stop concentrating on the holes and instead feel grateful to the person who is filling them.

It is helpful to have a picture or image of Siva in your room and put fresh white flowers in front of it. The image of Lord Siva, sitting in silence in a rigid position on Mount Kailas in the snowy regions of the Himalayas is a symbol for the state of complete silence and motionlessness that follows the destruction of emotional attachments and fears.

Om Sri Rama Jaya Rama

Om Sri Rama Jaya Rama Jaya Jaya Rama is a call to victory for the spiritual Self. *Rama* means one who delights in the consciousness of the spiritual Self. *Jaya* means "hail"or "victory." *Rama* represents the aspect of God as king and ruler of the universe. If you want to be God's servant, to carry out His will and accept Him as king, then chant this Mantra. It is used to evoke the power that leads to victory for the spiritual Self; that it may obtain realization of the God within.

Although not a literal translation, the words "I am Thine, all is Thine, Thy Will be done O Lord" are in the spirit of the Mantra. They are an example of following inner inspiration and intuition to give the meaning in a different language.

Swami Ramdas, a saint of modern India, who toured the West in 1954 and died in 1963, concentrated his search for God-realization in the chanting of the Ram Mantra. He initiated all his devotees into the name of Ram, and had a deep relationship with God in the aspect of Ram. He talked to Ram and in moments of danger would ask, "Now, Ram, how are you going to save me? Or are you going to destroy me?" One day he was commanded by God to write down his experiences, and they can be obtained from his Ashram in India.

There are different types of Mantras which have the purpose of achieving different goals. Some Mantras promise power or material benefits. For example, the verses of the *Ananda Lahari* by Sankara of the first century A.D.† are mainly a description and glorification of the Hindu Divine Mother, the female aspect of God. Saraswati is God as Divine Mother in the aspect of beauty, music and learning. The verses usually consist of four lines and each verse has a specific *yantra* (abstract representation of the Divine). Divine Mother's power is expressed on many levels: one verse may be recited to gain the power to foresee the future through dreams; another may bring immunity from famine and pestilence; still others will remove sterility, cure consumption, or charm snakes.

However, the Mantras which have been discussed in this presentation are Mantras of the heart that are used as short formulas to bring about single-pointedness of mind for the purpose of achieving Self-realization.

---

†*Translation and commentary by Swami Sivananda, 4th ed Rishikesh, 1949.*

Hari Om Hari Om

Chapter Eight

Mantra and Healing

There are many theories concerning healing, but your own observation and your own growing understanding will bring to you, your own unique insights. With our limited minds, functioning only on the three dimensional plane, we cannot really grasp all the law of the Divine, or the extended law of nature, nor understand the complicated causes of illness.

However, by chanting or praying with single-pointedness of mind, by reinforcing that concentration with action, by directing the will, healing will take place naturally within ourselves. Mantras can have a healing effect by releasing the emotions and bringing about a state of calmness and deep relaxation both in the chanter and in anyone listening. With the mind relaxed, the source of the disease and the hidden roots of conflict may come to the surface where they can be dealt with. But we must know what we want to be healthy for, what we will do with the remainder of life if health is restored. We must be single-pointed in our desire. There may be advantages to being ill which, although we might not admit them consciously, our ego wants to hold onto. By enforcing our will and giving strength to that part which wants to be well, this polarity of the mind can be overcome, permitting healing to take place.

There is a Mantra, *Aham Brahmasmi*, which means "I am Brahman" or "I am God." This may seem a strange thought but a person becomes what he thinks. If you think you are a failure, you will become a failure. Conversely, if you continually chant *Aham Brahmasmi* you will eventually realize your Divine nature and there will be little room for sickness at any level — physical, emotional or mental. If you are to chant this Mantra, it is important that you clarify in your own mind what the meaning of God is to you. You must also do serious self-purification, and the rest of your life must reflect this purification. You must develop the ability to surrender to the Mantra and to the energy that comes from it. You must have the humility to be able to ask for forgiveness and apologize to others if you are in the wrong.

Besides the ego's need for attention which perpetuates illness, and lack of humility which indicates a wrong attitude, there are many other factors which may interfere when you do spiritual practices for your own healing. You may have a lesson to learn, and so healing may not be what is best for you; you may be eating the wrong food, or violating certain laws of nature to which your body is subject. You may hold an unhealthy belief that you are too great a sinner to deserve to be healed. You may also lack awareness that you are hurting others and unconsciously punishing yourself for their pain. The complexity of the human mind and its capacity for pain is so tremendous that we must beware of over-simplification. Pain is a great teacher, but we must understand its message and deal with that before the way is clear for health to be restored.

All this must be remembered also in regard to the healing of others. It may be necessary for the person to experience pain or go through an illness in order to have the time to reflect, to develop humility and devotion, and to overcome selfishness. Perhaps a physical healing can take place only after the mind has been healed. You cannot know the purpose of an ailment, or its possible cause, nor can you know what is best for the person. But you may offer a prayer or chant Mantras, letting the power of the Mantra itself work. Chanting can be an expression of your sincere concern, although you must not decide how this help should be given.

When you chant or recite a Mantra for someone, visualize that person well and healthy. Do not picture the individual in a sick state, as such an image has remarkable power. Instead, invoke the image of Hari or Krishna or Siva or Jesus and, in full expectation, see the person standing in the radiance of Light. Let the healing force flow through you, never from you, and think of the energy of the Mantra as that healing Light. Wrap the individual in a spiral of this Light so that he or she becomes barely visible and let the image of this spiral move to the source of all Light.† Now focus all your attention on the chanting.

What takes place when we chant a Mantra? We attract spiritual power and we offer ourselves as a channel for this power, that it may work through us to the sick person and do whatever is necessary. We must not demand healing, nor tell God how to accomplish it — when, how quickly, in what way. We do not know what karma has to be paid off, or what lessons have to be learned. Healing is not a hit-or-miss affair, even though to human perception it may seem so.

Most spiritual healers find, for a variety of reasons, that not everyone benefits. Sometimes a person who appears to be a disbeliever is healed while a believer is not. This may be because the subconscious convictions of these people are exactly opposite to what they proclaim. The receptivity of the person to be healed is an important element.

The healer must surrender to God, to the Cosmic healing forces, making sure that no personal opinion is held, no judgment made. Only by invoking all the compassion of which you are capable will you be able to apply or direct or invoke the healing power of the Mantra.

How does one develop compassion? Observe yourself, practise awareness in order to gain understanding of yourself. Wrong conduct must be discarded, not condemned. When you see and forgive your own failures, you will be ready to forgive the failings of others and have more understanding for those you wish to heal. In the process of healing we meet ourselves. Jesus told us to forgive "seventy times seven." He meant us to forgive always, and not to sit in the judgment seat for ourselves or for others.

When you attempt to heal someone, first invoke all the feeling of compassion possible, chant the Mantra, and fill yourself with this vibration, attracting the forces of the Mantra and channeling them, directing them toward the sick person. If you feel that the vibration flows out from the tips of the fingers or the palms, you may hold your hands above the person. Or you can mentally open the doors of your heart and let it flow through. With this vibration flows your own love and this is evidence of your willingness to help. Always put sick persons at ease, helping them to accept themselves without the feeling of being burdened with sin. Healing will not take place with the attitude of "unworthy sinner."

Confidence will come with success, but do not become overconfident and think that healing will always take place. The Mantra could overcome anything if the person would recite it, or receive it, as a paying off of Karma, with trust in forgiveness, and a readiness to alter the course of their life and dedicate it to serving God. Even when a healing has come about, a sickness might come back with greater force if the person who was healed does not change a selfish or hurtful way of life. Gratitude to the Divine must be shown in charity or selfless service to others.

Record the results of your efforts in order to increase your understanding of the law of healing. When we call up the spiritual forces we attract through the vibration of a certain sound or a Mantra, one particular aspect of the Cosmic Light that is suitable for specific healing, but perhaps not for all. Much will depend on the makeup of the person who is ill. The influence of such a healing ray can be rejected by the one who is expected to receive it. This does not necessarily take place in the conscious mind but may be a subconscious rejection because of the idea of being unworthy, or of being too great a sinner to expect forgiveness. Sometimes healing is expected too quickly and we give up before it can take place. Not all healing can or should be instantaneous.

When we chant a mantra we definitely change the sick person's state of mind. We can relax them and gently probe into the depths of the soul or the mind to find out what resistance we may have to deal with. We can try to help to lift their burdens. Perhaps we can point out that we really can trust the Divine, that we have many good reasons to do so.

May all of you who read this become channels of help and healing and goodness to many others. Bless you all.

†The Divine Light Invocation, by Swami Sivananda Radha, Siva Press, 1966.

Chapter Nine

Mantra and Initiation

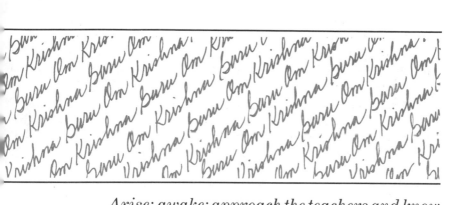

Arise; awake; approach the teachers and know the Truth.

The person who is blessed with a teacher knows the Highest.

He whose devotion to the Lord is great and who has as much devotion to the teacher (Guru) as to the Lord, unto him, that high souled one, the meanings of the sacred texts stand revealed.

— Quoted from the Upanishads.

All sacred texts and spiritual Masters emphasize the need for a teacher on the spiritual Path. When you think you have found your Guru, take time to examine yourself and your motives. Do not desire initiation unless you have made up your mind that you want to accept the Teachings and that you will listen and obey. Put aside all worry that you might become dependent on your teacher. A true Guru will lead you to the discovery of the Guru within — your own Higher Self.

Make no demands as to how your Guru should be and how you should be taught. Pray to the Divine that you will be led to a true Guru. Make a bargain with God: ask Him that the teacher who is your Guru by divine appointment will either say something special to you or greet you in a certain manner, giving you a particular present, leaf or a flower or a book, whatever you decide. But once you make a promise to God that you will accept that individual who comes to you with that special sign, you must keep your end of the bargain. The teacher will come when the student is ready.

When your choice has been made, if you feel that your Guru acts in a way that is not in accordance with your perceptions of spirituality and that you may have made a mistake, remember that the error may be in your perception. Say to the Lord, "I am confused. Is my time with this teacher over? Should I look for another Guru?" Then wait. If no sign comes, stay with the teacher you have, until the sign you have asked for is given.

A true initiation into a Mantra is like a spiritual marriage between Guru and disciple. It cannot be dissolved by the breaking up of the human relationship, it is only delayed and must be taken up and continued in another life, until the disciple has achieved Self-realization. Guru and disciple are always linked through the power of the Mantra. There is an obligation on both sides: the one who initiates accepts responsibility for the disciple, and the initiate must be ready to accept the guidance and authority of the Guru and feel that it is right to take the initiation. According to Swami Sivananda, although it is very difficult to find a teacher who will sincerely look after the interest of the pupil, it is also extremely difficult to find a disciple who will sincerely act according to the instructions of the Guru. His advice to aspirants is to equip themselves with the qualifications of sincerity, humility and devotion before approaching a Guru, and then not to use reason too much in the selection. For both parties the relationship is an intense one and, because of its duration and importance, must be cherished.

Only one who has practised intensively and has received the power of the Mantra can initiate. Otherwise there is nothing to pass on to the student, in the same way that a father can only bequeath to a child what he himself has already acquired.

Before the initiation, both student and teacher must examine their relationship to see if there is anything that could cause friction between them. These problems should be worked out first. Indeed the student should never accept an initiation until his or her worst weaknesses have been overcome. To again quote Swami Sivananda, "The reason for the early downfall of the majority of aspirants is that they imagine themselves to be qualified to adopt the highest form of Yoga at the beginning. The qualified aspirant will be humble enough to approach a Guru, surrender himself to the Guru and serve and learn from him."

In the initiation, or "Diksha," the Guru transmits to the student something of the power of the Mantra. Gurudev Sivananda says, "Initiation gives spiritual knowledge and destroys sin. As one lamp is lit at the flame of another, so the divine Sakti within Mantra is communicated from Guru to the disciple." This may be similar to a mild electric shock; it can also be experienced as ecstatic joy, like walking on clouds, lasting for several hours or even a few days. There can be various effects. The power of the Mantra becomes greater after the initiation and will become more perceptible to the disciple, increasing his or her sensitivity. The Mantra then becomes a self-generating force, propelling the disciple into union with the power of the Mantra. The effect on the recipient is dependent on the quality of love and depth of sincerity with which the power of the Mantra is transmitted.

The commitment that is involved in a Mantra initiation is not suitable or possible for everybody, but the ideals which it implies may be pursued just as earnestly by those who are not initiated. When you have received an initiation, there is a commitment to be frank and open with the Guru about the actions and plans of your life. This brings with it the positive aspect of the initiate having someone who cares and who will give advice in an objective manner. Many pitfalls and much pain are thereby avoided. But if this intention of a free exchange dies in the initial stages, it is an obvious signal to both parties that the relationship should be reassessed. There might have been, on the part of the initiate, false hopes of gaining powers or having exciting experiences. If this is the case, the sincerity of the decision must be questioned. Either the full meaning of initiation should be applied, or the relationship dissolved.

Karma will not take effect when there is agreement between parting individuals, assuring that there is no disappointment or pain to

either partner. This applies to ordinary marriage and we can therefore reasonably expect that it also applies, to some degree, to the mystical marriage of Mantra initiation.

A one-sided relationship is not really a relationship. There is no
better way of describing the purpose and effectiveness of Mantra than
in the words of the Parable of the Sower (Matthew XIII) in which
Jesus speaks of the seeds (of Mantra or power) which fall along the
path to be devoured by birds, those which fall on rocky ground where
the roots wither away, or among thorns where they are choked, and
the ones which fall on fertile ground where they grow and bring forth
a good harvest.

There are many misconceptions surrounding the idea of initiation. Mantra initiation can take many forms. In India it may be given
by a father or a mother to the child. This took place, for instance, in the
life of Papa Ramdas, the renowned saint of Southern India. In these
situations the parent is of high spiritual calibre and guides the children's steps with the aim of helping them find the same state of realization. This means that the home life is a highly spiritual one, with study
of scriptures, recitation of sacred texts and invocation of Mantra, as
part of daily living. The effect of such early training is deep and lasting. The parent who initiates a child does not have the goal of Sannyas
in mind. (Papa Ramdas was not a Sannyasi). It is a blessing for the
child and a different kind of Mantra is used.

Mantra initiation may also be given by a compassionate Guru to
help an individual, not always on the basis of the recognition of great
spiritual potential, but rather on that of need. There may be Karmic
conditions which are difficult to deal with, and which would make a
favourable birth in another lifetime questionable. One of the young
fellows in Sivananda Ashram had a record for theft. When I became
aware that he had been initiated by Swami Sivananda, I felt that this
had been unwise and was puzzled how a Guru could have exercised so
little caution. When I asked him why he would initiate such a person,
his answer was that by accepting the individual and giving him an
initiation he was helping that person to obtain better conditions in
another life, and also to give support in the present struggle to overcome weaknesses.

In order for this effort of the Guru to be worthwhile such a disciple
would have to possess true humility and a sense of gratitude. Unfortunately, this gratitude may be only temporarily expressed, soon to disappear as if in quicksand. It is clear that, regardless what the

problems are, the Divine Energies will always extend help and it is very foolish to allow pride to stand in the way of accepting and appreciating such a precious gift.

If a Mantra has been received in a dream, usually enough of it is experienced in the dream state to allow the aspirant to recognize the Guru. However, it is entirely at the discretion of the Guru whether or not an initiation will be given. There is no obligation for the Guru to give a Mantra in such cases. Nor is there an obligation just because of contact with a devotee for a number or years, even through living together in the Ashram of the Guru. It is not any kind of automatic promotion.

Sometimes Guru and disciple will meet again because of the promise of the Mantra. The disciple will also return when the Guru incarnates to help with the Work, to repay the time and effort that was spent with the disciple in previous lives. Before his death Ramakrishna indicated when and where he would come back. Those around him asked him jokingly how they would know him and he said that he would carry a hookah! One disciple remarked it would not matter to him because he was not going to return. Ramakrishna replied, "Oh, yes, you will. When the lotus flowers it brings along all the leaves, buds and flowers on the stem, for its completion." This illustrates the responsibility that also rests with the disciple, and makes it more clear why the Guru must be informed of actions, which may be contrary to the furthering of the Work.

The Mantra initiation is an essential first step if the aim is to become a Sannyasin. In Ashrams it is a rule of thumb that one is initiated by the Guru first into Mantra, followed a few years later by the Brahmacharya initiation, and then Sannyasa. The periods of time between these initiations are meant for intensive study, and for putting into practice what has been learned. The initiation into swamihood gives the right to teach Vedanta and there are different orders which have certain distinctions.

As an example of the inflated ideas some aspirants have of their qualifications, one student was under the belief that he could be a teacher because he already felt like one and resented that others did not see him that way. He thought that his saintliness and greatness as a Guru might be purposely retarded by God in order to maintain his interest in helping and guiding others. This is a perverted way of thinking and is an escape from possible criticism for not having the development necessary to be a Guru. Such misconceptions may arise from observing situations in which the Guru may purposefully joke or even pretend to be slow or stupid, in order to diminish the fear of some devotees. Or some may naturally, like Swami Purushotthamananda, be very childlike, able to take great joy in simple things and find humour in situations that would be unnoticed by others. The awe of the devotee is a hindrance for both Guru and disciple. In considering what qualifies one as a Guru, we can remember St. Augustine who was told "not yet" because there were a number of pleasures — women, debating — that he still enjoyed and was not willing to give up. He tells of this in his book, *Confessions of St. Augustine*.

The accusation is made that Gurus dangle initiations before aspirants. If this is done, there is a certain objective in mind. There may be the desire to collect many initiates for emotional or economic purposes, although I have not personally encountered this. As in anything which involves human beings, there will always be good and bad Gurus. The human mind is capable of exploiting anything — the wars which have been fought in the name of various religions is proof of that.

However, this kind of "stick and carrot" method is applied by many parents; companies dangle promotions before people, so the thought is justified. But if such a suspicion is in the heart of the devotee, the wisest thing would be not to seek initiation from that Guru.

Aspirants often ask what would happen to the world if everyone became an initiate, took Brahmacharya or Sannyas. There is no danger of the world dying out, because there are too many people who want to keep the old games going.

Chapter Ten

Mantra in Daily Life

Whatever you achieve through your Mantra practice becomes knowledge which is indestructible. You may lose your life, but the knowledge remains and will reappear in another lifetime. Its purity depends upon how pure a channel you have made of yourself, to what extent you have put your ego aside. Feed your mind the finest food, as you feed your body the most healthful food. Bring quality into your life, refine your senses so that you may become more receptive to the Most High. Do not seek to acquire powers. Whatever the Divine is giving you as a gift or as a signpost that you are on the right path, do not seek to increase that power for some personal end. Do not seek to have power over others. Be grateful and give thanks to the Gurus who have gone before you, because they have opened and prepared the way.

When you feel critical of yourself or others, counteract this by chanting a Mantra in your mind. Let the Mantra truly take over and purify the mind and you will see the blessings that come to you. That effort may sometimes seem beyond your capabilities. When you feel that way, resort to prayer and ask for help. This is an act of humility, to realize that you cannot do it all by yourself. Those who have achieved Cosmic Consciousness before you will respond and bring you also close to that state.

Do not hesitate to cry at the feet of God about your unworthiness because God will make you worthy. If you have received a Mantra initiation there must be some worthiness, but it is your responsibility and obligation to demonstrate it. God and Guru work with you but they do not carry you, they do not work for you. Yoga is the path of revelation and liberation. You have to open the door.

When you chant the Name of God the work you do becomes easier, more joyful; it is no longer a distasteful duty because the Mantra will be continuously in the back of the mind, bringing the attention back to God and to the thought that God is working through your mind and hands.

By chanting or reciting, aloud or silently, you carry the force, the power of the Mantra and this power will be a blessing wherever you go. But remember that it is from the Mantra, not your personality, that the blessing comes. By mentally repeating your Mantra when others come to you with their problems, you prevent the thinking process from obstructing intuition. However, do not think that you always have to have the answer. You may not be the channel for this person, or your silence may be their best lesson at this point.

For people living an ordinary life in the world, all the practice and work in self-development will build a foundation for the time when they can pursue a more intense search for higher values and the spiritual goal. It is good to chant a Mantra while engaged in such routine tasks as washing dishes, scrubbing floors, or cutting the grass, because in these the mind is left relatively free and much energy can be wasted in allowing it to drift. These tasks provide an opportunity for self-purification.

At the end of the day do not watch the news or have an argument, or, at this most susceptible time, you will take the anger and violence into your dreams. Instead take a positive message with you when you go to sleep by playing a Mantra tape or chanting your Mantra. You can train yourself to keep the Mantra with you all night during sleep. As you switch off the light, think that you are symbolically switching off all daily activity, then lie quietly and recite your Mantra. Soon the Mantra will take over because at this time, when the power of suggestion is at its strongest, the energy of the Mantra is most active.

Learn to keep the Mantra going in your mind at all times. Use the various forms of Japa — Likhita, Vaikhari, Upamsu, Manasika — alternating them with chanting, depending on the occasion, or to give your busy mind the variety it wants. It does not matter if others think you strange to be writing or whispering to yourself. Be God's fool — the "Pearl of Great Price" is worth the price.

Practice until you get results. Do not give up! Yogananda once said, "A saint is a sinner who never gives up."

Hare Om Hare Hare Om Hare

Chapter Eleven

A Disciple:
Faith Can Work Miracles

A Disciple — Faith Can Work Miracles
from *Japa Yoga* by Swami Sivananda Sarasvati

A great Guru who lived in a temple on the bank of a broad river and had many hundreds of disciples all over, once summoned his disciples, saying that he wanted to see them before his death, which was to take place soon. The most favourite disciples of the great Guru, who always lived with him, grew anxious and kept themselves close to him day and night. For they thought that he might disclose to them at last the secret which made him so great, and all of them fearing lest they should miss the great opportunity, watchfully awaited the moment when the secret would be revealed. For, though their Guru taught them many sacred Mantras they acquired no powers and hence thought that the Guru still kept to himself the method which made him great. Disciples from everywhere arrived every hour and awaited with great expectation.

Now a humble disciple who lived far away on the opposite side of the river also came. But the river which was in high flood was too turbulent even to allow boats to pass. However, the humble disciple must not wait, as in the meanwhile the Guru may pass away. He should not tarry; but what was to be done? He knew that the Mantra which his Guru taught was all-powerful and capable of doing anything. Such was his faith. So, chanting the Mantra with faith and devotion he walked over the river. All the disciples who saw this were surprised at his powers. And recognising him as the one who came long ago to their Guru and stayed but one day and went away after being taught something by him, all the disciples thought that the Guru had given him the secret. They sternly demanded of their Guru why he deceived them thus, though they served him in every humble manner for many years, and yielded the secret to a stranger who came there for a day, long ago.

The Guru, with a smile, waved them to be calm, and summoning the humble disciple to his presence, ordered him to tell the disciples what he was taught by him long ago. The anxious group of disciples was taken aback with amazement when they heard him utter the name of "Kudu-Kudu" with awe, veneration, and devotion. "Look," said the Guru, "in it he believed, and thought that he got the clue to all. And even so is he rewarded for his faith, concentration and devotion. But you always doubted, thinking that something remained unrevealed still, though I told you Mantras of great powers. This distracted your concentration, and the idea of a great secret was in your mind. You were constantly thinking about the imperfection of the Mantra. This unintentional and unnoticed concentration upon the imperfection made you imperfect."

The Disciple and the Temple

There was once a temple in a small mountain city near a holy river. The temple had a door that closed very firmly — and had no handle. The only way the door could be opened was by chanting the Lord's name. Every few years all the saints and sadhus were invited to come to the temple and take turns at sitting, chanting one of the names of God, before the temple doors. If God accepted their offering, He would Himself open the door.

Now, not far from the city was a cave, in which was living a very famous Mantra singer, and a young man, and they shared their practice time together. They slept the same length of time, ate together and spent their meditation time together. The cave was very small so it was necessary for them to coordinate their activities so as not to disturb one another. And as they both worshipped the same aspect of God there was a harmony between them as perfect as can be among spiritual people.

In accordance with tradition, they went to the temple and the opportunity to chant before the temple doors was given first to the older man. When his turn came, he sat before the door and sang his heart and soul out to God. After two weeks the doors opened with a bang.

So the younger man's turn came and he, too, sat before the temple doors and chanted. A week passed, two weeks, three weeks. According to the tradition no one was refused to sit before the temple door and chant, however long he may spend there. The young man chanted for a month, two months, and as the weeks went by three months passed. Then, suddenly, with a great clap of thunder, the doors of the temple burst open and everyone present was thrown to the ground by the shock.

The young man went home and sat under a tree and wept. He said, "Lord, am I so far away, so very far away from You that it has taken me this long to open the temple doors? What have I done? Please tell me." And the Lord granted His beloved devotee a vision and said, "Put aside all your worries, my child. I was so delighted with your singing that I forgot to open the door."

MANTRAS

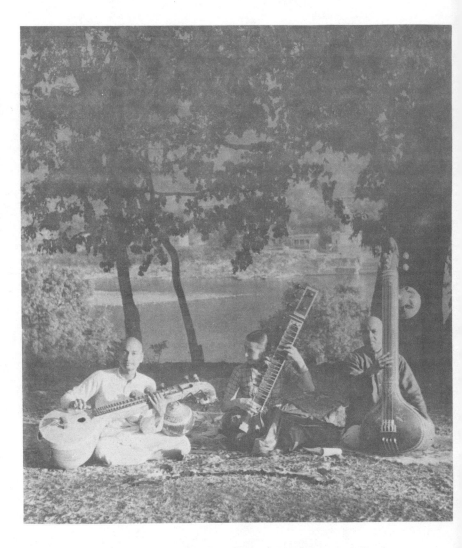

On the banks of the Ganges Swami Venkatesananda plays
the veena, Swami Radha the sitar and Swami
Nada Brahmananda the tambura. These Indian musical
instruments are mainly used while chanting Mantras
and Bhajans to help the singer keep the correct tune.

Om Namah Sivaya

Om Om Om Om

Hari Om

Swami Venkatesananda playing the veena for his guru,
Swami Sivananda. This seemed to be Swamiji's way of
"communicating without words."

Radhe Govinda

Om Krishna Guru

Krishna Invocation

Swami Nada Brahmananda instructing Swami Radha in the
use of the harmonium for chanting Mantras.

Ave Maria. . . Most Beautiful Mother

Namo Amitabha

Om Namo Bhagavate

Swami Sivananda playing a harmonium, a specially developed
instrument to bridge the gap between the scale of Indian music
and Western music. Gurudev liked to chant. He felt that
chanting was the greatest inspiration and also the best way of
glorifying the Most High and cultivating the emotions
into noble feelings.

Sri Rama Jay Ram

Om Sri Ram

I am Thine, All is Thine

MANTRAS
Guru & Disciple

Excerpts from the Writings
of Swami Sivananda Saraswati

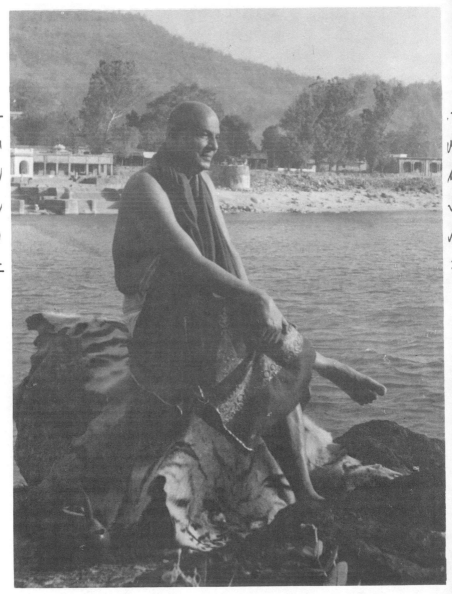

Swami Sivananda seated on a tiger skin placed over a rock
on the banks of the Ganges. Swami Sivananda later presented
the tiger skin as a gift to Swami Radha.

Excerpts from the Writings
of Swami Sivananda Saraswati

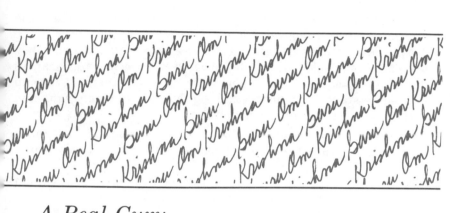

A Real Guru

Here are the characteristics of a real Guru. . . . He has full knowledge of the Self and Vedas. He can remove the doubts of aspirants. He has equal vision and a balanced mind. He is free from. . . egoism, anger, lust, greed, . . and pride. In his presence one gets Santi and elevation of mind.

India, the sacred land of Adwaita philosophy, the land which produced Sri Sankar, Dattatreya, Vam Dev and others who preached oneness of life and unity of consciousness is full of sectarians now. . . . it is difficult to count the number of sects that are prevailing now in India. . . . Hopeless discord and disharmony reign everywhere. . . . The disciples of one Guru fight with the disciples of another Guru. . .

Lord Chaitanya, Sri Guru Nanak, Swami Dayananda were all catholic, exalted souls. All their teachings were sublime and universal. They never wanted to establish sects or cults of their own. Had they lived now they would have wept at the actions of their followers. . .

A spiritual teacher should never establish a sect of his own. Founding a sect means creation of a fighting center to disturb the peace of the world. . . . He can have an institution with broad, universal principles and doctrines that will not conflict with the principles of others and that can be universally accepted and followed by all.

Some. . . made no Ashrams. . . gave no lectures. . . made no disciples, yet their names were handed down. . . as ideal, spiritual personages. They have created such an indelible impression on the minds of people by their exemplary lives. . . . The vibrations of a realized soul do purify the whole world even if he remains in a far-off cave in the Himalayas. . .

Can a patient gauge the merits of a doctor as soon as he enters the consultation room? Ignorant disciples who have no experience in the spiritual path at once begin to test and examine their Guru. They make hasty conclusions and inferences from external appearances and ways of living. . . . Even though you live with them. . . you can hardly understand their hearts and depth of knowledge. Jnana and spiritual experiences are internal states.

A young man with a little training. . . poses for a Guru. . . . Ignorant worldy people are deceived. . . . Ladies are very easily duped, easily attracted by sweet music and melody. . . . These Gurus. . . easily influence them. . . make them their tools or instruments. . . exploit them. . . . Open your eyes. . . . Use your reason. . . . Beware of posing Gurus. . . . Some make disciples to get services when they become old.

Devotion to Guru

Guru is Brahman Himself. . . . A word from him is a word from God. Even his presence or company is elevating, inspiring and stirring. . . . Living in his company is spiritual education. . . . He knows the spiritual path. He knows the pitfalls and snares on the way. He gives timely warnings to the students. . . . It is he who overhauls the old, wrong, vicious Samskaras of aspirants, removes the veil of Avidya, all doubts, Moha, fear, etc., awakens the Kundalini and opens the inner eye of intuition.

A thirsty aspirant who has implicit faith in his Guru and who is very eager to imbibe the teachings, can only drink the nectar from him. The student can imbibe from his Guru in proportion to the intensity and degree of his faith in him.

The Guru tests students in various ways. Some students misunderstand him and lose their faith in him. Hence they are not benefitted.

The student and the teacher should live together as father and devoted son, with extreme sincerity and devotion. The aspirant should have an eager receptive attitude to imbibe the teachings of the master. Then only will the aspirant be spiritually benefitted.

In the initial stages, an aspirant will have to face many difficulties and doubts on his path. He must have somebody whom he can approach to get his doubts cleared.

You should be careful in selecting the Guru. Do not be carried away by the belief that somebody is a great Mahatma. ... You should not change your Guru after choosing one. ... Live with them or move among them for sometime. ... If he puts forth a contrary view to the one you hold, listen to it by all means, but do not change your central, basic principle. ..

It is only the Guru who will find out your defects. The nature of egoism is such that you will not be able to find out your own defects. ... In the spiritual path you will have to take out your bones, crush them into powder and extract oil from it and burn the wick with this oil for several years. Only then, will God appear before you. ... What is the nature of your goal? It is immortality. To attain this should you not strive hard?

Karma Yoga is very necessary for man's evolution. ... Ethical perfection can only be got by following the instructions of your Guru and by selfless service. ... Work is worship for a Karma Yogin. ... This is the way to annihilate your pride and vanity and false notion of superiority.

Energy is indestructible. What I have said will not go in vain. When a sound is uttered, it is not lost. And those who are in tune with my vibrations will be benefited by my speech.

Guru and Disciple

As man is under the influence of beginningless ignorance, he needs the help of a Preceptor to have Self-realisation. Just as a man cannot see his back, so also he cannot see his own errors.

When you live with your Guru, you must be prepared to do willingly any work assigned by him.

An aspirant who attends on his Guru with great devotion in his personal services, quickly purifies his heart. This is the surest and easiest way for self-purification.

Intense devotion to one's Guru and faithful adherence to his teachings are the most essential qualifications of true discipleship. . . . Gurubhakti draws down the grace of the Preceptor and bestows ultimately illumination and bliss. . . . The grace of the Guru flows towards the disciple if the latter has a true receptive attitude and sincere faith in his Guru.

One's individual ego, preconceived notions, pet ideas and prejudices and selfish interests should be given up. These stand in the way of carrying out the teachings and instructions of one's Guru. . . . Do total self-surrender to obtain the Guru's Grace. . . . Love of Guru should engender love for the whole universe, because you must see him in all.

The spiritual path is not like writing a thesis for an M.A. It is quite a different line. The help of a teacher is necessary at every moment. Young aspirants become self-sufficient, arrogant, and self-assertive these days. They do not care to carry out the orders of a Guru. . . . They want independence from the very beginning. They apply in an absurd manner, with a perverted intellect, the Neti-Neti Doctrine.

If you cannot get an ideal Guru, you can take even a man who has been treading the path of realisation for some years who is straightforward and honest, who is selfless, who is free from pride, egoism, who has good character, who has good knowledge of the Sastras.

Beware of pseudo-gurus. . . will exhibit tricks or feats to attract people. . . . Do not be deceived by their sweet talk.

★   ★   ★

Guru and disciple should be well acquainted with the nature of the other. The student should be able to know thoroughly well the ideas and principles of his Guru and the Guru must be able to detect the mistakes and imperfections in the student. The Guru should be allowed to make a complete study of the aspirant's inner nature. . . . The disciple should lay bare all weakness and shortcomings. . . allow himself to be tested in the crucible of sufferings by his Guru so the Guru may have full confidence in him.

Guru and Initiation

It is better if you get your Mantra from your Guru. This has a tremendous effect on the disciple. The Guru imparts his Shakti along with the Mantra. If you cannot get a Guru, you can select any Mantra according to your own liking and taste, and repeat it mentally, daily, with Shraddha and Bhava. This also has a great purificatory effect. You will attain the realisation of God.

The method of initiation need not necessarily be the same for every aspirant. According to the yearning of the aspirant the Lord will arrange his guide suited to the temperament of the Sadhak.

Initiation, inspiration and the attainment of knowledge depend upon the aspirant's personal efforts and his earnestness. The Lord's grace descends on him at the proper time, when his patient and sustained struggle for realisation is no longer necessary.

Some like Yogi Milarepa have to serve their masters arduously for a long time whereas some get the initiation in a flash. It depends upon the spiritual Sadhana and evolution of the Sadhak. Yogi Milarepa underwent a series of struggles during his service of his Guru. He had to perform superhuman acts of heroism and bravery before he was initiated. Sages and Rishis of yore put their students to severe trials before they took them into their confidence. They intuitively knew whether a student was fit for initiation. The neophytes were entrusted with the work of tending the cow, bringing fuel from the forest for the Ashram, washing the clothes of the Guru and such other works which look like menial service in the eyes of the present day Sadhaka. For Sadhaks like Swetaketu, Indra, Satyakama and others every act was an act of Yoga or worship of the Guru. To them nothing was menial. They dedicated everything to their masters with unselfish motive. Therefore, they quickly attained Chitta Shuddhi, studied and mastered the Vedas and finally acquired the knowledge of the supreme Self.

Gautama chose four hundred lean weak cows and asked Satyakama Jabala, his disciple, to tend them and instructed him not to return before they became one thousand.

The aspirant, before he desires the grace of the master, should deserve it. The supply of divine grace comes only when there is a real thirst in the aspirant and when he is fit to receive it.

If a Bhakta-saint is approached by an aspirant who wants to tread the path of knowledge, the former may direct the latter to the proper Guru for initiation. . . But a saint of perfect realisation can give initiation in any path.

It is very difficult to know the particular Yoga by which the Guru reached perfection unless he himself reveals it to the aspirant out of compassion. No Sadhak will be bold enough to put this question to his Guru lest he should be considered impertinent.

Except in cases of advanced Sadhaks, initiation comes after a long and patient service to the preceptor.

The disciple should come in close contact with the Guru during his service and try to imbibe all his good qualitites.

If the fault-finding nature is strong in the disciple, he cannot pick up anything from the preceptor and his spiritual progress will be at a standstill.

In the absence of a realised Sad-Guru, senior aspirants who have trodden the spiritual path for a long time, who are above base desires, who have served their preceptors for a long time, and who are Sannyasins also can help a neophyte. . . . If one is not able to find such an advanced aspirant, one can follow the teachings contained in the books written by realised saints. . . keep a photo of such a realised Guru and worship the same with faith and devotion. Gradually the aspirant will receive inspiration. The Guru may appear in a dream and initiate and inspire him at the proper time.

The disciple becomes like his Guru after some time by following his instructions. . . . A disciple is he who follows the instructions of the Guru to the letter and spirit, who propagates the teachings of the Guru to less evolved souls in the path, till the end of his life.

Are You Really Qualified ?

The spiritual aspirant must have faith and devotion to Guru and the Lord. . . intense aspiration and dispassion. . . lead a contented life, and possess the three fundamental virtues — Ahimsa, Satyam and Brahmacharya. . . be gentle, humble and noble.

The aspirant has to. . . observe moderation in everything and lead a well-regulated, disciplined life of perfect celibacy and self-restraint . . . discipline the senses. . . possess a loving heart. . . never injure the feelings of others. . . not be jealous.

He has no right to compare his privileges with those of others. If a thing is refused to him he should not aspire for it again. Without the spirit of selfless service and self-denial it is very difficult to progress.

The Sadhak must speak gently, sweetly and truthfully... always be cheerful, earnest, vigilant and diligent.

He must possess adaptability, courage, mercy, generosity, tolerance, patience, perseverance and discrimination. He should bear insult and injury, have equanimity, fortitude and forbearance.

His speech must agree with his thought, and his action must agree with his speech.

Even for a single day he should not miss introspection and self-analysis.

He must stick to his ideal and should be ever aware of his goal.

Never despair; be hopeful always. Persist in your practice.

★   ★   ★

Even in the study of secular science and wordly matters you need the help of a teacher. You cannot understand science, mathematics, algebra, geometry without the aid of a teacher. ... Is it not much more necessary, then, to have a Guru in transcendental matters, when the aspirant has to walk along the rugged, thorny spiritual path?

Guru's Grace alone will sustain you in the perilous spiritual path which is as sharp as the edge of a razor.

Even Sri Sankara, Lord Krishna, Lord Rama, Sri Ramanuja, and Ekanath, had their Guru.

The Four Means

Warning:

A student who treads the path of Truth must equip himself with the four means of salvation or Sadhana Chatushtaya viz., Viveka, Vairagya, Shad-Sampat and Mumukshatva.† ... These four means are as old as the Vedas or this world itself. Every religion prescribed these four essential requisites for the aspirant. Names only differ.

Let me sound a note of warning here. ... Vairagya also may come and go if you are careless and mix promiscuously with all sorts of worldly-minded persons. You should develop Vairagya to the maximum degree. The mind is so constituted that it is waiting like a vulture to get back the things once renounced... you should take refuge in Viveka and in the impenetrable fortress of wise, dispassionate Mahatmas.

There are different degrees in Vairagya. Supreme dispassion comes when one gets himself established in Brahman. The Vairagya becomes perfectly habitual.

The desire for sensual enjoyment is deep-rooted or ingrained in the minds of all. The Rajasic mind is so framed that it cannot remain even for a single moment without thoughts of enjoyment of some kind or another. People invent various sorts of subtle enjoyments. Modern science has made marvellous contribution towards bringing forth refined ways of enjoyment. Modern civilisation is only another name for sensual enjoyment. . . hotels, cinemas, aeroplanes, radios. . . new dishes, new syrups, new drinks. . . fashion in dress. . . the hair. Even the man who is treading the path of Truth wishes to find lasting and intense sensual enjoyments by means of his Yogic practices. He wants to taste the nectar of immortality. . . hear the music of celestial nymphs. . . These are the subtle temptations. The sincere aspirant will resolutely turn his back from all sorts of refined, subtle, intense forms of enjoyments herein and hereafter.

†*Viveka — discrimination; vairagya — dispassion; shad-sampat — six-fold virtue bringing about mental control and discipline; mumukshatva — intense desire for liberation.*

Greatest Factor in Spiritual Realisation

A true disciple is concerned only with the Divine Nature of the Guru. The Guru's action as man, is not the disciple's concern. . . . Always remember that the nature of a saint is unfathomable. . . . Measure not his divine nature with the inadequate yardstick of your ignorance.

★   ★   ★

He who initiates Mantra is Diksha-Guru or initiatory Guru.

He who teaches the various forms of Sadhana and Yoga is Shiksha Guru or the teaching Guru.

Of these two, he is the supreme Guru from whom the great Mantra of Ishtadevata has been heard and learnt and by him alone Siddhi can be attained.

Competent disciples are never in want of a competent Guru.

The disciple achieves results in proportion to his faith in his Guru.

The possession of a university degree cannot entitle a man to be an examiner of a Guru.

It is the height of impertinence and foolishness on his part, blinded by the vanity of worldly knowledge, to test the spiritual knowledge of the Guru.

The Guru teaches through personal example. Learn it and act wisely.

The day to day conduct of the Guru is the living ideal to the disciple who is observant.

The true Guru is like a central power-house. He electrifies his disciples.

Mantra-Diksha is indeed a very rare and unique good fortune. Receive it with the utmost reverence and pure spiritual bhav.

A God-realised Sadguru never dies in the ordinary sense. He is ever present, as he has identified himself with the Immortal Cosmic Being. Worship the Guru always. . . . To sincere disciples, he can appear whenever he wills.

The highest form of worship of Guru is meticulous practice of his teachings and living by his example.

The relation between a Guru and disciple is real, sacred and everlasting.

Learn how to obey. Then only you can command.

Learn how to be a disciple. Then only you can become a Guru.

Listen to all but follow one. Respect all, but adore one. Gather knowledge from all, but adopt the teachings of one Master.

Correct understanding, non-attachment to wordly objects, serenity of mind, restraint of the senses, absence of base passions, faith in the Guru and devotion to God are necessary equipment with which the aspirant has to approach the Guru.

Satsang or association with the Guru is an armour and fortress to guard you against all temptations and unfavourable forces of the material world.

The mission of the saints is to save those lost in ignorance of the path leading to God.

The words of a saint go straight to the heart of hearers and cling there.

Saints do the great work of distillation. They raise the souls to purity, perfection, freedom and union with God.

The ink of a sage or Yogi is more precious than the blood of a martyr. A saint or a sage is a Teacher. He is a healer, harbinger of light, love, peace, strength and solace to the weary and heavy laden heart of humanity.

Stories

Our Wedding is Indissoluble!

"Sorrow not, my child. Sit down. In this world of phenomena such things do happen in the natural course of events. It is nobody's fault. When two minds come together, misunderstandings are natural. Sometimes quarrels do arise. Eventually the love of the heart overcomes all and cements the differences."

"It is not always possible for any two persons, however highly evolved they may be, to be always thinking alike and feeling alike. No two minds can ever agree. This is because each one is guided by one's own peculiar desires and cravings, ambitions and aspirations, and in so adjusting our conduct that their fulfilment becomes a joyous sacrifice on our part. If we have the spirit of service the very desires and ambitions in the other person would help us manifest our own spirit in a greater and greater measure."

"Inordinate attachment to things often causes an aggravation of disharmony."

"Such is the relationship between a Guru and his disciple... for it is on the plane where everything is Eternal. You and I have been together not only in this incarnation, but in so many of our past lives. Our relationship is irrevocable."

A Self-Sacrificing Disciple

Sri Gopala received his initiation from his Guru, Swami Santananda, in Benares. The Guru said: "Look here, my dear Gopala; you will attain Moksha by recitation of this Mantra. But do not reveal this Mantra to anybody. If you reveal it, you will go to hell."

Sri Gopala was an aspirant of a very large heart. He at once went to the market and recited the Mantra openly before a large assembly of persons. He spoke plainly: "You all can attain salvation through the recitation of this Mantra. It was given to me by my Brahma Nishta Guru. My guru told me that I would go to hell if I reveal it to other people. I am prepared to go to hell. But I am exceedingly glad to see that you all will attain Salvation."

Swami Santananda was passing along the market road. He heard the candid speech of his large-hearted, sympathetic disciple Sri Gopala. He was highly pleased with his sincere disciple and said: "My dear Gopala, you will also attain Moksha this very second. You are a noble, magnanimous soul. I want disciples of your description." Aspirants should develop Udaratta to a considerable extent. This will induce oneness, unity and cosmic love. It will generate Adwaitic feeling. It paves a long way to the attainment of Moksha.

The Technique of Perfection

Seekers of Truth!

The desire to seek help, to search for light, to look up to higher powers, is inborn in all beings. The incapacity to achieve the ideal of the aspirations that spring from the heart, the anguish which accompanies such incapacity, and the knowledge of the existence of superior powers, obliges individuals to take shelter under those that are endowed with the ability to lift them up to higher levels. The world is a dramatic scene of dependence of beings on others that can fill up what they lack. Love for God means the yearning to reach the highest, to become perfect, and this is not easy for all who wish to be so.

Perfection has its center in the core of the seeker himself and hence the difficulty of knowing the exact technique of realising it, which is God, Self, and all that is best. The key to the door that opens into the realm of truth and perfection does not lie in those who see through the intellect, but those who intuit the reality in integral comprehension, not as an object lying outside, but as rooted in the very meaning of the subject. These are called the seers or the sages, the Brahmanishtas who can communicate the spiritual consciousness even through a glance or a touch or through a single command. They are the Gurus or the Masters who teach the truth to and shower God-consciousness on the mortals. Patanjali Maharishi says that Ishwara himself is the greatest Guru, for he is the most ancient and is omnipresent and, being the seed of omniscience, he is the teacher of all teachers, unsullied by the changes of time. To surrender oneself to God is, therefore, to seek shelter under the origin of knowledge, the source of power, the Lord of creation itself. Guru is not the human personality. Guru is the Divine Being, the immortal essence that shines through the human person. The perishable body constituted by the physical elements should not be mistaken for the Guru. The real teacher is the one Brahman that manifests itself as and when it likes. Man can learn only from a human and hence God teaches man through a human body. The human body of the Guru is an occasion to worship his universal nature of supreme Light, a nail to hang the shirt on. The human side of the Guru is not what is important, it is the unseen but the only real Atman, the ubiquitous principle that underlies it, that is the true Guru. When we pray to God, we pray not to a body. When one resorts to a Guru, he does not do so to a material form. The dignified substratum of life, light and joy, the grand consciousness that soars above the paltry grandeur of the universe, that is what is to be seen in a Guru! "Hit it, O Somya," says the Upanishad. That is the target of meditation and the object of devotion, the teacher and the saviour, the support and the goal. Lord Krishna says, "Know me 'in truth'," where he emphasizes the fact that his form, the body, is not to be mistaken for the Eternal. Guru is God and God is Guru, and the Svetaswatara Upanishad says that the truth is revealed to that great-souled one who does not consider God and Guru as two different beings.

The sacred relation of Guru and disciple is a very ancient one. Even from Vedic times we hear of the necessity of the aspirants seeking Brahma-Srotriyas and Brahmanishtas being stressed. "Examining the worthless nature of the action-bound world the wise one should get disgusted with it, for the eternal cannot be reached through action. For the sake of knowing That he should resort to a Guru, well versed in spiritual lore and also established in Brahman-consciousness," says the Mundaka Upanishad. Though the Guru does not actually give anything not already possessed, he becomes the means which digs out the spiritual wealth that is buried under the ignorant mind of the aspirant. Since all experiences in the world are the effects of the interaction of the knower and the known, the spiritual experience too is in a different way the effect, as it were, of the union of subjective endeavour and the object presented before it, be it physical or purely psychical, be it embodied teachers or bodiless mental forms or ideas.

It is from the Guru that the seeker gets the influx of spirituality

and divine Bhava. What the aspirant receives, he intensifies and mul-
tiplies a thousand-fold through earnest Sadhana. This is the duty of all
aspirants. The Guru is the gateway to the transcendental Truth-
consciousness, but it is the aspirant that has to enter through it. The
Guru is a help but the actual task of practical Sadhana falls on the
aspirant himself.

In truth the Guru dwells in your heart. The Guru is ever by your
side. You have only to think of him with real Bhava and you will at
once feel his spiritual presence without fail. In proportion to the
effacement of the lower ego does the Guru manifest in you and appear
before you. Therefore be ever ready to receive him and empty yourself
of all contents so that he may fill himself in you.

Talks with the Aspirants

Is a Guru Necessary?

A Guru is absolutely necessary for everyone. In the initial stages
an aspirant will have to face many difficulties and doubts in his
path. He must have somebody whom he can approach to get his doubts
cleared. Even ordinary secular sciences have to be learnt from a
teacher. To learn the Science of science, Brahma Vidya or Self-
knowledge, the help of a Guru is absolutely essential. It is only the
Guru who will find out your defects. The nature of egoism is such that
you will not be able to find out your own defects. In the case of a very
few exalted souls, their own Self serves as their Guru and guides them
from within; but this is due to the fact that they have in their previous
births performed intense Sadhana with the help and guidance of
Brahma Vidya preceptors.

★　　★　　★

Only the man who has already been to Badrinath will be able to
tell you the road. In the case of the spiritual path it is still more difficult to find your way! The mind will mislead you very often. The Guru
will be able to remove pitfalls and obstacles and lead you along the
right path. He will tell you: "This road leads you to Moksha; this one
leads to bondage."

Some might find their own inner conscience is their Guru. It will
guide them aright. They, too, have ascended the steps of the ladder of

yoga through service of the Guru and through his instructions in their previous births. Their heart is so pure that doubts do not arise at all in them. They are, so to say, born Siddhas.

★   ★   ★

"Whom shall I choose as my Guru?"

He who is able to clear your doubts, he who is sympathetic in your Sadhana, he who does not disturb your beliefs but helps you on from where you are, he in whose very presence you feel spiritually elevated — he is your Guru. Once you choose your Guru, implicitly follow him. God will guide you through the Guru.

★   ★   ★

It is the duty of saints and elder Sannyasins to protect spiritually thirsting aspirants.

The aspirants of today need not renounce the world and run to the forest in search of a Guru. Some will, no doubt, do so; and they will eventually act as the spiritual guides to the rest of humanity. The vast majority would, however, have to learn at home and practise Yoga in their daily life, to learn and apply the technique of transforming their daily actions into Yoga Sadhana.

. . . The teacher and the seeker should meet half-way. This divine meeting place is a spiritual institution, Ashram or Math.

The worship and adoration of the Guru is the first step to Cosmic Consciousness.

The vision of the Guru will slowly expand. You will, under the wise guidance of the illuminated Guru, gradually perceive that Supreme Principle that resided in your Guru pervades the entire creation. When the inner consciousness expands, there will be nothing to obstruct it, no ego to limit its expansion. You will very soon realise Cosmic Consciousness. This is the Supreme secret of service of Guru, worship of Guru and self-surrender to Guru. First realise your God in your Guru. Then you will realise God in everyone. First serve your Guru selflessly. Then you will be able to serve the entire humanity selflessly. First worship your Guru with sincerity and devotion. Then you will worship the All-pervading Lord. Guru is the gateway to God-realisation.

Guru is the sacred altar at which you can willingly and lovingly sacrifice your ego.

★   ★   ★

It is the Guru who removes the veil of ignorance. Serve him with Bhakti. Then you will get his Grace. The physical form of the Guru will slowly vanish. You will realise the Atma in and through him. You will see your Guru in all forms, animate and inanimate.

★   ★   ★

Do not use your reason too much in the selection of your Guru. You will fail if you do so. If you fail to get a first-class Guru, try to follow the instructions of the Sadhu who is treading the path for some years, who has purity and other virtuous qualities and who has some knowledge of the scriptures. Just as a student of an intermediate class will be able to teach a student of the Third Form when a Professor with M.A. qualifications is not available. . . this second-class type of Guru will be able to help you.

★   ★   ★

The greatest service that I can do to humanity is training and moulding of aspirants. Every Yoga student, when he is purified and elevated, becomes a centre of spirituality. He will draw to himself through his magnetic aura thousands of baby-souls in spirituality for transformation and regeneration.

If you think that I am worthy enough, you can take me as your Guru.

★   ★   ★

Realised souls are not rare. Ordinary ignorant-minded persons cannot easily recognise them. Only a few persons who are pure and embody all virtuous qualities can understand realised souls and they only will be benefitted in their company.

Testing a guru is highly difficult. Do not use your intellect here. Have faith. The real aspirant is quite free from such questions and doubts. You will be miraculously helped if you believe in my words.

I am neither a Guru nor a Sat-Guru. I take great delight in serving others.

★   ★   ★

Fail not to observe the vow of celibacy at any cost.

★   ★   ★

Every Sannyasi, every Yogic student has some defect or other. It is only a full-blown Yogi or a Jnani who will be absolutely free from evil qualities and defects. . . are rare. . . . Slight friction is bound to come between friends, at times between Sannyasins too. One must excuse the other, must reunite and forget the past. You must have a tendency to grasp only the good in others. . . . Everyone has some virtues. No one is entirely bad. Remember the point well. After some time you will find good only in others. . . .

★   ★   ★

If you cannot get a suitable Guru, you can select any Mantra according to your inclination and repeat the same with great faith in the power of the Mantra. Any Mantra is powerful. Stick to one and to one form. Do not change. . . . Aspirants who have no faith in the Mantra, after some practice, jump to another. To avoid this, it is advised to get a Mantra from a Guru. Further the Guru imparts his special power to the disciple through the Mantra at the time of Diksha.

. . . I continuously work, read and write. I never go to hill-stations or sea-side for a holiday, change of work gives rest. Meditation gives abundant rest.

★   ★   ★

. . . I am a strange mixture of service, devotion, Yoga and wisdom. I am a follower of Sri Sankara. I am a Keval-Adwaita Vedantin. I am not at all a dry lip-Vedantin. I am a practical Vedantin.

I practise and advocate the Yoga of Synthesis. I practise Ahimsa, Satyam and Brahmacharya.

★   ★   ★

Renunciation of egoism alone constitutes the renunciation of all. Doership or enjoyership arises through the idea of 'I'.

★　　★　　★

The word Guru contains two letters — *Gu* and *Ru*. *Gu* means darkness and *Ru* means the dispeller. Being the dispeller of the darkness of ignorance, the teacher is called Guru.

Guru and Diksha (Initiation)

Yoga should be learnt from a Guru. It is he who will recognise the class to which the aspirant belongs and prescribe suitable Sadhana. The reason for the early downfall of the majority of aspirants is that they imagine themselves to be qualified to adopt the highest form of Yoga at the beginning. The qualified aspirant will be humble enough to approach a Guru, surrender himself to the Guru and serve and learn from him.

Diksha is the giving of the Mantra by the Guru. Initiation gives spiritual knowledge and destroys sin. As one lamp is lit at the flame of another, so the divine Sakti within Mantra is communicated from Guru to the disciple.

Initiation tears the veil of mystery and enables the disciple to grasp the hidden truth behind scriptural texts. The Guru only, by Diksha, will give the right perspective in which to study the scriptures. He will flash his torch of Self-realisation on the truth within them.

Siddhi

Siddhi is perfection. A Siddha is one who has attained perfection or Self-realisation through Sadhana. Literally Siddhi means success, achievement, attainment and fruition of all kinds.

One may attain Siddhi in speech, Mantra, Yoga, etc. The greatest of all Siddhis is liberation or Moksha, freedom from the cycle of births and deaths and union with Para Brahma or the Supreme Being.

The aspirant should not pursue siddhis, as he may misuse the powers. He should ignore them as they are obstacles in the spiritual path.

I Am Pain: Thy Teacher

I

O Man! You curse me, blame me,
You hate me and frown on me,
You think I am cruel and heartless;
You try to slay me with anaesthetics,
With Chloroform and Bromides;
You attack me with anodynes,
Sedatives and opiates;
You phone to the doctors
And run to the hospitals,
You fly to the Vienna and hill stations,
You wire to your friends and relations;
You approach the saints of Himalayas
For Buties or herbs;
You do Mrityunjaya Japa and Havan,
You burn incense and pray —
To kill the Teacher
Who warns you,
Who comes to help and bless you!

II

I am not your enemy —
I am your sincere friend!
I am a messenger from God,
I am an Angel from heaven —
To teach you wisdom,
To instill in your heart
Mercy and dispassion,
To turn your mind towards God,
To destroy your intense clinging
To things mundane —
That are perishable and illusory.
I am your guide and silent Teacher!
I am pain, the best thing in this world!
I am an eye-opener, soul-awakener,
I am an inspirer and thriller;
I came to remind you of God,
To point to you the Divine Path,
To make you desist from evil ways,
To make you practise virtues, good habits.
You have really misunderstood me.
I am a mental Vritti in the mind-lake,
I am only absence of pleasure,
I co-exist with pleasure —
I am the other side of the coin of pleasure-pain.
I am the cause of the starting of philosopy,
I am the cause for man's Purushartha —
I am the cause for man's aspiration:
I set the mind of philosophers to think,
I make the Yogis to start Sadhana,
I make the sages to practise meditation,
I make a worldly man a Super man.

III

You failed to observe the laws of health —
The rules of hygiene and right-living,
You took Rajasic and Tamasic foods,
You were not regular in doing exercise,
You did not practise Pranayama and Asanas,
You did not pray and meditate;
You were immoderate in your food —
You did not take a balanced diet,
You did not bask in the sun,
You slept in ill-ventilated rooms.
You took too much of sweetmeats,
You drank impure water,
You hated and injured your neighbours,
You were lustful, malicious and greedy,
You took meat, fish and eggs
And developed gout, rheumatism and albuminaria;
You married a third wife,
You were a heavy smoker in the club,
You drank liquors in the hotels;
You took bribes and cheated in business;
You twisted the truth in the courts,
And by clever advocacy
Sent innocent men
To the prison and the gallows
You injected water into the veins
And charged heavily for injections: —
And so, I come to you
To heal, teach and guide!

IV

Understand now at least
My secret and good nature,
My interest in your well-being.
Lead a virtuous life,
Practise simple living and high thinking,
Lead a natural life,
Observe the laws of health and hygiene —
Eat simple food, a well-balanced diet,
Take only vegetarian diet;
Practise Ahmimsa, Satyam, Brahmacharya,
Lead the Life Divine,
Remain as a Brahmacharin,
Or better still, take to Sannyasa
After equipping yourself with 'four'.
Attend the Sadhana Weeks,
Practise Sadhana in Ananda Kutir,
And the Training Courses,
Go through the "Divine Life" magazine,
Study "Spiritual lessons," "Aphorisms,"
"The Necessity for Sannyasa"
And practise the precepts contained therein;
Remember Lord Viswanath always,
Take bath in the Ganges and purify.
Then I will depart and leave you,
I will not trouble you any longer.
Love me, believe me, heed my message
I will give you peace, bliss, immortality,
I will surely bless you:
This is my definite promise, friend!
Good bye, comrade! Be cheerful!

MANTRAS
Questions and Answers

Om - Om
Hari Om Hari Om
Hari Om Hari Om Hari Om
Hari Om Hari Om Hari Om
Hari Om Hari Om Hari Om
Hari Om Hari Om Hari Om
Hari Om Hari Om Hari Om Hari Om Hari Om Hari Om Om
Hari Om Hari Om Hari Om Hari Om Hari Om Hari Om Hari Om
Hari Om Hari Om Hari Om Hari Om Hari Om Hari Om Hari Om
Om Hari Om Hari Om Hari Om Hari Om Hari Om Hari Om
Om Hari Om Hari Om Hari Om Hari Om Om Hari
Hari Om - Om Hari

Questions and Answers

Interview with Swami Radha

Q. *Swami Radha, let us begin at the beginning; what is a Mantra?*

A. A Mantra can be many things, but at the start it is enough to say that my own Guru, Swami Sivananda of Rishikesh, defines the Mantra as a "sacred syllable or word or set of words through the repetition and reflection of which one attains perfection or realization of the Self."

Q. *Is a Mantra, then, always associated with the Divine, with the name of a Deity?*

A. Not always, or not directly. The three Mantras that we often chant at the Ashram, "Om Krishna Guru," "Hari Om," and "Om Namah Sivaya," are associated directly with the Deity, the first two with Krishna and the last with Siva. But "Om" can also be chanted alone; it is indeed a Mantra and many volumes have been written on its meaning.

Q.   I know that to be effective the Mantra must be repeated many times; can you tell us how many?

A.   There really is no limit; I myself have chanted five hours a day for two years. Later I continued to chant for only two hours, because by that time I had built up what is called "Mantric Power," which is necessary before one can give another person a Mantra initiation. Why would I have to chant for five hours at a time? Because it takes that long for the mind to become single-pointed. There have been some spiritual giants in India who have chanted ten hours a day for many years. Obviously, the more you put into it, the more you will achieve.

Q.   This seems extraordinary to the Western mind. What can one really achieve through chanting? What good is it likely to do me to repeat the same thing over and over?

A.   Yes, I can understand that it may not seem rational, but I know from my own experience that there are certain immediate results. First, the ability to concentrate is much increased; then control of breath and emotions is gradually achieved. After this first stage of development, when emotions have been refined into true feelings, the influence of the power of the Mantra becomes very subtle. The image of the Deity, with which you start, will disappear as perceptions attain greater clarity and a state of purity unknown as long as they were overruled by the senses. The most important goal in chanting is the attainment of perfection, the realization of the Self.

Q.   Before we get into that, perhaps you might wish to tell us of your own experience. Did you know anything of Mantras before you went to India to meet Swami Sivananda?

A.   Not at all. As a child I had many out-of-the-ordinary experiences and perceptions and, although I did not think of it that way, I used to sit in meditation — deep, deep in thought looking at one spot. My mother tried to discourage these strange ways and interest me in doing the things young girls usually do. I never read any books on the subject of meditation, Mantra or Yoga while I was in Germany and do not know if any were available. When I came to Canada I was so busy trying to learn English for my job that I had no time to read.

When I came to India I heard about Mantras and the marvelous power they have. But I was Western and very skeptical, and remarked to my Guru, "I cannot question it because I do not know enough, my questions would only be on the level of assumption." I realized that the only thing for me to do was to practice chanting the Mantra so I would have something substantial to ask about. As a result, through my practice of Mantra and keeping notes — I would record most of the times when I reached "impasses" as I called them, times when I just did not know why I was doing this practice — I recognized the rebellion of my mind. It complained of carrying on something that seemed useless. But I continued — five hours a day, seven days a week, for seven weeks.

Swami Sivananda told me that I should intersperse the chanting with worship. When I said that I came from a Protestant religion and had no interest in ritual, he suggested something very simple and very beautiful, that I grow white flowers and place them on some form of altar when I chanted to Lord Siva. He said that I should always designate the same spot in my house as a holy place, and when I placed white flowers there, by the law of thought association, they would put me in touch with the spirit that is expressed in the symbol of Lord Siva. Then I was to grow blue flowers to associate with Lord Krishna, and roses or any colourful flower for Divine Mother.

By this time Sivananda had explained the male-female duality in the pantheon of the gods and goddesses of the Indian religions. To help me understand, he compared this to the family unit in the villages where one always know the mother of a child, but not always the father. One can always recognize the power manifest — the female aspect, Divine Mother, or Sakti — but one cannot always recognize power unmanifest, the symbol of the male, Lord Siva. I reflected on this, "Yes, I can incorporate that into my thinking. When I grow white flowers for Siva I will remember that white has no colours, or has all colours, and Siva is energy, power. It is hard to think of energy, but the very fact that I know that it is energy will help me. Sivananda is not asking me to worship an image of Siva." I had the insight that the meditation on Lord Siva did not need to end with His image, that the image just became a focal point for my mind until I understood on a deeper level, intuitively, the principle of energy as such.

I did not feel strong in my spiritual practice, my meditation; my concentration was on a teeter-totter. An image helped me to focus on something that was a little strange; although it was a human figure I could not mistake it for any person I knew. In particular, the symbolic meaning of the bent position of Lord Krishna was helpful — "I am lenient with you, I am aware of your human failings. You keep forgetting your Divine nature on account of the body, but I will remind you."

I thought in the same way about Divine Mother, and then I began to understand that a religion that has both the male and female aspects is bound to survive. I could see why the Buddhists had the Mother of Mercy, and why the Catholics had placed so much emphasis on Mary.

It was not easy, but I learned many things. As I had not had time to read books, what I did learn came to me from my own experience. I became aware of the impasses of the mind, the obstacles that the mind creates. I became aware of habit; habit had suggested to me that I would not be able to accomplish this chanting, that I would reach an impasse. If I had not made this suggestion to myself, or had not accepted the disparaging remark of someone I looked to as an authority, I might have had less difficulty.

I also had the problem of being sure that I had completed an accurate number when I chanted my Mantra. So I took a box of matches, I had my mala with 108 beads, and every time I finished one mala I would throw one match on the floor. When I had finished 10 malas I thought, "Well, I have done 80 extra Mantras. What shall I do with them?" I decided to make it 1100, simply to overcome the resistance of my mind. Slowly I got hold of myself. The side effects of this were remarkable.

My very depressive moods, seeing no purpose in life, all lifted. I had been given every material thing I wished for but did not find it worth living for that. Nor did I find it worthwhile to live for a marriage, when I saw all the problems of married life. But I felt there must be happiness somewhere and I wondered — there were so many stories that we have descended from heaven — is it possible for anyone to think of anything that has not existed at some time in the past or might exist at some time in the future? The story of Icarus in Greek mythology came to my mind, the man who wished to fly. I thought that this may have been the beginning of the airplane. Maybe these things have to be imagined and desired in the mind to bring about the manifestation. The same principle Sivananda had told me about — power unmanifest. What can I manifest? What will sound manifest? Do sounds manifest at all?

I was probably very hard on myself. I would sometimes get up and walk around the Prayer Room to stop myself from falling asleep, until I had finished my practice. I had not known about such a spiritual practice until I went to China. The monks there often walk for as much as 16 hours, but I was only walking to keep myself awake until I had finished my Mantras.

I became aware of numerous things; that when someone pronounces my name, from the resonance of the voice I know if that person is friendly, if that person likes me, or is only socially polite, cool, reserved and distant. So many people are unaware of the messages they give, even in a simple word, how they give themselves away. So I began to understand that there was something in the practice of chanting Mantras, after all.

Then some very beautiful things happened. I saw clouds of colours — lovely shades of blue. I thought of what blue meant — the blue Monday when people are depressed and not very active; the beautiful blue of the sky that makes everyone happy. Lord Krishna is presented as blue, and this shade of blue has become anchored in my mind as Krishna blue. The fleeting thought came to my mind that I must study symbology. I noticed that after I had seen these beautiful shades of blue when chanting I was elated for a long time.

After some time I became aware that I was becoming indulgent, and I said, "Oh, my God, I am looking forward to something like spiritual movies. When will I ever stop looking for entertainment, comfort?" That is disastrous. Then one day I had an experience in which I maintained awareness. The sounds became like huge soap bubbles and they were spinning around; they had a kind of colour and yet they didn't. Suddenly the desire surged up in me, "I wish I could sit on one and travel into space." At that very moment I saw myself move into space. That experience was a discovery for me that there is more than one way of leaving the body. I never had the connection of a silver cord or anything like that, as I had heard of in others' experiences; there was nothing tugging at me. And I began to wonder if my experiences were genuine, but then I stopped making comparisons, remembering again my Guru saying, "Competition is not desirable, although it is tolerated in business; but it should not exist on the Spiritual Path."

These experiences became a tremendous foundation and source of strength to help me to carry on when my mind became restless, when it tried to revolt against this new discipline. My Guru, my great Guru, was a wonderful inspiration. I wanted to make real changes in myself and any pain and any effort were worth it.

Q. It is very good to have this information of how you felt personally in your early days of chanting Mantras. Perhaps now we can discuss in more detail some of the reasons for undertaking this practice.

A.   Well, then, let me first say a few words about developing the quality of single-pointedness, and about overcoming self-will. In the beginning, while I was chanting, I would be sitting there asking myself, "Am I an idiot? What am I doing here? What is going to come of all this? I could be doing so many other things, and being of help to so many people, instead of just sitting here all this time chanting." These are typical thoughts, typical complaints, and what you are going through is a tug-of-war with your mind which wants to force your Higher Self out of control. When I say "mind" or "ego" I do not necessarily mean pride and vanity; I mean rather, a body-mind which has been the ruler, and when we encourage our Higher Self to exert mastery over us through the practice of Mantra Yoga, we suddenly become aware of all the personality aspects which have ruled our lives. These personality aspects, when threatened, put up a fight; they do not want to lose their hold on us.

The ego or personality aspects of the intellectual will put up a greater fight than those of the rather naive person. The latter is more able to say, "Yes, I see where I was wrong; I won't do that again," while the intellectual is still stubbing his toes, thinking up rational explanations to justify mistakes.

This is one of the dangers facing the follower of Jnana Yoga, the yoga of the mind; he will look down on the practitioner of Bhakti Yoga, the yoga of love and devotion. This only indicates that he has not used his mind to develop true discrimination. Many swamis and yogis in India told me that they hoped that in their next lives they would be reincarnated as women because women have true devotion, true humility, and this is the path to liberation.

You see, to overcome the ego we must practice surrender. We must be able to surrender to the Mantra itself and to the energy of the Mantra, and this requires purification. If we cannot surrender, that energy will feed the ego and we will become real ego-maniacs. That is why many disciples prostrate themselves at the feet of their Guru; it is an aid in developing humility. The disciple will, in fact, be prostrating himself to the Divine Spirit that is in the Guru, and in all of us.

Another important aspect of chanting is that it will help us to understand and control our emotions. And this will come about as you become more aware of your own voice. At the beginning, in order to help develop single-pointedness, when you notice that your mind is just not able to be still, you allow it to be active, but you keep it within the framework of your activity by going into all the small details. Think, "How does my voice produce a sound? What is necessary for it to do so? How do I create a higher sound?" and so on. Even an exercise such as this to maintain single-pointedness can lead to many insights.

You will find in the course of time that you can sing as you have never done before and that your range has expanded; you can sing both higher notes and those that are lower. You will notice that when the breath flows evenly, the voice is smooth. You will hear the expression of anger or disappointment in your voice, as well as all other emotions. But you must learn when to stop, when to think, "All right, that is enough now; I do not need to continue or I will be indulging myself." When you find that your emotions are extremely difficult to control, then you address the Divine Energy at a very personal level, saying, "YOU! I'm not responsible for all of this. Why did You give me all these emotions? Why did you not give me the strength and insight to handle them? I want You to come here now and do something about it; open the door or pull the curtain back so that I can see why I feel this way." You may not consider that to speak like this to the Divine is a form of prayer, but it is. It is all right for you to address the Divine Energy at a very personal level, even though you understand intellectually that when you say "Lord" or "You" there is no other being, but the intelligence that created you as a personal unit is both personal and impersonal. To recognize the need for help and to be willing to ask God for that help, this is humility.

It is interesting and a little sad that most people can only be single-pointed when they are in distress; when they are joyful they will be single-pointed for an instant, but then they begin to scheme to keep that joyful mood, and of course the scheming destroys it. But when you are chanting in the single-pointedness of your despair, then you let go and you give it all back. You can say, "Well, I'm sorry, but I have to admit that I am like a baby that can't even walk. You must come and pick me up. You have to wait until I can walk. And if You want me to walk, if You don't want me to always be a spiritual baby, then You must come now and help me." There comes a time when each seeker must take off the spiritual baby shoes, but for a while do not be too proud to be God's little child.

Q. Could you tell us now how Mantras were created and something about the history of this practice?

A. The goal of all yogas is revelation, union with the Divine. Different paths of yoga have been followed in different ages, or "yugas" as they are sometimes referred to. In each yuga the goal of yoga is fulfilled in the best possible way suitable to the individual in that particular age. In the Satya Yuga, for example (satya means purity), it was not necessary for the aspirants to do very much Hatha Yoga, or Bhakti or Jnana Yoga, the emphasis was on meditation. In the Treta Yuga sacrifices were recommended. These did not need to be the sacrifice of life; it might be the sacrifice of the desires for life, desires that are not really deep and that would have meant fulfillment on a particular level of life. In the Dvapara Yuga all forms of worship were encouraged, prayers, conversations with God, worship in the highest form.

Each yuga had certain yogis, teachers, saints to show the Path, holy people who have understood the emphasis of their particular time. We are now supposed to live in the Kali Yuga, the Iron Age, the last of the four yugas, the evil age. Evil forces and immorality are supposed to prevail, and it would certainly seem to be so. At this time, the chanting of the Lord's Name, and the Mantra or Mantra Yoga is supposed to be the best development for the individual. There is a saying, "Kali Yuga Keval Namah Adhara" — in the Kali Yuga the Holy Name is the boat to cross the ocean of Maya, illusion. The Name of God is the weapon with which to conquer the mind.

Tradition says that the Mantras were given to us by the Rishis, the great seers, holy ones and teachers who lived in times past. They, in turn, are said to have picked up the Mantras, or tuned into them, on the etheric level. The Mantras were created from the subtle vibrations of many millions of people who have cried out in their distress across the centuries. They are, so to speak, the essence of all those cries, but the Mantras are more than that; they are the answers to those cries.

Q. You have described some of the benefits of chanting a Mantra and told of the possible origin of the Mantra. Does the Mantra have any power of its own, or is all the benefit to be gained just from the repetition?

A.   That is a very good point to bring up, though here again, the Western mind may find it a little difficult to accept this concept. Consciousness may be perceived as energy. Subconscious, superconscious, all is energy, a vortex of energy, and it can be compared to the funnel you might see in a tornado. Actually, the funnel does not exist; it is the air current picking up the dust and forming a funnel. When the tornado is gone, the energy goes somewhere else and manifests in the same or a different way. Compare consciousness to that energy — consciousness is indestructible.

To give another example which may lead to the understanding of the power of the Mantra, I read sometime ago of a very curious incident in England, when the call letters of a television station in the United States were picked up on the receiver of a television studio. What was really curious was not that the call letters had travelled such a long distance, but that that particular test pattern had not been used for several years. So the energy that had been manifested in those call letters had drifted about in space for five years at the rate of 186,000 miles per second and then apparently by chance, had come back to the planet earth.

Now, if you think of all the people in India over the years who have chanted the name of Krishna or Siva, or all the Christians over the centuries who have repeated or chanted the name of Jesus, you can see that this constant repetition would create a tremendous reserve of power and that the truly devout person who chants the name of a particular aspect of the Divine will eventually tap into that power.

It is important to understand the meaning of the Devata, the presiding deity of the Mantra, the informing power, the personified aspect of God. If you think of a diamond as representing Cosmic Intelligence, where the Light falls on the diamond that which is reflected becomes visible. A diamond that has many facets will reflect many rays of Light at the same time. But one particular ray will appeal especially to you as you begin your way on the Spiritual Path. The full power of God or the Divine Energy is just too much for the human mind to grasp and so it needs to have the link established in a personal aspect such as Krishna or Siva in the Indian religions, or Jesus or Mary in Christianity. Adults who are still spiritual children need to have a personal concept of God until they can see the Divine Energy in its pure form.

But there is still more that can be said about the power of the Mantra. There is, for example, the Kilaka, the very fine thread that links the disciple to the Mantra, to the power of the Mantra, to the Guru, and to the Deity — and also to all who have ever chanted the Mantra, or are chanting that Mantra at that time throughout the world.

Q.   Could you give an example?

A.   I will tell you of a very beautiful experience that came to me when I first started the Ashram in Burnaby, in Vancouver. There was so much work to be done and the young fellows who were at the Ashram at that time did not always sympathize with my desire to be alone for spiritual practice, or my wish to do spiritual practice rather than be always helping with the painting or the carpentry. So one day I was in the garden with my mala and my box of matches, and I was aware of all the opposition and I thought, "Perhaps this is not the right time for me to do it; I should perhaps wait until I am older and there are more young people here to do my work." So I opened my eyes. My mala was on the ground and there were some matches around which I gathered together.

When I looked up I was amazed to see that there was a whole circle of people sitting around. They were all reciting Mantras, moving their beads, moving their lips, looking at me, smiling, nodding encouragement. This vision gave me the impetus to carry on. I knew then that I had contacted other souls who had gone through the whole thing before me and who said, "Come on, stick it out, carry on, come on, we sit here with you." And I often had the feeling that other help was given to me.

The struggle to know where my first duty was, to the physical work of the Ashram or to my own spiritual practice, is similar to the conflict which may occur within the family setting. This experience was the answer to the intense conflict within myself over this problem.

The Mantra has what I call a self-generating power. If you were to chant quite regularly now, abandon the practice and then perhaps 20 years from now you suddenly found yourself in some crisis, the Mantra might come automatically to your lips and you would continue to repeat it as if you had never ceased.

Q.   Supposing I had never heard of the practice of chanting or repeating Mantras, but instinctively, or perhaps after reading something about Coue, I might begin to repeat to myself some phrase like, "I am growing into greater spiritual awareness," or I might take a phrase from the Bible such as, "The Lord is my Shepherd" or "My soul doth magnify the Lord," and constantly repeat this phrase. Would it have the same effect?

A. If you were persistent, yes, it would. Because you would first of all develop single-pointedness of the mind, and then the constant repetition of these phrases would fill your being with very positive thoughts. These would help you to erase all the negative garbage that you had allowed to accumulate over the years. You might not receive any outside help in the same way that you would if you were to chant "Hari Om." But I cannot really say even that, because if your devotion is sincere and you continue your practice, God is sure to hear you.

Q. *What about the Lord's Prayer? Would it be possible to recite it as a Mantra?*

A. No, it is too long and there are too many different ideas within it, so you could not achieve single-pointedness.

Q. *Would there still be anything to be gained by repeating the Lord's Prayer many times, aloud or silently?*

A. Oh, yes. The Lord's Prayer is very much like a hymn. It has many aspects. First there is the statement, "Our Father, who art in heaven." Then there is a request, "Give us this day our daily bread." Although these induce a variety of thoughts, feelings and emotions, leading us away from true single-pointedness, the repetition of the prayer will bring your mind into some concentration if it is done with sincerity and meaning.

I have done this and have gained many insights. I have realized, for example, that "Give us this day our daily bread" does not refer just to the bread we eat or even to spiritual bread. "Bread" can refer to anything that may happen to you, both positive and negative. You can absorb only so much as you now are, unless you make a very special effort to extend the perception of your senses. You might have an overpowering experience of the Christ Consciousness and this could be a terrifying experience if you did not know what it was. So when you ask that you may receive your daily bread, ask also that you be not given more than you can handle, or be given additional strength, additional perception to meet whatever comes your way. Thus, each phrase of the Lord's Prayer could be considered as a Mantra.

Now if you take the name of Jesus and focus on that, through repetition you can achieve single-pointedness. It is like focusing all the rays of light through a magnifying glass, so that you can achieve one very bright, very powerful point of light. Jesus has said, "I am the Light." So, the name of Jesus can be called a Mantra because it is a symbol of power and energy. I think there are perhaps 500 million Christians alive today in the world, and there have been many more who have walked the earth since the time of Christ. Their belief in Him, the belief in His name, gives that name tremendous power, tremendous energy.

Another way to look at it is to think of one drop of water which will accomplish very little, but 500 million drops can cut through rock or, indeed, change the face of the earth. Think again of all the people who have achieved God-consciousness through the chanting of the name of Krishna, Siva, or Jesus, and think of the power of their achievement being present in the combined energy of the Mantra, and you will have some idea of the force that is there.

Q.   *You stress the power that comes through the repetition of the Name. It seems to me that there would be a danger that I might mispronounce the name of the particular Deity whose Mantra I had chosen to chant. The English version of many Biblical names is different than the Hebrew, and the same must apply to other Eastern names. What influence would this have?*

A.   It is true that in India many people are concerned with this and when I was there, comments were made that as a Westerner I could not possibly know how to pronounce the names of God correctly. But I did not allow myself to become emotionally involved with this problem. I learned much just by sitting back and watching the people who came to see Sivananda. They came to him from all over India, from different states, speaking different languages and dialects. Some would call him "Shevananda," some would call him "Shivananda" with the accent on the third syllable.

One day I went and asked Gurudev how his name was correctly pronounced. The question startled him and I continued, "Well, if your name is pronounced in so many different ways and the first part of your name, Siva, comes from Lord Siva, and I am repeating the Siva Mantra, is it possible that if I do not pronounce Siva correctly I will have no result? And yet," I continued, "I notice that you listen to me whether I address you as Gurudev, or Sivanandaji; you answer my questions, and so perhaps God does the same."

Swami Sivananda replied, "Yes, your sincerity and what is in your heart and mind are more important. There are thousands of people who pronounce words correctly, but they have not yet become saints. In the same way, the interpretation of the law can become a preoccupation and we can miss what the law is all about."

So I tell other Westerners who wish to practice Mantras not to worry if they do not know exactly how certain names are to be pronounced. Even in the West, English, French, German, Italian, all come from Latin, and yet today nobody knows if "Cicero" is pronounced with a soft "c" or with a hard "c." I feel that if the power of the Mantra depends only on correct pronunciation then that power cannot be very great. Rather it is your love of God, your persistence and devotion, and your intentions that will bring results.

Q. Well, then if the correct pronunciation is not so important, how important is it to use the correct melody? I find some of the higher notes difficult after awhile, could I not sing them an octave lower?

A. No, no. The Raga* is extremely important and must not be altered. The singing voice can be changed, whereas it may not always be possible to form the sounds for correct pronunciation, but we must make some effort. My own music Guru at the Ashram in Rishikesh, Swami Nada Brahmananda, went to great trouble to help me to increase the range of my voice. I am sure that if it were not so important to sing the correct note at the correct pitch he would not have taken so much time and trouble. He was always happy to be able to report to Gurudev that I was able to sing another tone or two higher. When I could chant the Krishna Invocation, he was overjoyed.

You see, sound is vibration. Sounds and images have a very close relationship. In his book *Japa Yoga* Swami Sivananda gives several examples of singers who could produce images simply by singing a certain note or combination of notes. By creating a particular sound, some material on that same rate of vibration may either come together again or, if the rate of vibration is stronger and higher than that of an object, the object breaks. In high school we made experiments with sound breaking glass. In the Old Testament there is the story of the sound of the trumpets bringing down the walls of Jericho. Today everyone has heard unhappy stories of youngsters who suffer a loss of hearing because they listen to rock music that is played far too loudly.

Raga or Ragini: the correct Indian term for melody or key, but includes much more than our idea of tune. Literally *raga* means love or passion. In Indian music it is that kind of sound composition which consists of the melodic movements that colour one's heart.

The Raga of a Mantra is primarily a monophonic one, a sequence of single sounds without harmony. In the teachings of Pythagorus it is pointed out that Music, as it was then understood, is linked to arithmetic. This view has been expressed in more recent times in the writing of the late P. D. Ouspensky. The term "Music of the Spheres" belongs to the Greeks as well as to the Orient. The Greeks linked sound and music with astronomy. Aristotle in his *Poetica* states that language, rhythm and sound together make up poetry. However, he points also to another element which has neither name nor form; he gives great emphasis to the power of the word and the power of sound both influencing human thought. The yogic teacher goes on to say that this influence is more far-reaching than it is generally believed to be. Music is not only an orderly system or arrangement of sounds, but power that can and does have an effect on the hearer. Confucius, like Aristotle, claimed that music will influence people and lead them to either right or wrong action.

It is interesting to discover that the Greeks also made a point that the established melody must not be changed because such "lawlessness" leads to destruction.

There is another aspect of the Raga that is very important and to understand this we must consider the two Sanskrit words, "Shabda" and "Bija". Shabda is the name given to the primal sound, the nuclear sound, or OM, from which all things are created. Bija means seed and it is the self-generating power of the Mantra. If you think about the meaning of these two words, you will see that through constant and correct chanting of a Mantra, you will be helped to release greater energy within your physical, mental, emotional and spiritual bodies. With this increase of energy you will also be helped to get in touch with the Divine within you, your true Self, your Higher Self.

Q.   *Is there a special Mantra for me? How would I go about choosing a Mantra?*

A.   Yes, there is a special Mantra for you, but this does not mean that no two people will have the same Mantra. There is a particular sound or vibration to which your spiritual body will best respond. In the beginning, many people feel they need protection and the Siva Mantra may be the answer to that first impulse. To worship Lord Siva it is sufficient to utter his name while dropping clear water over a Siva stone. The early Rishis perceived the various aspects of the Divine and Siva was recognized as the originator, the Sakta, the Lord of Kundalini and

Hatha Yoga, which are very active practices demanding discipline. But for those who do not have that ability, calling on Siva's name while pouring a little water over a stone representing Him is adequate.

Worship of other aspects of the Divine may be more elaborate, burdening the worshipper with details to the exclusion of the finer feelings of gratitude for knowledge of what this personalized aspect of the impersonal power truly represents.

The subtlety of the psychology of these procedures, concepts and attitudes may be more easily understood if we remember that at the time of the development of such systems, mechanical clocks did not exist, so the inner clock in human beings had to be developed. That practice alone, when done with precision, could lead the devotee to remarkable understanding. The early yogis then realized that this was not the only way in which the mind could be trained, in fact its powers could be vastly extended. The desire to make oneself accessible to those powers, using the methods developed, can bring about an experience of greater Reality.

Hari Om, a Mantra to invoke Lord Krishna, is not as different from Om Namah Sivaya as it appears to the beginner, It leads to an understanding of the greater Oneness by a different aproach. Krishna is like a lover luring the devotee into a personal relationship with the Divine by the haunting sound of His flute. Here the devotee is lead by an inclination to romance into a partnership with Krishna, thereby easing feelings of loneliness.

In each situation the natural inclinations and temperament of the devotee are met. Is that not what we see everywhere in life? Each person is drawn to that which is most attractive desirable and satisfying. The division between the power and meaning of Mantras will disappear as the spiritual aspirant matures. Understanding of Eastern psychology takes on greater and greater subtlety until the aspirant is finally no longer dependent on the personal aspect of that awesome Power called by these various names.

Each Mantra will lead to God-realization, to the top of the spiritual mountain, but each one will take a slightly different path.

There are many ways in which a Mantra may be chosen. You may be fortunate enough to find your Guru who will choose a Mantra most suitable for you; you may give the message to your Guru, or it may be given by the Guru in a moment of inspiration.

Q. Does it ever happen that someone will write to you, perhaps some-one you have never met, telling you that they wish to follow the spiritual life more fully and would like to begin the practice of chanting a Man-tra? If they wish to choose a Mantra, what advice would you give them?

A. In such a case I make them aware of the existing record or tape that I have made giving samples of three or four Mantras. One way to make a choice is to stretch out in a comfortable position with closed eyes, listen and see if there is any response, any intuitive indication. It might, for example, be "Most Beautiful Mother" or the name of Jesus Christ chanted to "Hari Om." This then would be the Mantra.

There is always the possibility that in the course of time another Mantra will come to the surface quite naturally. The melody may just come up by itself. But I would make detailed inquiries into this, to ascertain that the new Mantra was not just due to the restlessness of the mind. I would not want anyone to change a Mantra until they had some experience of the power of the first one. It is not until a later stage of development that several Mantras can be used simultaneously, because all of them are active within you. You must start with one Mantra and lay a good foundation. Then, when your comprehension has grown and you understand that all power is indeed one, there is no confusion. You can take another Mantra and recite it to know the difference in experience. You will want to help others, and be able to help them from many angles.

Q. So then, if a housewife were to write to you requesting help in chant-ing Mantras, would you suggest that she choose one of the Mantras on the tape and then repeat this when she is doing her housework, washing dishes and so on?

A. Yes. Washing dishes and scrubbing floors are good tasks to be doing while reciting a Mantra. They are also good for self-purification. I would also suggest that a new student keep a daily diary, record experiences and obstacles encountered and write to the Ashram for advice. I would also suggest chanting or reciting the Man-tra in some quiet place at a regular time each day, as this is very important.

Q. Where should I keep my concentration while I am chanting? On the third eye?

A. No, not necessarily. If you are washing dishes you cannot keep your concentration on the third eye, but you can hold the mental image of the power of the Mantra personified in a deity, and so spiritualize your housework. You can also listen to the sound of your voice, watch your breath, and you can create a desire and a liking for the Mantra. Do this by thinking of what a Mantra is, what the mystery and power of a Mantra are, how you create sounds, what happens to them, and whether the energy of the sound you produce disappears when it can no longer be heard. Jesus has said that we are responsible for every word that we say, so we must think about that. We may then become aware that much of the sound that has come from our lips has not been the best. We will learn this through chanting, and by using the power of the Mantra we can undo any wrong we may have caused.

Q. *I do not quite understand you.*

A. Very well. Let us take an example on a personal level. Let us say you have been doing some negative talking about someone and suddenly you catch yourself. How can you undo it? It is done, you have said it. You can do two things. First, on becoming aware of your mistake, quickly chant a Mantra and surround the person with Light and with the power of the Mantra. Use the Divine Light Invocation† and put the person you spoke negatively about into the Light. As you become more aware you may say, "Oh, I don't want you to think this is all there is to him; there is also another side to his personality. I do not want you to have a one-sided picture that is all negative; in fact, I would prefer that you forget what I said." In this way you can try to undo what happened in a moment of carelessness.

Now, if you think that there have been more moments of carelessness than you are aware of, it is a good idea to do the same thing for others you know; put them in the Light, chant a Mantra and ask that your weakness will not affect them and that you will be forgiven. The great Aurobindo has said that even the most advanced yogi may make a mistake in a moment of forgetfulness or unawareness. It is difficult to be on guard 24 hours a day. To protect yourself while sleeping, fill your mind with the Mantra before falling asleep. If you wake with the Mantra, it is likely that you have been with it throughout the night.

Q. *You have mentioned that we might chant while doing some household tasks, but I think you have also recommended chanting or repeating the Mantra while engaged in Hatha Yoga. Could you comment on this?*

A. Yes, this is a very good idea. Of course, I learned this approach from Swami Sivananda. He would make me sit in an asana and chant Mantras, and I would certainly advise you to begin this practice. I would suggest that you start with some asana that you are fairly comfortable in. You might sit in the Spinal Twist, for example, and repeat "Om Namah Sivaya" ten times, first on one side and then on the other. Then you can go through your body and think, "How many bends are there in my body, what else is my body doing at this time besides just bending?" From there you can investigate thoroughly, trying to understand the psychological and symbolic or spiritual meaning of each asana.

Let us take the Peacock Posture (Mayurasana), as another example. There are certain things you know already about the peacock; it is associated with vanity. There is the famous painting of Narcissus, a young boy stading naked in front of a mirror, holding peacock feathers behind him. And so the colours, the feathers, make it clear that he is admiring himself and showing off. But that is quite an obvious message. You will also read in Iyengar's book, *Light on Yoga*, that this particular asana is beneficial for removing toxins from the body. Iyengar tells us that just as the peacock kills snakes, so does this asana "kill" toxins. But there is also the peacock that is the vehicle for Lord Subramanya, and the peacock that is used in Christian iconography to represent the glory of heaven. And you may think, perhaps, of the position of the asana, how you are balanced with the elbows pressed against the abdomen in the region of the navel. You meditate on all the meanings of these suggestions.

Q. To return to the housewife for a minute. I can imagine that if she were very enthusiastic, or perhaps felt a little uncomfortable about chanting by herself, she might just put on a tape of you singing the Mantra over and over — "Hari Om," for instance, or "Om Namah Sivaya" — is this a legitimate practice?

A. Yes, it is. It is always beneficial to have the Mantra tape playing in the background, preferably the same Mantra. If you are doing something else, or if you are very tired and you do not feel that you have the will power to sit down and chant yourself, it will always help to listen to the Mantra.

Let us look at it another way. Suppose that before you go to sleep you watch the late news on television. Then everything that you see or hear would be taken into your sleep and you might have nightmares.

Or if you have an argument with someone before you go to bed, you will take the anger to bed with you and it will manifest in your sleep. The unconscious will try to free itself from the feeling and will work it out in a dream.

But if you play a Mantra tape, you are doing several things; you are displaying a certain weakness and a certain power. The weakness to be overcome is the ego and the inborn laziness that says, "Why should I do this?" But, by even switching on the tape you are giving in to the higher desire, "Really, I must do something!" So you read the newspaper to satisfy the carnal mind, but you exercise a control or mastery over it by listening to the Mantra. If there are negative things in your reading, the Mantra will help to counteract them and, by continually playing the tape, and chanting whenever you have a few moments to yourself, the habit will gradually become stronger and stronger in the day-to-day events of your life.

The habit of keeping the Mantra close to the surface will become stronger with practice. When I hear a fire siren or an ambulance I immediately say, "Om Namah Sivaya — somebody is in need, let there be help." If you see a picture of people killed in a battle in the Middle East, or anywhere in the world, and you become aware of how much suffering there is, do the Divine Light Invocation. Think of the lonely people dying in hospitals. If you wonder what you can do about such things, before going to sleep, spin a cocoon of Light around yourself and say, "Let the soul go out, the body is at rest, the house is taken care of, let the Higher Self do what needs to be done, many things that I cannot do, even if I want to, sitting here by day."

Q.   This will be very inspiring for the individual in the city who aspires to the spiritual life and undertakes to chant the Mantra, repeat the name of God, and so on. Are there any other aspects of this practice that they should know about? For example, at Satsang at the Ashram I have sometimes seen people break down and weep for no apparent reason and I feel that this might also happen to someone in the city. Can you comment on this please?

A.   Tears are not easy to accept. We have been brought up in the West to believe that tears are just an emotional outlet and perhaps something to be ashamed of, but this is not really the case. When chanting we often get in touch with emotions we did not know were there, tears held back from childhood. There can be tears of self-pity, or tears of regret at having wasted so many years, maybe even lifetimes, in pursuits that did no more than feed the ego.

Sometimes these tears can be a spiritual bath, a rejuvenating force that can refresh by washing away an accumulation of sadness. Life can then take on, little by little, a different meaning. Swami Sivananda had suggested that at such times I say, "All right, here are my tears. I have symbolically collected them. My tears are very precious to me and I don't want to cry them senselessly. With them I wash the feet of Divine Mother." But do not indulge yourself. Do not let yourself think that you are making great progress because you shed tears. Only a little progress!

Q.   *I have also seen people quite literally pass out while chanting. Is this a usual phenomenon?*

A.   Yes. There are several reasons. You can become unconscious if you have poor blood circulation and you chant by yourself over a long period of time; then you just faint, and this has no particular after-effect on you. However, it is also possible, particularly in group chanting, that someone will collapse, but this is because the atomic structure of the brain has to be changed to adjust to the new vibration to which it is being exposed. The same experience of a sudden loss of consciousness can be caused by the Divine Light Invocation, or any similar spiritual practice.

Now, if it is a genuine response to the power of the Mantra, and not just due to poor circulation, there will be a noticeable change in the personality of the individual; there will be a tendency to rethink many concepts, new ideals will be established. There will be a growing desire to break free from limitations. There will be a conscious striving to be on the Spiritual Path. However, the student must be taught how to control this power that has so suddenly manifested.

Q.   *How can this be done?*

A.   There is a very simple method. It is necessary only to feel the feet placed firmly on the floor and to remind oneself that one is here, now. Because, you see, we have to be here. Man is the bridge between two worlds, the world of the physical, material body, and the unseen world created by the mind, which also manifests something of that which is created through our belief in it.

There is also another technique to help control the sudden rush of this new energy, or energy newly experienced: it is explained more fully in my record on *Guided Meditation on the Light*, but briefly it consists of seeing a beautiful golden Lotus at the base of the spine and then gently but firmly placing the Light within the spine back in that Lotus where it belongs, and closing the petals securely around the Light. Again, remind yourself by an act of will to be here, now. The control of will is a very fine decision; when to surrender and when to exercise will is one of the secrets of being succesful in yoga.

It is very important not to indulge emotions, not to seek experience, not to try to bring on a similar experience by chanting very quickly or trying out some fancy breathing technique. Two things will happen if you give in to this temptation. First of all, you will soon doubt if any experience is really a manifestation of the Divine and not just an artificial production of your own imagination. Secondly, you will be caught up in the desire for experience, for sensation, and not look beyond to see the true Light.

As a small child is given little rewards each time it makes greater effort to walk or master some other skill, so the Divine will give us some reward, some beautiful experience, as we endeavour to make our first, faltering steps on the Royal Highway that leads us back to our true Home. At a later date in our spiritual practice we will be faced with another temptation, the lure of "siddhis", the powers that will develop within ourselves, powers of extrasensory perception, powers of foretelling the future. At times, of course, we can use these powers for good, but too often they are only a temptation to the ego, giving it an excuse to exercise itself after we have kept it under control for so long. If we give in to this temptation we may fall back even further from our spiritual goal than we were before we started the practice of chanting Mantras!

Q.   I think I understand you correctly that I should not use any energy that I may manifest through chanting a Mantra for the gratification of my own ego, and that certainly makes sense. But how can I safely use this energy to help others?

A.   You can chant for others when you are prompted by your own intuition, the Guru within. You must be sure that you are acting out of compassion and not just sympathy, in which you identify with the problem of the person you want to help. Be aware of any desire to influence events or of any strong emotional response. In chanting for others we must keep our own will out of the way, surrendering to the power of the Mantra, to the Most High.

Q.   If I were chanting and my mind began to wander, would it be alright to chant each Mantra for a different friend or relative, as well as people I might remember having met on the street or in a shop, or seen in a restaurant?

A.   Yes, but you should not keep your mind on the person. It is like writing a letter, except that you write only the address. You may address many different envelopes, but you send each person the same message. At the beginning of each Mantra you may mention the name of the person for whom you chant, but you try to concentrate on the Mantra itself, the different tones, or the image of the deity connected with it. Do not think of the image of the person you are chanting for, because by doing that you may interfere with that person and this we must not do.

Q.   At different times we have talked about Hatha Yoga, Jnana Yoga, Bhakti Yoga, as well as Mantra Yoga. Where does Mantra Yoga fit into the overall picture? Is Mantra Yoga as important as the others? I suspect from what you say that it is one of the most important yogas.

A.   Yes. It is like this. Think of a rose and then take the rose apart. Are the outer petals important, or the inner petals, is the very centre important, or is the stem? The whole thing together is important. Each part is important and the rose becomes imperfect without some of the petals, for example, or without the stem.

It is the same thing with yoga. It is very difficult for us in the West to really understand any of the yogas. When you do Hatha Yoga, for example, what we call Hatha Yoga is nothing more than a few asanas ripped out of a very complex system. When you do the various asanas you are also meant to stimulate the inner glandular system for the posture to be really effective. And as I have already said, you should then, at that time, recite your own Mantra, the one you have chosen or that has been given to you, the one you feel comfortable with.

Q.   I have heard reference made to Nada Yoga and the Science of Thaan. Could you explain the connection with Mantra?

A.   Nada Yoga is the Yoga of Sound and you can say that Mantra

Yoga and the Science of Thaan are both systems with Nada Yoga. The Indians have for centuries made a very detailed study of the effects of sound or, more correctly, of vibration. They are well aware of the power of sound in healing and in awakening the Cakras (the centres of consciousness) in the Kundalini system.

Q.   *I have heard it said that Mantra has an effect on the subconscious and I would think that one of the most common criticisms of Mantra or Japa is that it is a form of hypnotism. What would be your answer to that?*

A.   I can understand how people would think that. It is a natural reaction. However, I do not think it is possible for anyone to hypnotize themselves into becoming holy. There would be a deep conflict and either the mind would one day become deranged or the individual would go back to the old way of living.

We should also consider that for a long time we have indeed hypnotized ourselves and thereby set up limitations which prevent us from seeing and making use of our full potential. Television is only one of the most obvious forms of hypnotism. We are constantly bombarded with the idea that we must have a new car or that our bodies have an odour which must be concealed. In more subtle ways we are told throughout our life that we must have a good job, make money and that we must be married. All this is hypnotism. I would rather consider the chanting of Mantra as a process of dehypnotism because greater awareness and understanding are achieved, however slow the process may be.

If we think, too, of the aspect of reincarnation, then we have to consider that for many lifetimes we have hypnotized ourselves into what we are today, into the strong beliefs that have become prejudices. These prevent us from seeing the beauty and the truth of the Divine, not only in others, but in ourselves. And so, even if the chanting of a Mantra were a form of hypnotism, by focusing on the name of God and the power of God within our being, the practice works to counteract these preconceptions.

I once met a young man who wanted to become the youngest millionaire. He achieved that. That was his goal and he put all his efforts into that. The result is that he had totally neglected the higher aspects of consciousness; he does not realize that man is the bridge between this world and a very different one that cannot be bought with any amount of money; where money, in fact, has no meaning whatsoever.

Now this young man can serve as an example. We can become what we put into our mind, and therefore if the intense effort, the drive and the power of the emotions are put into becoming the youngest millionaire then that can likely be achieved. If the same amount of energy is put into becoming Self-realized, that is worth the effort. After Realization there is probably very little left to wish for, but after one has become a millionaire there is a whole new set of problems and desires: how do I keep the money, how can I make more money, how will I find friends who love me for what I am and not for my money. But if one becomes Self-realized then all are friends, because one can see the Divine in everyone.

Q. I suppose the young man who wanted to be a millionaire would have been better off if he had chanted to Lakshmi! This brings me to another point that we really have not touched on. You have said that there are Mantras for Siva and Mantras for Krishna and Mantras for Lakshmi, and these all have separate ragas and achieve slightly different results. But are there other forms of Mantra? Some seem to me to be much longer than "Hari Om" or "Om Namah Sivaya."

A.   There are, first of all, the Mantras dealing with Light, purity, reality. This is the highest form of Mantra leading to purification and Realization. These Mantras are given by the Guru to the initiate, and you will find very little written about them.

Then there are Mantras dealing with the changing quality of nature, filled with restlessness, and those who wished to satisfy more worldly desires, having lots of money, giving birth to a son, and so on, would resort to these.

Lastly, there are Mantras reflecting ignorance, inertia, darkness, all that perishes and these would be used for selfish purposes, such as revenge. The Mantras which lead to Self-realization will obviously take the longest time to come to fruition.

The four-line Mantra, however, promises the attainment of a particular specified power. Shankaracharya has written in the 11th century a treatise called "The

Mantras of Ananda Lahari," which means "waves of bliss." It can be consulted for more information about those which are used for different purposes. He has discussed some 140 Mantras and dismissed many others as insignificant or quite useless. With the four-line Mantras, of course, there are also different forms of worship and different forms of "Yantras," the allegoric designs associated with a Mantra.

There is one four-line Mantra that we recite at the Ashram. It begins, "O Divine Mother, may all our speech and idle talk be Mantra." Now, if you recite this Mantra a thousand times a day for 45 days you will attain the power that is in the Mantra, in this case the knowledge of all scriptures.*

There have been many books written about four-line Mantras, and if you were to read them all you would learn a great deal. But what you learn would be as nothing in comparison to the experience you would have by reading nothing and instead just chanting Mantras.

Salutations And Gratitude To All The Gurus
Who Have Prepared The Way.

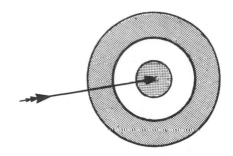

See following page.

O Divine Mother!
May all my speech and idle talk be Mantra,
All actions of my hands be Mudra,
All eating and drinking be the offering of oblations
unto Thee,
All lying down prostrations before Thee;
May all pleasures be as dedicating my entire self unto Thee,
May everything I do be taken as Thy worship.

Suggested Reading

ANDREWS, DONALD HATCH. *The Symphony of Life.* Lees Summit, MO: Unity Books, 1966. 121p.

BLOFELD, JOHN. *Mantras: Sacred Words of Power.* New York: Dutton, 1977. 106p.

EASWARAN, EKNATH. *The Mantram Handbook.* Berkeley: Nilgiri Press, 1977. 260p.

FRENCH, R. M. trans. *Way of the Pilgrim.* London: S. P. C. K., 1930. 125p.

HAMEL, PETER. *Through Music to the Self.* Boulder, CO: Shambala, 1979. Translated from the German. 228p.

KHAN, HAZRAT INYAT. *The Mysticism of Sound: the power of the word; cosmic language.* vol. 2. Geneva: Servire Wassenaar, 1962. 262p.

LALITA. *Choose Your Own Mantra.* New York: Bantam, 1978. 212p.

RADHA, SWAMI SIVANANDA. *Kundalini: Yoga for the West.* Kootenay Bay, B. C.: Timeless Books, 1978. 356p.

——— *Mantras, Songs of Yoga.* (cassette or record). Kootenay Bay, B. C.: Yasodhara Ashram Society, 1973.

——— *Power of Mantras.* (cassette tape). Kootenay Bay, B. C.: Yasodhara Ashram Society, 1974.

RAMDAS, SWAMI. *In Quest of God.* Bombay: Bharatiya Vidya Bhavan, 1961. 168p.

SIVANANDA SARASWATI, SWAMI. *Concentration and Meditation.* Himalayas, India: The Divine Life Society, 1975. 416p.

——— *Japa Yoga: a comprhensive treatise of Mantra-Sastra.* Himalayas, India: The Divine Life Society, 1972. 192p.

——— *Music as Yoga.* Rishikesh, India: The Yoga Vedanta Forest University, 1956. 121p.

SRI AUROBINDO. *The Mother.* Pondicherry, India: Sri Aurobindo Ashram, 1928. 62p.

TYBERG, JUDITH M. *The Language of the Gods.* Los Angeles: East-West Cultural Centre, 1974. 297p.

WHORF, BENJAMIN LEE. *Language, Thought & Reality,* selected writings. Edited by John B. Carroll. Cambridge, Mass.: M. I. T. Press, 1956. 278p.

ZUCHERKANDL, VICTOR. *Sound and Symbol: music and the external world.* Translated from the German by W. R. Trask. (Bollingen Series XLIV). Princeton, N. Y.: Princeton University Press, 1956. 399p.

Mantras, Bhajans, Songs at Yasodhara Ashram. Kootenay Bay, B. C.: Yasodhara Ashram Society, 1979. 27p.

Other Books by the Author

Swami Radha's books and recordings focus on interpreting the ancient teachings so that they can be understood and applied in the daily lives of westerners:

Kundalini: Yoga for the West is a profound and lucid presentation of the path of Kundalini Yoga. Clear directions for exercises and practices are given for those who wish to co-operate with the evolution of their consciousness.

Aphorisms of Swami Sivananda Radha is a beautifully illustrated book of insight and inspiration, containing positive statements of spiritual wisdom and guidance gleaned from her books, lectures, and workshops.

The Divine Light Invocation presents detailed instructions on a powerful spiritual practice of healing and regeneration.

For those who wish to experience Mantra through the medium of sound, a number of cassette recordings of Mantras for meditation chanted by Swami Radha are available, as well as other tapes on the subject of Mantra.

Index

Hollywood in the Information Age

Passion Pit Puddles Mud and debris frame a deserted drive-in located near Springfield, Oregon. The dramatic decline of drive-ins (once known as "passion pits") has been generally attributed to the popularity of video-cassettes, although some operations in warmer climates have survived by adding more screens. In 1991, there were 908 drive-ins operating in the USA. *Photograph by Carlos R. Calderon*

HOLLYWOOD IN
THE INFORMATION AGE

Beyond the Silver Screen

Janet Wasko

University of Texas Press

Texas Film Studies Series
Thomas Schatz, Editor

First published 1994 by Polity Press in association with Blackwell Publishers, UK

First University of Texas Press edition, 1995

Requests for permission to reproduce material from this work should be sent to
Permissions, University of Texas Press, Box 7819, Austin, TX 78713–7819.

This book is printed on acid-free paper.

ISBN 0–292–79093–7
ISBN 0–292–79094–5 pbk.
Library of Congress Catalog Card Number 94–60642

For Carlos & Scruffy Joe

Contents

List of Plates

Acknowledgements

Some sections of the book are based on previously published material.

Some of the issues considered in chapter 3 were presented (with Thomas Maher) as "Hollywood Silicon: The Advent of Post-industrial Filmmaking," University Film and Video Association, University of Southern California, Los Angeles, California, August 1985.

The discussion in the section "Setting the Scene" in chapter 5 is based on the article "New Methods of Measuring Media Concentration" in Vincent Mosco, ed., *Policy Research in Telecommunications*, Norwood, New Jersey: Ablex Publishing, 1984.

A version of the section of chapter 5 entitled "The US Cable System in the Nineties" was previously published in Andrew Calabrese and Janet Wasko, "All Wired Up and No Place to Go: The Search for Public Space in US Cable Development," *Gazette* 49, 1992, pp. 121–51.

Chapter 8 represents a version of Janet Wasko, Mark Phillips and Chris Purdie, "Hollywood Meets Madison Ave.: The Commercialization of US Films," *Media, Culture and Society* 15, no. 2, April 1993.

Chapter 9 is based on a paper presented at the Political Economy section of the International Association for Mass Communication Research, August 1990, in Bled, Slovenia, and later published as "Hollywood, New Technologies and Europe 1992," *Telematics and Informatics* 8, no. 2, 1991.

Many people contributed to this book in many ways.

My thanks to Mark Phillips, Chris Purdie, Tom Maher, and Andrew Calabrese for their collaboration on some of the material used on product placements and tie-ins, film production and cable television. Research assistance for different pieces of the study also came from Victor Muniz, Suzanne Julber, Scott Hampton, Alice Slaughter, Marc Jaffe, Denise Wallace, and Wendy Barbour. Special thanks to Thomas Guback, Vincent Mosco, and Eileen Meehan for their insightful and helpful comments, as well as the continuing inspiration that their own work provides. More thanks to Susan Davis, Dan Schiller, Deanna Robinson, and Bill Willingham, who also read versions of the manuscript, and to Sean Axmaker for his insights on the home video business.

The Directors Guild of America (especially Selise Eiseman) provided support to attend their Educators Workshop in August 1991, giving me the opportunity to confront Hollywood insiders on their own turf. Funds from the School of Journalism and Communication at the University of Oregon allowed me to attend the National Association for Television Programming Executives (NATPE) convention, January 1993, in San Francisco, California, where I was able to observe the buying and selling of entertainment programming first hand.

The people at Polity Press have been a joy to work with. Everyone has been extremely patient and quite professional, but a special thanks to John Thompson who supported the book from the beginning.

Finally, Carlos Calderon not only deserves credit for most of the photo work, but for providing a huge measure of inspiration and vital support which made it possible to ultimately finish this project.

1

Introduction: Hollywood and the Culture Industry

The Entertainment Age

Over the last decade or so there have been dramatic changes in the technologies employed for the production and distribution of entertainment and information. Computer systems have been introduced in a wide range of situations, from factories to offices to homes. New communication channels, such as cable television, home video, and satellite systems, are in use in most of the USA and much of rest of the world. Other developments, such as high-definition television (HDTV), direct-broadcast satellite systems, fiber-optics systems (or "electronic superhighways"), etc., are promised in the near future.

The confluence of these technological developments – the number and variety of technological devices and processes introduced or employed at one time – is perhaps unprecedented, and has prompted discussion and analysis of a new age: the *information* age.

An information society has been claimed by many to be more dependent on information and service industries, and thus organized and characterized fundamentally differently from previous eras. It is further argued that information has become a commodity – bought, sold and traded in marketplace situations.

Yet, in many ways, the notion of an information age is inherently problematic, and rather than embracing the concept, this study serves to challenge it on several fronts.

First, the myriad of technological changes that have prompted discussions of a new age of information has been introduced into societies which remain fundamentally the same. In other words, there is as much continuity as change in our "new" age. This fundamental concept is at the heart of this study, which provides an example by looking closely at one sector of our society – the entertainment business – to examine the extent of the change or continuity that has accompanied these technological developments.

Second, it might be noted that many of the new technologies associated with an information age have been introduced and employed for leisure-time activities or entertainment. In other words, many of the *information* technologies have been promoted for their *entertainment* components, and it would seem that people's everyday lives are influenced as much, if not more, by these entertainment and leisure-time activities as by new or enhanced information channels.

Although it could be argued that entertainment is as characteristic of this age as information, we have heard little about a new *entertainment* age. And, come to think of it, both information and entertainment have existed in other historical periods, so why a new age at all?

Still, it is interesting to consider why discussions of an information age frequently neglect analysis of the entertainment component of information technologies.

One explanation is that the business of entertainment is often not considered *serious* business by economists and other proponents of an information age. More often emphasis is placed on business and military applications of information technologies, such as telecommunications and computers, rather than on consumer communications products, such as home video and cable, that merely provide diversion.

On the other hand, technological components or economic characteristics of entertainment are less important to many media scholars or cultural analysts, who are more interested in studying entertainment products as texts or measuring audiences or the effects of entertainment messages, thus missing the possible connections to fundamental components of this (supposedly) new technological era.

Revenues from the media/entertainment business may not compare to other "information age" industries and other sectors of the economy. For instance, Standard & Poor's Industry Surveys for 1993 reported domestic sales for the electronics and computer sector at over $287 billion in 1991. The film industry's domestic box office revenues for the same year were a mere $4.8 billion. Comparisons also might be made with the aerospace industry's total sales, reported at $134 billion in 1990, and the chemical industry's sales of nearly $300 billion in 1991. These sectors easily dwarf the revenues of the entire media and entertainment sector, as indicated in table 1.1.

Table 1.1 Domestic filmed entertainment revenues, 1986 and 1991

	Revenues ($M)		Annual growth rate (%)
	1986	1991	
Consumer spending			
Movie box office	3,778	4,803	4.9
Home video	5,015	10,995	17.0
Basic cable	5,225	11,080	16.2
Pay cable	3,325	4,715	7.2
Consumer total	17,343	31,593	12.7
Advertising			
Broadcast TV networks	8,342	9,435	2.5
TV stations	13,085	14,675	2.3
Barter	600	1,275	16.3
Subtotal	22,027	25,385	2.9
National cable	676	1,530	17.7
Local cable	179	455	20.5
Subtotal	855	1,985	18.3
Advertising total	22,882	27,370	3.6
Total spending	40,225	58,963	7.9

Source: Veronis, Suhler & Associates, Motion Picture Association of America, McCann-Erickson, Wilkofsky Gruen Associates. From: *Standard & Poor's Industry Surveys*, 11 March 1993, p. L17.

Nevertheless, the media/entertainment industry has grown considerably during the last few decades, and increasingly attracts the attention of financiers, investors and companies outside the traditional entertainment world. New technologies introduced by some of these companies, plus the integration of media and information systems, continue to expand the markets for entertainment commodities.

Furthermore, these media industries distribute important ideological and cultural products, with significance for the representation and reproduction of social norms and values. It would seem, therefore, that economic and technological developments in these industries would be not only of passing interest, but crucial in understanding the cultural role of these media and communication products.

Beyond the Silver Screen

At the heart of the entertainment business in the USA (and, indeed, much of the rest of the world) is a set of corporations commonly referred to as Hollywood. At one time, these companies were primarily involved in the production and distribution of motion pictures in the USA and abroad. Many still think of Hollywood in these terms.

However, films are seen today in many places other than theaters: most often, in people's homes on television monitors, via over-the-air television stations, networks, cable and pay-cable channels, or home video systems; but also in airplanes, hospitals, schools, universities, prisons, even in dentists' chairs. Popular films often initiate or continue an endless chain of other cultural products. A film concept or character often leads to a TV show, with possible spin-offs, video games, and records. Merchandising efforts also include toys, games, T-shirts, trading cards, soap products, cereals, theme park rides, coloring books, magazines, how-the-movie-was-made books, etc.

The major Hollywood corporations are transnational conglomerates, often involved in all of these activities. Thus it becomes increasingly more difficult to distinguish the film industry from other media or entertainment industries. Indeed, Hollywood – or those corporations collectively referred to as Hollywood – can be considered one of the focal points of the culture industry, to recall a term popularized by the Frankfurt School, and no longer as merely involved in the traditional production, distribution, and exhibition of movies. Thanks to technological developments, commercial motivations, and globalization trends, Hollywood has moved . . . beyond the silver screen.

From Production to Exhibition: Promises and Myths

New technologies introduced since the 1970s have influenced the way that motion pictures are produced, distributed and exhibited. Some claim that the adoption of new techniques, especially in the area of production, has been relatively slow, thus reinforcing Hollywood's reputation as technologically backward.

Nevertheless, there have been important changes in the structure and policies of traditional Hollywood activities. New computer and video techniques are employed in the production of motion pictures, providing new possibilities for manipulating sounds and images. Distribution channels have expanded, with the proliferation of cable systems, home video, and satellite technology. And exhibitors are increasingly being forced to consider new projection systems or distribution methods, such as HDTV.

These technological developments have been, as historically media technology has been, accompanied by predictions and promises, in this case for filmmakers, the film industry and movie audiences. Three main promises can be identified: (1) more competition, (2) increased industrial conflict, and (3) more diversity and access.

First, more opportunities for independent production, or in other words, more competition, has been anticipated for the film business, with independent production sources proliferating. Consequently, the new technologies have prompted claims that there will be intense industrial rivalries and conflicts, as the film industry battles with the television industry and both confront the cable industry, etc. The third, and possibly more prevalent, prediction pertains to the availability of cultural products. Better quality and more spectacular films have been promised through the "magic" of new production technologies. And consumers have been promised more convenient access and more consumer choice or program diversity. Thus, with more information and entertainment, a better informed, more educated, and happier public is portrayed.

Through a series of questions and careful analysis, however, these promises become merely myths. We might ask, for instance, what the latest technologies have actually changed about the production and distribution of motion pictures, the traditional foundation of Hollywood entertainment? Have the structures and policies of corporate Hollywood actually changed? In other words, is discontinuity or change the only operating principle applicable in this entertainment or information age, or is there also a good deal of continuity observable in the industry's structure and strategies? To answer these questions, technological change in Hollywood, as in other areas of the communications sector, must be analyzed historically.

Other important questions relate to who is in control of technological development, or in other words, how are decisions being made about what new technologies will be innovated and introduced, and what products will be delivered via these new technologies? How are changes in the production and distribution of film related to other media products? And, finally, is the public offered more choice and better quality entertainment, or just more of the same?

To answer these questions and more fully understand these developments, this book will present a political economic analysis of Hollywood and the latest technologies. It presents a survey of the newest technological developments since the 1970s in the traditional production, distribution and exhibition of motion pictures. It is essential to look beyond the technologies themselves, however, and consider how Hollywood has reacted and adapted to more general economic and political changes.

The main points delineated throughout this book are:

1 The major Hollywood companies have been interested and involved historically in a variety of media and other commodity forms beyond film.
2 Hollywood as an industry means more than film production, distribution and exhibition; it also has incorporated promotion, merchandising, theme parks, and other media forms, such as television, cable, home video, etc. In other words, Hollywood does not merely represent the film industry, but crosses over traditional industrial boundaries and engages in transindustrial activities.
3 The changes and continuity in Hollywood must be understood in light of general economic and political contexts, i.e. deregulation of media sectors such as cable, privatization and commercialization tendencies in global markets, etc.
4 Hollywood's relationship to new technologies must be seen in light of these other contexts.

Chapter 2 will consider historical treatments of Hollywood and technology, with a brief discussion of specific periods of technological development in film history. Chapter 3 presents an overview of some of the technological developments in the production of motion pictures, while chapter 4 details the activities of the dominant Hollywood corporations that link film production with distribution. Major outlets for the distribution of Hollywood products are considered in the following chapters: cable (chapter 5), home video (chapter 6), and theatrical exhibition (chapter 7). Hollywood's marketing and merchandising strategies are detailed in chapter 8, while global activities are outlined in chapter 9. Based on these discussions, conclusions will be offered in chapter 10.

2

The Way We Were:
An Historical Look at
Hollywood and Technology

Hollywood and technology? How about Charlie Chaplin's assembly line in *Modern Times*, Hal, the misbehaving computer in *2001*, or R2D2 and Robocop? While Hollywood has produced these vivid and memorable depictions of future technologies, there is more to this relationship than the images that appear on the silver screen. After all, film *is* technology and the motion picture industry has exploited technological developments throughout its history.

But recently such developments have come under more intense scrutiny as new distribution outlets, such as cable, pay cable, and videocassettes and discs, have challenged the traditional distribution outlets of theaters and over-the-air television. Interestingly, the attention directed at film technologies has churned up some myths that have long been associated with the US film industry. An example is the following statement by George Mair in his recent book on Home Box Office (HBO):

> Hollywood has never grasped the importance of new technology. It fought against the talkies, against color, against radio, against television, against cable TV, and, most recently, against the videocassette and home video. Hollywood ended up profiting from all of these new technologies, but only after it tried unsuccessfully to kill them. Hollywood always views a new way of doing things as a threat, instead of as an opportunity.[1]

Mair is not alone in this opinion, as evidenced by the following comments by Jack Valenti, head of the Motion Picture Association of America (MPAA):

> Major technical developments in the audiovisual field generally make
> their initial appearance as esoteric laboratory curiosities, innocuous and
> benign. But many rapidly metamorphose from cute chicks to voracious
> vultures. To survive and prosper, our industry has had to develop not
> only coping skills, but more important, the ability to anticipate and man-
> age change. This has not always been the situation.[2]

Mair and Valenti are echoing the received history of Hollywood's
technophobia.[3] Historians have repeatedly reported the reluctance of
US film companies to anticipate and accept new technological innovations, from the introduction of sound film to the home video "revolution." This chapter will explore the challenges to this myth represented
by more recent work on the history of film technology, but argue that
there are still some problems with these newer approaches.

The Myth of Hollywood's Technophobia

First, it might be noted that the image of Hollywood as technologically
backward does not seem to apply to technological development within
the film industry itself, i.e. lighting, cameras, film stock, etc.[4] Film histories abound with detailed accounts of developments in these areas,
with praise heaped on Hollywood producers for a wide range of special
effects techniques.

However, major technological changes outside the traditional parameters of motion pictures have been labeled by many as beyond Hollywood's vision. Specifically, some historians have observed that the
introduction of important new communication media, such was radio,
television, and more recent video technologies, have been only reluc-
tantly accepted by the film industry. The studios are even accused of
resisting sound film, which was introduced by forces mostly outside the
industry.

But how was it possible that these large, profit-seeking film corporations were as myopic as reported in these histories? Could they have
been unaware of the competitive threat posed by these new media, and
uninterested in the profit potential or promotional possibilities represented by these new technologies?

A good deal of evidence in recent historical accounts leads us to
believe that they were not. Furthermore, this recent research indicates
that there were a variety of reasons why the industry was not always
successful in initially dominating or controlling these new technologies,

but there was nearly always great interest in the possibilities of exploiting them and some successful efforts to do so. A brief look at the introduction of sound film, radio and television will illustrate the point.

Sound film While the introduction of "talkies" in the late 1920s was a technological achievement eventually utilized within the parameters of the film industry itself, there have been claims that the industry resisted the initial innovation of sound film. One of the reasons for this interpretation may have been the fact that the technology needed to integrate sound and pictures was developed by companies outside the industry, primarily AT&T and RCA. But, in many ways, this was not unlike other technological developments for the early film industry. As Janet Staiger notes,

> Although the major film studios claimed to have their own "research departments," most were small-scale design and machine shops. No studio could afford the research facilities of a General Electric, a Union Carbide, or a Western Electric. . . . The most basic and significant research was performed by the manufacturers and suppliers of materials and equipment. In an important sense, Hollywood filmmaking only became a modern industry when it joined forces with corporate research.[5]

Although the larger studios (Paramount and Loew's) initially may have resisted the move to sound film, there was a deliberate and co-ordinated effort to adopt the new technology after smaller companies in the industry had proven its viability by introducing sound features and newsreels around 1927–8.[6]

At least two smaller Hollywood firms were involved with the innovation of sound at the technological level. Warner joined AT&T's efforts in 1925, producing vaudeville shorts for the Vitaphone system. Meanwhile, the Fox Film Corporation had formed a subsidiary to exploit the Case sound system, using it to release Movietone newsreels beginning in 1927. Both companies enthusiastically pursued sound film and were able to rise to the ranks of the majors because of their success.

When these two companies had proven the viability of the new sound systems, the other studios quickly adopted one of them (AT&T's). As Douglas Gomery notes, "once the decision was made, the actual switchover occurred rapidly and smoothly."[7] And they were not disappointed – substantial and immediate profits were gleaned by the major companies from the transition to talkies.

So, while the largest firms in the industry may have hesitated at first, their strategy ultimately paid off. Other Hollywood companies did not appear to resist the new technology at all, and actually played important roles in its innovation, thus challenging the myth that Hollywood had resisted the transition to sound.

Radio Interesting by-products of the development of sound film were the corporate links forged between the radio and film industries. Besides the previously mentioned alliance between Warners and AT&T, the phone company formed a subsidiary (ERPI) to deal exclusively with its film activities.[8] Meanwhile, RCA became directly involved in the film industry through its formation of RKO in 1928 and through its intimate ties with the fully integrated studio until the 1940s.[9]

Nevertheless, there is a long-standing myth that Hollywood and the radio industry had nothing to do with each other. For instance, in his classic history of radio, Erik Barnouw states uncategorically that Hollywood ignored radio until the 1930s.[10] As Michelle Hilmes observes, most other film and broadcasting historians either agree with Barnouw or refer to radio only in terms of its threat to film.[11]

In addition to the previously mentioned corporate ties, there were numerous examples of radio aficionados among studio executives. Samuel Rothapfel ("Roxy") was an early radio enthusiast, organizing live broadcasts as well as writing about the future of broadcasting. The Warner brothers also were involved with broadcasting and set up radio stations in Los Angeles and New York. Harry Warner even proposed a radio network to publicize Hollywood films.[12]

Meanwhile, other film companies participated in the radio boom, including experiments with the transmission of pictures via radio, thus also challenging the myth that the film industry was not interested in television until it was too late. In the late 1920s, Paramount Pictures and MGM announced radio chains. Although neither studio followed through with their plans, it seemed clear that a move towards diversifying corporate activities was clearly the aim. Paramount later became involved with the formation of the CBS network (but ultimately withdrew), and MGM briefly experimented with radio programs called "teleshorts," based on the studio's recently released films. Hollywood's interest in radio reached its peak in 1927. Hilmes explains: "Although the 1930s and 1940s would bring heavy Hollywood involvement in production for the radio networks, after 1927–28, Hollywood potential for actual 'control' of the medium diminished rapidly."[13]

Recent historical accounts have speculated that the demise of these activities was due to the impending introduction of sound, radio's potential threat to exhibitors, the precarious financial standing of the companies involved, and the Federal Trade Commission's suit charging the film industry with unfair methods of competition.[14] Thus, Hollywood retreated to the role of talent and program supplier, developing a symbiotic relationship with the radio industry. Even the ban in 1932 (when the studios prevented their contract talent from working for radio), although cited by historians as evidence that the two industries were bitter rivals, was actually only a partial arrangement, not universally supported, and lasted only about nine months. Meanwhile, Hollywood was actively involved in radio programming through the supply of variety, dramatic and gossip shows, in addition to radio adaptations of movies.[15]

Radio also contributed to film activities, as radio personalities became film stars and radio programs inspired motion pictures during the thirties and forties. An obvious example was Orson Welles' activities in both film and radio, but other radio/film stars, such as George Burns, Gracie Allen, Bing Crosby, Bob Hope, Rudi Vallee and Eddie Cantor, also come to mind.

Thus, it is clear that the film industry was not a stranger to radio (and vice versa) throughout this historical period. And while it certainly was the case that Hollywood was not able to dominate the industry in its formative years for a variety of specific historical reasons, there were definite attempts to exploit the new technology in one way or another.

Television A similar misconception exists for Hollywood's involvement in early television development. The heads of the major studios are often seen as resistant to the possibility that television would offer a real threat to their business.[16] It is typically assumed that Hollywood executives dug their heads in the sand, wishing that television would go away, until it was clear that they had to compete with the new medium in order to survive.

Yet, there is strong historical evidence that film companies were involved much earlier in television's evolution. As previously mentioned, some of the studio executives demonstrated interest in television experiments as early as the 1920s. Later, in the thirties there was much discussion of the industry's preparation for the new medium. In 1938 the Academy of Motion Picture Arts and Sciences requested its Research Council to study the film industry's preparation for the inevitable introduction of television, while numerous articles discussed the subject.[17] Around the same time, the Motion Picture Producers and Distributors Association (MPPDA), the industry's trade association, also investigated the role of the film industry in the forthcoming television business.[18]

Meanwhile, concrete evidence of such interest is represented by Paramount's purchase of half ownership of DuMont (including the DuMont Laboratories, where much television experimentation was carried out) in 1938.[19] In addition to the stations owned by Dumont, Paramount itself received licenses for two television stations (KTLA in Los Angeles and WBKB in Chicago), although the studio had applied for 13 licenses from 1940 to 1948. Other studios, including MGM, Warners, Disney and Twentieth Century Fox, actively vied for early TV stations.[20]

But film companies also were involved in attempts to introduce alternative television systems, i.e. not supported by commercial sponsorship. Paramount invested in theater television as early as 1941, using an intermediary film system produced by Scophony (owned by Paramount). Twentieth Century Fox became involved with a similar system through General Precision Laboratories, as well as purchasing the rights to the Eidophor system in 1949. These systems competed with RCA's direct transmission process and enjoyed some success until around 1953, when home television's rapid growth overwhelmed plans for further theater TV development. The systems also suffered from problems with transmission, intensified by lack of Federal Communications Commission (FCC) support, as well as with other details, and these seemed to doom theater television by 1953.[21]

Meanwhile, experiments were conducted with subscription or pay television. And, interestingly, Hollywood (in the broadest sense) was involved in both the initiation of and opposition to some of these early efforts, despite the claim that the film industry ignored developments in this area.

From about 1949, several companies actively experimented with pay television. One of these companies was Telemeter, a cable system which eventually offered three channels using a scrambled broadcast signal. Films were viewed by placing coins in a box on a television set, which then descrambled the picture. Paramount Pictures owned 50 percent of Telemeter.

Another system was developed by Matthew Fox, "an entrepreneur with a long history of involvement with the movie industry."[22] Fox also received the help of IBM to develop a system called Subscribervision, which used a punch card and scrambled broadcast signals. RKO General became involved with this system when WOR-TV was given permission to test the Subscribervision system in 1950.

While these various systems were tested during the early 1950s,

Telemeter attracted the most attention in 1953, when the company provided a community antenna system, plus special programs for extra fees, to homes in Palm Springs, California. While some of the theater owners cooperated with the experiment, others fought it, charging Paramount-Telemeter with violation of the recent antitrust suit against the majors. While Telemeter claimed to be a success with over 2,500 subscribers, the system apparently buckled under the threat of governmental restriction.

Meanwhile, another system operated by Southwestern Bell Telephone and Jerrold Electronics was drawing attention with its pay-TV experiment in a small town in Oklahoma. The local theater chain was part of the project, thus avoiding one source of opposition. While the experiment received a good deal of press attention, the service apparently was charging too much and encountered problems with costly telephone lines, thus came to a close in 1958.[23]

Opposition to pay-TV came from the theater sector of the film industry, as well as broadcasters and other groups. Ironically, it pitted Paramount Pictures (with its Telemeter experiment in Palm Springs) against United Paramount Theaters, which had recently been divested from Paramount and merged with ABC Television in 1953.

While various experiments were carried out in the early 1960s, broadcast and theater forces lobbied extensively to defeat pay television. A state-wide referendum in California in 1964 was directed against a system called Subscription Television, initiated by Pat Weaver, former president of NBC.[24] Although the referendum was eventually declared unconstitutional, the extensive publicity around the ballot measure and its success seemed to seal the fate of pay television, at least during this period in history.

Indeed, most of the experiments in pay television seemed to have failed by 1965. Hilmes argues that the decline of these systems was due to the FCC's support of the existing broadcast system, as well as the recent attention the film industry had received from the Department of Justice in the Paramount decrees and other cases.[25]

It also might be noted that the Hollywood companies moved in the wrong direction with their subscription experiments. It seems that it was just too early for pay systems that did not offer a regular schedule of special programming for which audiences felt it was worth paying an extra fee. For whatever reason, the Hollywood companies failed or gave up and their interests shifted to other profitable endeavors. (For more on Hollywood's involvement in cable TV, see chapter 5.)

While the film industry failed in its opportunities to dominate the television industry, it is important to at least set the record straight as to the efforts by Hollywood to attempt such involvement and to again acknowledge the interaction of these two industries. As Hilmes concludes,

> Opposition from exhibitors and from established broadcast interests, backed by FCC protectionism and the lack of alternative distribution systems, would once again block film industry plans to move into television broadcasting in a substantial way. And again, as in the case of radio, broadcasting and film interests would establish a system of accommodations by which Hollywood's influence over the forms and structures of broadcasting would become stronger than ever before.[26]

In summary, then, it might be possible to conclude that, contrary to commonly held beliefs, the film industry has been interested and actively involved in technological developments pertaining to new distribution and promotional outlets for their products.[27] However, because of specific historical factors in each case – sometimes incorrect decisions about the future of the technology concerned; at other times, lack of support from regulatory agencies – Hollywood did not initially succeed in dominating these new profit arenas. Yet ultimately, the film industry was able to capitalize on their successful innovation.

The Problems of Technological Histories of Film

Why has the Hollywood technophobia myth been perpetuated? One basic problem has been access to accurate and relevant evidence. The problems of documenting film technology's history are similar to those of studying its economic activities. Corporate decision-making often is veiled in secrecy, which only frustrates historical inquiry. Add to that the chronic problem of finding good, accurate information about the film industry. Morris Ernst was not the first or the last to complain about Hollywood's "infantile skittishness in respect to statistics."[28] Meanwhile, it is not surprising that historical myths are built and perpetuated around the business of Hollywood. Indeed, the industry seems to thrive on them.

However, with the growth of the academic study of film and especially more attention to film history and economics, some of the age-old Hollywood myths have been challenged. A brief look at the various ways that film technology has been studied may be instructive at this point.

Numerous film scholars have delineated approaches to the study of film history, in general, and film technology, in particular. Similar to other technological histories, many accounts of film technology have traditionally focused on inventors and inventions. Edward Branigan describes an "adventure" version of film history, while Robert Allen and Douglas Gomery refer to the more familiar "great men" theory of history.[29] Meanwhile, Eileen Meehan refers more generally to an instrumental approach to media history, which emphasizes individuals.[30]

A technological preoccupation also has been prevalent in film history, as in communication history in general. Branigan refers to technological histories of film, while others have discussed technological determinism applied to cinema.[31] A similar approach is identified by Stephen Neale, who describes simple chronological histories or "one technology after another": "There are no real determinations on this process. Aesthetic, economic, legal or political facts and factors will from time to time be acknowledged and discussed. But they will tend to be accounted for in piecemeal fashion and at a purely local level, thus in effect depriving them of any general, systematic significance."[32]

While these approaches have been appropriately critiqued, other types of historical analysis have developed within film studies. While these new historical approaches are not without their own limitations, they offer some welcome relief from the previous great man and technological determinist versions of film history.

Film scholars have finally taken seriously the charges that cinema history has typically neglected economic factors and the industrial nature of Hollywood filmmaking. An industrial model has been introduced, exploring the invention, innovation, and diffusion of technologies and emphasizing management decision-making and cost-reduction strategies. This approach draws on the industrial organization model in economics, as a branch of neoclassical economic theory. While the approach has been promoted most strongly by Douglas Gomery, other film scholars have accepted and implemented an industrial model.[33]

The managerial emphasis of such industrial analyses provides interesting insight into how technologies have been introduced, often supplying important primary documentation. The approach also traces the uneven development of the film industry, documenting the inevitable concentration and monopolistic tendencies inherent in a market system of film production and distribution. Yet, the answer to these problems, implied if not overtly stated in much industrial/management analysis, is to simply fix the system – eliminate excesses and monopolistic tendencies, and everything will be fine. In other words, there is a strong reliance on the neoclassical conceptualization of corporate behavior, which underestimates power relations and emphasizes rational management decisions geared to maximizing profits and reducing costs. While these are certainly motivations for corporate behavior, there are other motivations as well. As Geoff Hodgson observes, "the firm is an institution of power, rather than one that survives due to its cost-cutting efficiency."[34] Generally, then, the industrial model uncritically accepts a corporate model as the dominant form of filmmaking activity.

A closely related treatment of the film industry is represented in the work of Michael Storper and Susan Christopherson, who use an historical overview of the film industry to support a theory of flexible specialization.[35] From their base in urban planning, but drawing again on neoclassical economics, the authors argue that the film industry has been restructured from the integrated, mass-production studio system of the thirties and forties (a Fordist model) to a disintegrated and flexible system based on independent and specialized production (a post-Fordist model). Thus the film industry provides an example of flexible specialization's viability for other industrial sectors to emulate.

Storper and Christopherson describe some important changes in the "entertainment industrial complex" that is the US film industry of the late 20th century. Yet, their analysis is severely handicapped by their emphasis on the production sector, neglecting the key roles played by distribution, exhibition and financing. As Asu Aksoy and Kevin Robins point out in their critique of Storper and Christopherson, "For them, the major transformation in the American film industry is centered around the reorganization of production, and, more particularly, around the changing relationship between technical and social divisions of labor in production. It is as if the Hollywood industrial story begins and ends with the production of films."[36]

As with the industrial model mentioned previously, the flexible specialization thesis relies on a characterization of corporate behavior based primarily on rational decision-making and cost reduction. Thus, Storper and Christopherson actually misread the dynamics of Hollywood, misrepresenting the autonomy and flexibility of independent production, and underestimating the power and domination of the Hollywood majors. And, as we shall see, rather than disintegration, the US film industry has experienced a process of re-integration in the late eighties and early nineties.

Another recent approach to film technology has been referred to as an ideological model, emphasizing economic and ideological analysis. This approach has been most often associated with the work of Jean-Louis Comolli, who concluded in his influential essay in *Cahiers du Cinéma* in 1971, "It is to the mutual reinforcement of an ideological demand ('to see life as it is') and an economic demand (to make it a source of profit) that cinema owes its being."[37] In other words, Comolli insists on linking technology with economics, which is thus linked with ideology. This model has been scrutinized and discussed during the last decade in film studies and found by many film scholars to be an improvement on previously mentioned historical models.[38] However, little or any actual historical analysis has accompanied the theoretical debates. In addition, it might be argued that the level of abstraction represented by some of these discussions often serves to mystify, rather than inform, the history of film.[39]

While Comolli's work is identified as "an avowedly Marxist perspective,"[40] a more recent attempt to use Marxist terminology in the analysis of film technology is the exhaustive (and exhausting) study of classical Hollywood cinema by David Bordwell, Janet Staiger and Kristin Thompson.[41] Their discussion of the activity surrounding the introduction and evolution of film technology covers territory often neglected by other historians, especially the role of engineers, trade associations, and other institutions in technological development. Yet, the primary and overarching concern of the book's authors is the role of technology in film style. For instance, they frame their section on technology with the following question: "How can we explain technological change in Hollywood in relation to the classical style of filmmaking and the Hollywood mode of production?"[42]

The use of the Marxist terminology by Bordwell et al. has an interesting twist, as well. While they insist on employing terms such as "mode of production," etc., the scope of analysis defies such use. In a rather stinging critique of these authors, Andrew Britton observes that

> they suffer (as Hollywood histories generally do) from the author's assumption that it is possible to extrapolate the object "Hollywood" from the social history of 20th century American capitalism as a whole. . . . she [Staiger] treats "The Hollywood mode of production" and its development as if this mode were a thing in itself which can be studied independently of the culture within which the development took place . . . Ms. Staiger derives no more from her excursion through Hilferding, Mandel and Sweezy than "new methods for analyzing the film industry": the wider world is acknowledged to exist, but it only confirms the autonomy of the object which has been detached from it.[43]

The study is preoccupied again with film analysis, as though a study of the industry and its technological development is only important to the extent that it contributes to the close examination of film texts.

While this is definitely an important contribution to film history, there may be other implications and consequences that are neglected by turning such analysis back on stylistic or textual readings, rather than outwards toward the rest of society. In addition, by focusing primarily on the production process, the important role of distribution is diminished. In other words, there are no real challenges to the actual power structure of the industry, and thus, ultimately, despite the radical rhetoric, the study offers little in the way of a truly critical approach to its subject.

Conclusions: Challenging the Future through the Past

While the newer versions of film technology challenge some of the old Hollywood myths and present useful, important historical insights, there are still limitations to their contribution to critical historical inquiry.

Studying film for film's sake   A good portion of the academic study of film typically has been insular and self-contained, with little regard to interrelationships between media or media and social context.[44] Hilmes, for instance, has argued for the need to analyze the film and broadcasting industries "in a new light":

> For various reasons having to do both with differentiation in product and organization maintained by the institutions themselves, and with the reception accorded them in the academic institution, film and broadcasting have been traditionally regarded as inherently separate, having little to do with each other except in discrete and unusual circumstances. Most accepted historical accounts on both sides of the topic routinely ignore any overlap between the two industries, particularly during the early period of network radio.[45]

Despite the competition within and between industries, the radio, television, electronics and film industries historically have been intertwined, often working collectively. It seems undeniable that the media business has increasingly become even more concentrated and unified. Corporate mergers and diversification activities have dramatically intensified this trend. But the fragmentation of academic analysis further perpetuates the myth of separation within the media/entertainment industry. While such academic segmentation is breaking down in some ways (the addition of television studies to film programs, academic journals and organizations), there is still much work to be done accounting for the interrelationships between media, as well as other forms of popular culture, as well as setting the entire consciousness industry in its overall social context.

The romance of Hollywood   By accepting the myths or concentrating primarily on aesthetic aspects of film technology, corporate influences on film activities, as well as the actual power structure of the industry, can be obscured. In addition, the emphasis on production technologies skews analysis away from important changes in distribution which have implications for the way that people experience film and the relationship of the industry with other social institutions.

While executives cannot always predict the future or act wisely in light of it, corporate imperatives have guided the film industry from its inception. The image of the typical Hollywood mogul has sometimes been exempt from the usual characteristics of the ruthless, calculating corporate executive. After all, these men were creating dreams, and Hollywood, after all, is a unique industry. Although the image of the studio mogul responding only to the seat of his pants may be part of the legacy of Hollywood, recent histories have challenged such myths in light of more careful, less romantic historical inquiry. But it might be argued that there is still a preoccupation with aesthetic and stylistic factors, thus obscuring the social consequences of technology developed according to a corporate imperative.

Status quo film history, or the way we were   In most of these recent histories, there is an acceptance of the Hollywood model as inevitable (i.e. film production/distribution and technological development guided by a profit motive). It may be useful to remember that the history of film technology, like any other history, has been influenced by the visions of the people who have written it. Along these same lines, a group of historians from MARHO, the Radical Historians' Organization, has noted that "We live in a society whose past is given to us in images that assert the inevitability of the way things are."[46] The new histories of film technology, then, may represent different approaches to film history, but their visions still basically support "the ways things are." Thus, by accepting the "the way we were," we may be undermining the possibility of different futures.

But, before we venture into the future, the task at hand is to understand Hollywood in the present. To do this, this study argues that we must:

1 seek to discover the actual history of the film industry and its relationship to other institutions, rather than merely accepting the received myths;
2 study the film industry in its entirety, production through exhibition, as well as how it relates, interacts and sometimes merges with other media and consumer activities;
3 analyze changes in film within its actual social context or, in other words, within corporate structures of power and control;
4 study technological development in the film industry, as in other arenas, as determined and changeable, not as determining and inevitable.

While this book does not direct its attention to ideological readings of texts, nor explore audience members' reactions or resistance to the products of the culture industry, the analysis is deliberately focused on assessing the industrial context in which a good deal of American popular culture is produced and distributed.[47] The proliferation of these products, both in the USA and other countries around the world, would seem to argue for this type of analysis as a base for further studies which may then incorporate these other relevant factors.

The next chapter will examine some recent technological changes in production activities, and that is followed by some snapshots of the companies that dominate Hollywood – the major production/distribution corporations.

3

Film Production in the Information Age

The US film industry has continuously integrated new technological changes into the filmmaking process. While some changes are obvious to audiences, others go unnoticed but have profound effects on the production process.

Over the last few decades, many of these developments have been aimed at resisting the move to video. While video has yet to replace film as the medium of distribution for theatrical presentation, the use of video technology contributes in many ways to the production process. And, as in other areas of life in the 1990s, computers are used during the pre-production, production and post-production of Hollywood motion pictures. This chapter will focus on changes in the production sector primarily related to video and computers (see table 3.1).

Pre-production

Even before a Hollywood film script is written, marketing research sometimes takes place to estimate audience interest in a film idea. Thus, as in other consumer markets, computerized marketing surveys are used more often these days in Hollywood to make decisions about the viability of film projects.

Computers also play a role in script preparation, as screen writers employ various software programs, such as Power Scriptor, Scriptor, Movie Master, Scriptware, or Final Draft to assist in formatting scripts, etc. Software for the preparation of story boards also is available, as are computerized story boards which make it possible to visualize a scene

Table 3.1 Examples of video and computer applications in the film production sector

	Pre-production	Production	Post-production	Other
Video	Video casting	Shooting on video	Video editing	
	Location scouting	Video assists Video dailies	Special effects	
Computerization	Scriptwriting		Studio management	Animation
	Storyboarding		Editing	Colorization
	Production management		Sound editing /effects	
	Talent bases		Special effects	
	Casting networks			

while writing a script or before shooting begins. Other programs make it possible to visualize space to be used in a film, thus making it possible to design and light sets, block shots, plan camera moves, etc. Such programs allow more careful planning for difficult shots, such as those filmed underwater, explosions, etc. An example is the Virtus Walkthrough program, which was used in planning for the film *The Abyss*.[1]

Production control has been simplified with software packages, such as Associate Producer, Movie Magic Budgeting and Scheduling, Filmworks Scheduling & Budgeting, Turbo, and The Remarkable Film and Video System, which assist film producers in planning budgets and coordinating production schedules. Computers also are employed for a wide variety of production activities, such as payroll, budgeting, financial records on daily production costs, etc.[2] Casting also has been affected by computer and video developments, as actors and actresses are able to find out about potential jobs through computerized casting networks, and then present casting directors with video audition tapes or video résumés. In addition, talent agencies, such as William Morris Agency Inc., are using computer networks and databases to store and access information about talent availability and other information.[3] Even the process of scouting locations has been influenced by video, as distant sites can be considered for scenes without additional travel expenses.

Studios and the corporations that own them have been affected by new computer technologies and telecommunications systems. Generally, such information systems are similar to those of other corporate sites, although special needs may exist to service the diversity of activities taking place (everything from the sale of clothing to film production to theme park rides), as well as the customized management structure of each corporation.[4]

Production

Film versus video   While it has been rumored for nearly two decades, the electronic process of video has yet to replace the chemically based process of film for the production of feature films and dramatic television programs. Some of the resistance has to do with traditional "film people" simply refusing to change. But other reasons have to do with technical differences and economic advantages.

Traditionally, video has most often used several cameras, while cinema typically uses only one, thus lighting effects are more carefully controlled on a shot-by-shot basis. In addition, video has been plagued by technical problems with more "down time" waiting for electronics, as well as presenting storage problems (video disintegrates faster than film negative and video systems change quickly).[5]

Shooting logistics often favor the portability of film. As an example, a video engineer referred to the problems of shooting video from a helicopter. Charles Eidsvik has even suggested that some technical changes in film production technologies have been made to enhance film's advantages for on-location shooting, thus ensuring film's role as the dominant shooting medium.[6] These new developments include faster film stocks for shooting in low-light situations, faster and sharper lenses, and more efficient lighting equipment, as well as more portable and flexible cameras and mounts (such as the Steadicam, Skycam and Louma Crane) and improved sound technology which allows unwanted location sounds to be electronically replaced in post-production.[7]

Yet the most often cited difference between film and video is the quality of the image. Specifically, film offers better resolution and dynamic range (or a better contrast ratio). In 1984, an Eastman Kodak executive explained, "There is no technology on the horizon capable of making video-taped images look like filmed images."[8] While some experts argue that HDTV (high definition TV) quality is close, video's technical limitations also have been pinned to problems with video monitors, which cannot reproduce the texture of film. The conclusion of a video engineer in 1991 was that "you still cannot make film on television look like a print."[9]

Video experimentation Over the last decade, several directors have experimented with different video processes. *Harlow* was shot in 1965 using a system called Electronovision, but with less than satisfactory results. Since then, several other films have been shot in video. For instance, a system called Image Vision has been used to tape concerts utilizing a video process with increased resolution. The tape is then converted to film for editing and theatrical release. (Examples include *Monty Python Live at the Hollywood Bowl* and *Richard Pryor in Concert*.)[10]

A few directors have experimented extensively with electronic film-making, including Michelangelo Antonioni and Francis Ford Coppola.[11] Coppola developed new technological innovations at his Zoetrope Studio, creating such novelties as a video storyboard and congruent edit system which was used, for instance, in the production of *One From the Heart*.[12]

Higher quality video Recently the hopes for video have focused on high definition television (HDTV), which involves high resolution video images (1,125 lines, for most HDTV systems, versus the US current standard of 525 lines) at a similar aspect ratio to film (1.78:1, rather than TV's current 1.33:1), with enhanced color fidelity and range, and digital sound. There is no doubt that HDTV would improve the technical quality of current television systems, yet there are still questions about which standards are to be adopted and how systems will be implemented, as well as whether or not HDTV is an essential technology, for television or film.

While HDTV systems have been on the drawing board for over a decade, the larger picture involves far more than just the film industry. HDTV may be used with computers in a wide variety of industrial and military settings, as well as its various applications in the communications industry. Consequently, the Electronics Industry Association has estimated that the market generated by HDTV will exceed $150 billion during the 1990s and into the next century. Peripheral products will add another estimated $400 billion.[13] Thus, the stakes are high to control the new technology, pitting nations, international organizations, industries, and corporations against each other.

While the battle over standards continued in the early nineties, "Hollywood and the major networks have sat on the sidelines, waiting for all the technical stuff to be resolved."[14] Japan started broadcasting HDTV signals via satellite in 1991, using the 1,125-line system, which also has been adopted in Europe and approved by the SMPTE (the

Society for Motion Picture and Television Engineers). Meanwhile, in early 1993 the USA had still not completed a five-year process of considering different standards, including digital HDTV systems which are thought to be superior because of the ability of interact with computers.[15]

Though home HDTV systems are distinct possibilities, the process may be utilized first in motion picture production and, possibly, exhibition. There are already examples of television programs and films shot in HDTV and transferred to film for exhibition. For example, in 1991 Viacom shot the TV movie *Perry Mason* in high definition, while Columbia Pictures' production of *Hook* used Sony's high definition video for eventual transfer to film.[16] In light of Sony's ownership of Columbia (see chapter 4), there may be more examples at the studio in the future. Sony has been working on HDTV since 1981, developing cameras, projectors, transfer equipment, etc. Not too surprisingly, Sony's High Definition System (HDVS) Center is located on the Sony/Columbia lot in Culver City, where the technology has been used primarily for commercials, titles, animation, and computer graphics.[17] Brian Winston points out, however, that even though Sony has targeted the production community, the company backed an analog rather than a digital system, thus offering "the wrong solution to the wrong problem at the wrong time."[18]

Several other Japanese electronic companies are promoting HDTV, including Matsushita, the owner of Universal Pictures (see chapter 4). Although they saw Hollywood as an ideal proving ground for the potential of high definition video, they have encountered a good deal of resistance, as well as increased competition from film suppliers. Harry Mathias, a cinematographer and HDTV expert, claims that high definition video "is desperately trying to solve a need in the motion picture industry that simply doesn't exist."[19] In response to the HDTV challenge, 35 mm color film technology, the industry standard for six decades, has advanced significantly in recent years, giving movie makers considerably more flexibility in creating visual images. Competitive pressure from the Japanese high definition video systems has also led the Eastman Kodak Company, the leading supplier of film to Hollywood, and other companies to develop sophisticated new editing and special effects capabilities.[20]

HDTV has still received praise for the creation of composite images and special effects, saving time and money as well as providing creative flexibility.[21] Recognizing that movie makers are not rushing to dump the 35 mm standard, the proponents of the new technology are concentrating for now on HDTV's advantages as a tool for special effects and editing. A few small companies in New York, such as Rebo High

Definition Studios and Captain of America, Inc., have taken advantage of these attributes, shooting high definition productions for commercial clients and building libraries for future use when the new technology finally takes hold.[22]

But the real revolution for Hollywood companies may come with HDTV "films" distributed directly to HDTV-equipped theaters or homes, which will mean serious changes in film distribution. While relatively few in Hollywood (except those involved with the Japanese electronic companies) displayed interest in the new process at the beginning of the nineties, predictions are that "Tinseltown will eventually play the HDTV game." (Future possibilities involving HDTV exhibition will be discussed in chapter 7.)

"The smell of the sprocket holes"[23]   In spite of these new video developments, many film workers and technicians stubbornly cling to "the film look," arguing that it will never be replaced by video.[24] For instance, many filmmakers say that "for all the crystal clarity of the images it produces, high-definition video cannot come close to film's ability to capture the moods, the richness of color, the contrasts and shadings that collectively give a story visual life."[25]

Ultimately, video may be accepted as the standard medium by the Hollywood production community, although some observers argue that this will not happen automatically as the quality improves, but when the cost of video production and equipment comes down. As an industry insider has noted, "The impetus to kill film is the dollar."[26]

It has been suggested, however, that film's superior quality has been deliberately mystified by the industry. As Eidsvik notes, "Driven by the nightmare of hearing the phrase 'we could just as well have done it on tape,' the film community made its internal power accommodations and promoted its mystique of quality in order to survive in the higher budget ends of the industry."[27] Winston makes a similar argument: HDTV's potential to cut costs may not be necessarily persuasive, in that "Hollywood has used technology, either because of its complexity or its cost or both, to limit competition by creating barriers to entry."[28] In addition, Winston echoes the concerns of others about the wisdom of introducing current HDTV systems when more advanced technologies may be on the horizon.[29]

Video assist   Although video has yet to replace film as the production medium for theatrical films or dramatic television programs, it has been integrated into the production process in a number of ways.

Many film crews utilize video assist units on the set, using cameras which shoot both video and film. The video signal is fed to a monitor controlled by a video assist operator.[30] While the recorded video is not used in the later editing process, video assist systems can be useful for checking the look of a shot or for continuity purposes (making sure that shots match from one day to the next). Although only one camera currently incorporates video assist into the camera system and there are no color systems perfected, some predict that all cameras will have such features in the future.[31]

While some directors rely heavily on the video assist images, viewing scenes as they are shot via video monitors, others may virtually ignore the video process except for the reasons noted previously. Although it is possible to play back every scene, the process is time-consuming and can present problems, especially when actors/actresses become involved in determining their best take.[32] In discussion of the utility of video assist units, the video versus film debate again surfaces. As cinematographer Haskell Wexler noted in response to the question of color video assists: "I am not in favor of a color tap. No matter how good it ultimately could be, it is not film and will not look like the film the camera shoots. This could make for faulty judgments and, in general, there are too many photographic 'experts' on the set already."[33]

Even when a film is not edited on video, a three-quarter-inch video copy of film dailies is often made at a video company, followed by a half-inch version for screening by studio executives.[34]

Post-production

The most pervasive uses of recent new technologies in the production of motion pictures have been computer and video systems to edit film, and for the creation of special effects.

Electronic time codes   As a kind of intermediate step between film and video, a motion picture can be shot on film using a time code that corresponds to videotape. In other words, rather than a 24-frame-per-second standard, the film uses a 30-frame-per-second standard. Kodak introduced this type of film stock in 1982, calling it Datakode and boasting that it automated the labor-intensive elements of production and post-production. While these systems allow for quick, pin-point accuracy in locating footage, some editors agree that the "old-fashioned" manual method is preferable.[35]

Computerized and electronic editing systems   Computers have been used for logging footage as well as other editing tasks.[36] But computers combined with video editing systems represent a profound change in the whole process of film editing.

Early videotape editing was a tedious and tricky matter. Until a time code system was developed in 1967, a cut-and-splice method was used with mostly miserable results.[37] With electronic editing systems, the job has been drastically simplified and, some argue, rivals film editing systems for efficiency and flexibility. As an *American Cinematographer* writer explains: "No elusive little trims all over the floor . . . just a few book-sized videotapes within arm's reach of the editor, who no longer needs an assistant. . . . The existing and soon-to-arrive technology is capable of saving the producer vast amounts of precious time and money."[38]

By 1988, 80 percent of network prime-time TV programs were shot on film, but 60 percent were post-produced electronically.[39] Editing feature films on video has been much more slowly accepted, as the "top end" pictures are still cut on film.[40]

While several different editing systems have emerged in the industry, the process of editing video is basically the same (see figure 3.1). The original film negative is transferred to video on equipment such as the Ran Cintel. The editor then views the video footage, recording decisions via a computer, which then allows preview edits without actually making a recording. Thus, electronic editing systems incorporate the use of video and computers. Popular systems include the Montage, Ediflex and CBS/Sony systems, which employ videocassette playback machines, and the EditDroid and Chyron CMX 6000 systems, which use laserdisc players. Others have included the Eeco Emme, Laser Edit, BHP Touch Vision, and Spectra Image. These systems have been fiercely promoted within the industry by the companies manufacturing them, with free training courses offered.[41]

Electronic editing systems may present advantages for some, but problems for others involved in the post-production process. One basic consideration is the cost of these new systems. For example, in mid-1991 a Montage system could be rented for $2,000 per week. It is unlikely that some small production companies are able to afford such rental costs, much less the purchase cost of such equipment.

Editors already have to deal with an increasing amount of footage due to new smaller cameras and other technologies. A two-hour feature may involve 20 times the amount of film eventually used. While an editor must manage all this footage, new editing systems give the director

Figure 3.1 Example of electronic production process: Pacific Video Electronic Laboratory™ Post Production Flow Diagram

Source: (Adapted from) Laser-Pacific Media Corporation, Hollywood, California. © Laser-Pacific Media Corporation.

even more possibilities for becoming involved in the cutting of a film.[42] It is even possible that certain editing personnel will no longer be necessary, thus greatly reducing labor costs in post-production.[43]

Apparently, everyone agrees that the new systems are faster than the old film routines: "No film editing system can match the electronic editing system's speed in making numerous versions of an edit, comparing different edits, reviewing coverage, and making changes. This speed translates into either a lower ultimate editorial cost, or the ability to go further in editorial perfection, or a combination of the two."[44]

While the new systems may be attractive to producers (for the lower costs) and directors (giving them immediate gratification and more control during the editing process), some editors are not quite as enthused. They claim that the systems may even be "too fast," not allowing time to think about cuts, or leading to complex problems too quickly.[45] Hollywood's technological conservatism, or the mystique of filmmaking crafts, also has been blamed for the reluctance of editors to convert to new cutting systems.[46]

Even some directors, enthralled at first with the new editing technology, sometimes return to the film process. Bernardo Bertolucci recognized the irony of returning to film editing after using the Chyron CMX 6000 system: "When there were just the 20 laser discs, I missed the smell, the touch, the vibration of the film . . . With laser disc, you see the film on the monitor as if it were on TV. OK, we know that's the destiny of all our movies at the end."[47]

Special effects Perhaps the most obvious use of new technology, at least for the audience, is in the area of special effects. With their bag of technological tricks, special effects experts now can create new worlds, alien creatures and previously dangerous or impossible actions on film. One visual effects supervisor has noted that "now virtually anything can be done visually. If you can describe it, you can do it."[48]

The aim of special effects has been to create things that do not actually exist. Some of the techniques used by the earliest filmmakers, such as double exposures and miniaturized models, are still employed. *King Kong* (originally released in 1933) represented a landmark in special effects and incorporated many of the same techniques used by today's special effects teams: models, matte paintings for foreground and backgrounds, rear projections, miniature or enlarged props and miniaturized sets, combined with live action.

However, the use of computers, robotics and digital technologies over the last 20 years has added to the sophistication of the effects process, and also enhanced the filmmaker's ability to create nearly anything imaginable on film.

There is a wide variety of optical or special effects, which are constantly changing as every film has its own set of unique requirements which inspire effects masters to create new techniques. Only a few of these techniques can be discussed here.

First, the use of computerized cameras has made stop-motion techniques smoother and more believable, while image compositing has become more complex.[49] Examples include everything from the flying sequences in *E.T.* to undersea shots in *The Hunt for Red October* and aerial combat footage in *Flight of the Intruder*. A more obvious recent example, however, is *Who Framed Roger Rabbit?*, in which computer-driven camera methods were used extensively to allow cartoons to interact with live actors.

Meanwhile, computers have been used not only to assist in manipulating images, but to create new ones. Computer Generated Imaging (CGI) has reached a new level of sophistication, as characters, objects and settings can be created and then composited with real images (or live-action). The spectacular results were apparent in the top-grossing film for 1991, *Terminator 2*, which perfected techniques called "morphing" (short for metamorphosis) to meld film and computer-generated images through digital compositing, and "making sticky" to graft the characteristics of one image onto another.[50]

With the 1993 film, *Jurassic Park*, new heights in special effects were reached with the creation of computerized images of ancient creatures. In addition to full-size models, the film includes about six and a half minutes of digitized dinosaur footage, which required 18 months of work by 50 people using $15 million worth of equipment.[51]

Other types of effect can be achieved through digital image processing, including manipulation of color, contrast, saturation, sharpness and shape of images. Certain elements of images can be removed, making it possible to repair damaged film, or eliminate unwanted parts of scenes. Examples are the flying sequences in *Hook*, which utilized heavy cable guides which could be electronically "painted" out of each shot.[52] One prediction is that stunt people will be unnecessary when "real" actors are (seemingly) able to accomplish these difficult feats.[53]

Another possibility is to create situations that seem real, but are actually computer enhanced. Rearranging scenes from famous films or newsreels is not only a possibility, but a reality, as illustrated in films such as *Zelig* and *Dead Men Don't Wear Plaid*, as well as the 1991 Coca-Cola commercial, featuring images of Humphrey Bogart and Louis Armstrong in the same scene with Elton John and other contemporary players. Some have predicted that these manipulations will become games of the future. A photo accompanying a *Discover* article features Clark Gable and Cher in *Casablanca*, stating that "in 2001 we'll be toying with old movies on personal computers, changing actors and story lines to fit our own cinematic taste."[54]

For some films, the number of effects can be staggering. For example, the underwater setting and alien creatures in *The Abyss* generated 290 effects shots covering 21 minutes of film, while one shot in *Back to the Future II* required compositing nearly 100 effect elements.[55]

Yet, some of these techniques and technologies actually save time, as effects can be done quicker and involve fewer people. One software program, Quicktime, uses digital and video compression to produce an inexpensive version of an effects sequence or edit.[56]

Computerized human images also have been integrated into films, for example, the villain in *RoboCop 2*, the skeleton images in *Total Recall*, and various images in *The Lawnmower Man*. The possibility of synthetic actors has attracted the attention of many filmmakers. George Lucas predicted in the late eighties that "more advanced technology will be able to replace actors with 'fresher faces' or alter dialog and change the movement of the actor's lips to match." While these possibilities may raise serious ethical questions, the problem may not be an immediate one for the acting profession. One of the drawbacks of computer-generated images has been the high costs involved. And, even though the price was falling rapidly and progress was being made at the beginning of the nineties, it was still impossible for synthetic actors to be mistaken for humans. In other words, morphed cyborgs may be one thing, but most experts agree that a fully computer-generated, "normal" human is somewhere in the future.[57]

The special effects boom has led to the creation of a few new companies. An example is Apogee Productions, which was formed in 1977 by a group led by John Dykstra, who had worked on the special effects for *Star Wars*. Its first project was the television series, *Battlestar Galactica*, but it went on to produce "spectacular images, models, mechanized props, and/or optical composites for over 50 feature films and television programs."[58]

Apogee also serves the varied interests of the entertainment business, designing and manufacturing a wide array of special effects devices and theme park attractions, as well as producing commercials, feature films and television movies.

However, one company seems to dominate the special effects scene. Industrial Light and Magic, formed by George Lucas while producing *Star Wars*, claims to do more business in the special effects field than its

five major competitors combined.[59] The company has worked on six of
the top ten box office hits in history and has created some of the most
spectacular effects in the industry, including those in *Jurassic Park,
Terminator 2, The Abyss, Back to the Future(s)* and *Star Trek(s)*. ILM
must be doing well: they reportedly spent $3.5 million on new equipment
for work on *Terminator 2* and used $15 million worth of equipment for
Jurassic Park, as noted previously.[60]

Sound   Sound editors also are assisted through the use of computerized storage of sound effects, as well as the manipulation of sound via
computers. New developments in sound reproduction have been introduced during the last two decades, in particular Dolby Audio Recording and various digital sound systems.

In the late eighties, 70 mm prints of *Dick Tracy* were distributed with
a six-track system called Cinema Digital Sound. The company responsible
for the new system is partially owned by Eastman Kodak and promises
digital sound for 35 mm prints (thus suitable for screening in most
theaters) in the next ten years.[61]

Music composition and performance also has been influenced by
computerization. Just as scriptwriters are able to employ computers to
assist in their work, music composers are also using software to aid in
the composition of screen scores. In addition, there is the possibility of
the electronic origination of music, via sophisticated synthesizers.

Other Production/Post-production Activities

Animation renaissance   Computers have been integrated into animation work, making it possible to complete drawings more efficiently and
clean up animated frames, but also to create scenes from new perspectives based on original drawings.

Because of these technical developments and marketing factors, there
has been a renaissance in animation.[62] A good deal of animated programming is completed by lower-paid workers in Europe and Southeast
Asian countries. Not only can animated features be accomplished more
quickly, efficiently and cheaply, the films tend to be popular with a wide
range of audiences, making them particularly suited for international
markets. As a recent *New York Times* article concluded, "Like so much
else in Hollywood, the renewed interest in animated films after decades

of general neglect stems largely from a hunger to duplicate some very impressive boxoffice numbers."[63]

From 1986 through 1990, it was estimated that animated films grossed more than $400 million domestically.[64] Some of the really successful animated films (and their box office revenues) that have wet Hollywood appetites have included: *Who Framed Roger Rabbit?* ($154 million), *The Little Mermaid* ($84 million), *Oliver and Company* ($52 million) and *An American Tail* ($47 million). Meanwhile, *Beauty and the Beast* set a record by selling more than 14 million videocassettes, while *Aladdin* provided even more treasures for the Disney company. The goal is to attract young and old audiences over and over again through perpetual re-releases and video distribution, and to capitalize on merchandising possibilities. In other words, other companies are trying to emulate the Disney model. (For further discussion of Disney, see chapters 4 and 9.)

Color me richer   While special effects and other new processes have received little but raptured awe from the popular press and Hollywood fans, another process has attracted nothing but controversy. A computer software system developed in the eighties can differentiate between shades of gray in black and white images, making it possible to select appropriate colors and thus colorize previously black and white films.[65] While the technique apparently had been available for a few years, it wasn't until the mid-eighties that a company called Color Systems Technology was able to find anyone interested in the process.

Even though films have been altered in numerous ways for television since the fifties, colorization immediately drew the wrath of Hollywood's creative community, legislators, and critics. The debate became especially heated after 1986, when Ted Turner purchased the libraries of MGM, RKO and pre-1950s Warner Brothers films and television programs. Turner immediately arranged for 100 films (including *Casablanca, Father of the Bride* and *The Maltese Falcon*) to be colorized by Color Systems Technology. The Hal Roach Studios also started colorizing films in the public domain (including *It's a Wonderful Life* and *Topper*) at its (partially-owned) Toronto-based company, Colorization Inc.[66]

For the most part, the Hollywood community was outraged. The strongest complaints came from directors, who wanted to draw a strict line between art and commerce. Fred Zinneman cried that it was "a cultural crime of the first order."[67] Martin Scorsese called colorization a "desecration," explaining that "*Casablanca* is art. You don't mess around with it."[68] In addition to directors (and the Directors Guild of America) and film stars, other groups opposed to the process included

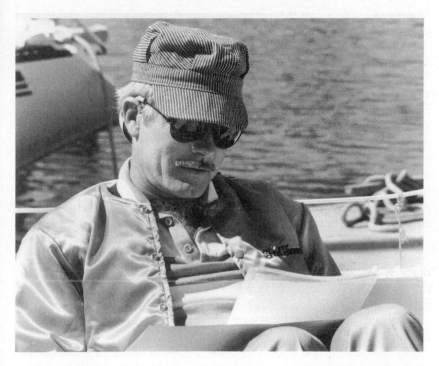

Plate 1 The Rebel with a Cause Ted Turner has contributed his share of business innovations to the film and television business during the last decade. Turner shocked many film celebrities by releasing colorized versions of classic MGM films which he held from his purchase of MGM in the mid-1980s. From his base in Atlanta, Georgia, he developed WTBS as a superstation beamed around the country via satellite, as well as expanded Turner Broadcasting to include important cable channels such as CNN, TBS, the Cartoon Channel, etc. (See chapter 5 for more on Turner's holdings and alliances with other cable companies.) *Photograph by Carlos R. Calderon*

The American Film Institute, the Writers Guild of America West, and the American Society of Cinematographers. During congressional hearings on the issue, the AFI stressed the cultural role of film, while the "moral rights" of artists – the right to approve *any* changes made in completed films – eventually became the issue.[69]

Those who colorize, however, saw the issue differently. A film can be changed from black and white to color for as little as $1,500 a minute, although $2,000–3,000 is probably more common.[70] A colorized film can then be sold to syndicated television and cable channels and released on videocassettes for a tidy profit. Color Systems is said to have attracted contracts worth more than $20 million around 1985.[71] As one colorizer explained, "We're talking about making them viable in today's television and cassette market."[72]

And, indeed, the market did seem to respond: *It's a Wonderful Life* sold a total of around 10,000 copies in the original black and white version in 1985–6, but between 55,000 and 75,000 copies had been sold of the colorized version by November 1986.[73] As Ted Turner finally concluded, "The vast majority of people really don't give a hoot whether you colorize movies or not. It's a handful of elitists in Hollywood that don't like it."

While the head of the Directors Guild claimed that classic films were "bastardized by people intent on squeezing the last possible penny out of marketing those pictures," others pointed out that Hollywood film companies were making the deals.[74] Turner not only insisted on his right to do anything he wanted with the films he owned, he also stressed the business side of filmmaking that the directors wanted to ignore: "Movies were made to be profitable. They were not made as art, they were made to make money, and any moviemaker who did make movies for art's sake is out of business. Anything that could make more money has always been considered to be OK."[75]

Crude, perhaps, but ultimately ownership rights and business sensibilities ruled. *Casablanca* appeared in its colorized form in November 1989, and around the same time, *Citizen Kane* was on its way to the computerized paintbrush.

Reflections on the Production Process and New Technologies

Labor issues   The question of new technological development ultimately involves a wide range of questions concerning the future of film workers.

Many of the developments discussed in this chapter have the potential for eliminating jobs in the film industry. Will workers be replaced by new technological developments or will their jobs become easier and more efficient? As noted previously, some editing positions are threatened by video editing techniques. In addition, musicians also may be replaced by increased use of synthesized music and computers also may threaten the craft of cinematographers. And, it is even possible that computerized actors or robots may one day replace real-life actors and actresses.

Other problems relate to the rivalries between workers and unions over jurisdictional problems. Film editors replaced by video technicians have resulted in skirmishes between the two technical unions in the industry, the National Association of Broadcast Employees and Technicians (NABET), which typically, organized video technicians, and the International Alliance of Theatrical and Stage Employees (IATSE), which generally organized film technicians. Another example cited by Michael Nielsen is the controversy between sound technicians and film editors using electronic editing, which allows sound and picture editing simultaneously.[76]

Another question has to do with education and reskilling. Who should be responsible for training film workers to use the newest technologies? Production companies, trade unions, equipment companies, universities, the government, or employees themselves? Nielsen cites an example of a state-sponsored job retraining program to prepare film editors for electronic editing techniques.

Other issues pertain to creative decisions, as the potential for shifting control of a film's creative elements is influenced by many of these new processes. For example, with electronic editing systems, there is the potential for less influence by film editors, even on the first cut of a film.

While unions and guilds should be able to protect jobs and the control of the work process, the labor organizations in the film industry generally have not represented a united front against technological change. As Nielsen concludes, "The net result of this dissension among the craft unions involved in broadcasting and film is that the producers have continued to have the upper hand in all negotiations. The unions seem too concerned with their immediate organizational needs to recognize fully the potential impact of new technologies."[77]

Independents/competition   With the addition of new technologies in production, the ability of independents to produce the slick, sophisticated look of the major production companies becomes more difficult. To compete, independents must locate the capital needed to use these new (and often expensive) techniques and equipment. Otherwise, they are relegated to making lower-budget films or cheaper versions (or, perhaps, satires) of the more expensive, blockbuster films.[78]

Yet the rhetoric from the Hollywood crowd is still that you do not really need the technology to make a successful film. We are told over and over that despite computer storyboards, shiny new editing machines and elaborate special effects, movie making still demands storytellers, and the industry is in need of imagination and talent.[79]

Technological genres   It might be argued that these technological developments also influence the types of film produced by Hollywood companies. Certainly, the number of science fiction or space epics have increased with the evolution of sophisticated special effects techniques. Indeed, seven of the top ten hits of the eighties were "effects" movies.[80]

The box office successes of action films incorporating special effects and spectacular stunts entice filmmakers to not only continue using such techniques, but to reach even further into their special effects bag with each film. It may even be possible that many audience members may reject films without such high-tech adventures and action, finding them slow, uninteresting and even boring.

Shooting for television   More definite effects can be assessed when it comes to changes in the way films are shot. As Bertolucci noted in his assessment of electronic editing, it is assumed that a film will eventually appear on television. Thus, "[m]ost cinematographers today put marks in their cameras' viewfinders so that they can frame a scene for the theater, but make sure everything important is 'safe' for video."[81]

When shooting in wide screen formats, compromises increasingly are made so that a film is tolerable in both theatrical and television releases. For instance, when David Lean made *A Passage to India*, HBO co-produced the film and demanded that it be shot at a 1.83:1 aspect ratio, so that it would be acceptable for viewing on cable.[82]

More discussion of the consequences of shooting for television will be presented in chapter 6, after we have explored these new forms of exhibition. However, it is important to point out that the way a film is shot and edited definitely has been influenced by new distribution outlets such as video and cable.[83]

Technological conservatism   It has been argued that technological change in film production over the last few decades has been mostly conservative and defensive; in other words, film attempts to resist the video revolution. As Charles Eidsvik observes,

> the majority of technical developments in the film industry have been aimed at facilitating extant production practices rather than at changing the 'look' or sound of commercial films ... there is very little that is esthetically revolutionary in the new technologies, and nothing that would upset the basic film-making power structure. Changes have been

conservative, a defense against inroads and threats brought by very rapidly evolving video technologies.[84]

Eidsvik's point is important in light of the perceived changes in the Hollywood production process. Whether or not film is prepared through a chemical process or an electronic one, or involves computerized techniques or video editing processes – the relations of production have changed little, if at all. Indeed, those technological changes – apparent or promised – may actually be detrimental to some of the traditional crafts people in the film industry and independent filmmakers.

Hardware for sale   In the past, the Academy of Motion Picture Arts and Sciences contributed to developing new technologies through its Technology Council.[85] Apparently that role has been diminished recently, in light of the competing companies involved in technological development.[86]

Meanwhile, the large hardware manufacturers have attempted to lure Hollywood into their electronic web. For instance, Sony and Apple have made generous contributions to the American Film Institute. The AFI-Apple Computer Center, complete with $1 million hardware and software donated by Apple and other companies, allows Hollywood filmmakers to work out the bugs in new programs and systems, to be developed by these manufacturers and sold to the industry.[87]

It is not surprising that the electronics companies have been interested in selling their new electronic and computer wares to production companies. But Hollywood's production activities represent a relatively small market, except where linked with consumer products (such as HDTV). Indeed, consumer products such as videocassette recorders (VCRs) and home electronic systems have been the primary target of the electronics companies, and these new technologies have attracted the electronics companies to the film industry, which they now partially own.

Indeed, it is in the realm of new *distribution* technologies where the most dramatic changes have appeared during the last decade. To understand the background and significance of this move, we need to look more carefully at the development of these home entertainment technologies, as well as the companies which control them. Thus, the major players in the entertainment industry – the Hollywood majors – are the focus of chapter 4.

4

The Big Boys:
The Hollywood Majors

"Who Are Those Guys?"

Film production often attracts the greatest attention to Hollywood, as the popular press, encouraged by the Hollywood promotional machine itself, focuses on new stars, hot directors and exciting scripts.

But the glamour of movie production is often closely wound up with the business of film distribution, as production teams often work directly for major production/distribution companies and "independent" production companies must deal with them if their film is ultimately to appear in theaters and video stores around the country and the world. So, to discuss film production, one must ultimately talk about distribution, and thus ultimately confront the Hollywood majors.

One way to depict Hollywood is as a "three-tier society." At the top are the big studios, or the majors – Paramount, Twentieth Century Fox, Warner, Universal, Disney, and Columbia. The second tier includes the smaller or less influential production and/or distribution companies, or minor majors, including MGM/UA, Orion, Carolco, and New Line Cinema. And at the bottom are the much smaller and often struggling "independent" distributors and production companies. As a recent industry survey concluded: "The large studios have the advantages of distribution profits, enormous film libraries and sheer size."[1]

The production of filmed entertainment is dominated by these large companies, which regularly receive over 90 percent of the revenues from the domestic theatrical market (see table 4.1). But they also supply the bulk of television programming to the major networks and syndication market (independent television stations). For instance, the first and

Table 4.1 Distributor shares of domestic film rentals, 1987–92 (all figures %)

Distributor	1987	1988	1989	1990	1991	1992
Columbia[a]	4.5	3.5	8.1	4.9	9.1	12.5
Disney	14.0	19.4	13.9	15.5	13.7	19.4
Fox[b]	8.7	11.6	6.5	13.1	11.6	14.2
MGM/UA	4.2	10.3	6.3	2.8	2.3	1.2
Miramax	NA	NA	NA	1.2	1.4	1.1
New Line	1.8	1.9	1.3	4.4	4.0	2.1
Orion	10.4	6.6	4.2	5.6	8.5	0.2
Paramount	19.7	15.2	13.8	14.9	12.0	9.9
TriStar[a]	6.2	5.8	7.9	9.0	10.9	6.6
Universal[c]	7.2	9.8	16.6	13.1	11.0	11.7
Warner	12.5	11.2	17.4	13.1	13.9	19.8
Total	89.2	95.3	96.0	97.6	98.4	98.7

NA: not available
[a] Currently owned by Sony Corp.
[b] Currently owned by News Corp.
[c] Currently owned by Matsushita Electric Industrial Co., Ltd.
Source: *Variety*, presented in *Standard & Poor's Industry Surveys*, 11 March 1993, p. L22.

second largest suppliers of network prime-time programs (not includ-ing movies) for 1991 were Time Warner and Disney. More than half of the 1991 Fall prime-time schedule was produced by the seven major Hollywood companies. These prime-time programs eventually reach the cable market in the form of syndicated programming. In addition, as we shall see, the majors supply the bulk of programming for home video and cable, as well as participating in other diversified activities (see table 4.2).

One of the problems in outlining the activities of these corporations is the on-going restructuring and realignments which take place as fin-anciers and investors merge and un-merge various corporations and their subsidiaries, and boards of directors, managers and their bankers make decisions to move into different markets, trying best to predict what products will be the most lucrative and profitable. (See table 4.3 for a financial summary of the majors for 1992.) Interest in Hollywood firms became especially intense at the end of the 1980s with a "frenzy of consolidation."[2] On the one hand, international markets for enter-tainment products continued to expand. And, on the other hand, for-eign interests were attracted to Hollywood conglomerates for many of

Table 4.2 Diverse entertainment operations and assets of major film and TV companies

Area	CBS	Capital Cities /ABC	Disney	Gaylord Entert.	General Electric	Matsushita	News Corp.	Paramount Comm.	Sony Corp.	Turner Broadc.	TeleComm. Inc.	Tribune Co.	Time Warner	Viacom
New movies			•			•	•	•	•				•	
Film library			•			•	•	•	•	•			•	
Theatres						•	•	•	•					
TV shows	•	•	•			•	•	•	•				•	•
TV station(s)	•	•	•	•		•	•	•				•	•	•
TV network	•	•			•	•	•	•				•		
Basic cable network(s)	•	•			•					•	•		•	•
Pay cable network(s)			•										•	•
Cable systems				•							•		•	•
Recorded music			•	•		•			•				•	
Theme parks			•	•				•					•	
Pro sports			•					•		•		•	•	
Publishing		•	•			•	•	•				•	•	
Audio players					•	•			•					
Video players					•	•			•				•	•

Mention of some relatively minor operations may be excluded.
Source: adapted from *Standard & Poor's Industry Surveys,* 11 March 1993, p. L17.

Table 4.3 Hollywood majors' parent companies' financial summary, 1992–93

	Assets ($m)	Sales/revenue ($m)	Net income ($m)	No. of employees	Report date
Paramount	7,054	4,265	261	12,200	10/31/92
Disney	10,862	7,504	817	NA	9/30/92
News Corp.	26,221	10,189	501	27,250	6/30/92
Time Warner	27,366	13,070	86	41,700	12/31/92
Sony	39,050	34,422	313	119,000	3/31/93
Matsushita	9,018	7,450	133	242,000	3/31/92
MGM	2,414	937	−271	NA	12/31/92
Orion		491	−312	NA	1992

NA: not available.
Source: Based on Form 10K reports from the corporations, as reported by *Disclosure 1993*, and *Moody's Industrial Manual*, New York: Moody's Investors Service, 1993.

the same reasons that Hollywood increasingly is looking to international markets: new technologies, deregulation of previously regulated markets, and the opening of new markets (in Eastern Europe, Soviet Union, etc.). (For further discussion of international markets, see chapter 9.) The profiles that follow, therefore, represent the Hollywood majors at the beginning of the 1990s.

Paramount Communications Inc.

Paramount represents an interesting example of corporate trends for the major Hollywood studios during the post-war period. Engulfed by Gulf + Western (G+W) in 1967 (with substantial assistance from the Chase Manhattan Bank), Paramount became a subsidiary of a larger, broadly diversified conglomerate, involved in financial services, publishing, sugar production, etc.

However, in the 1980s, G+W began narrowing its interests towards its entertainment and communication-oriented activities, culminating in a corporate name change in June 1989 (from Gulf + Western Inc. to Paramount Communications Inc.) and the sale of its financial subsidiary (The Associates) in October 1989. While the shift has been attributed to a change in leadership at G+W (with the death of G+W's founder, Charles Bluhdorn, in 1983),[3] the change also reflected the recognition of lucrative markets for entertainment and information products in the

1980s. As its 1991 Annual Report boasts: "Paramount Communications is a global entertainment and publishing company with exceptional creative and distribution capabilities and extraordinary financial strength."[4]

Entertainment operations include the production and distribution of motion pictures and television programming. The company produced more than 700 hours of original programming in 1991 for the networks, cable and first-run syndication, including eight weekly programs and five first-run syndication series. The company distributes television programming to 110 markets, where sales doubled between 1986 and 1991. Paramount also holds an ownership interest in Zenith Productions, one of the UK's leading independent TV program companies. In the USA, Paramount was influential in boosting the first-run syndication market with the success of *Star Trek: The Next Generation*, followed by *Star Trek: Deep Space Nine* and *The Untouchables*, thus contributing to (or taking advantage of?) the decline of the major networks' prime-time domination.[5]

Paramount also owns six television stations (the Paramount Group) in markets representing nearly 10 percent of US television households. An indication of the company's interest in television was evident when the television group's headquarters were moved to Paramount's Hollywood studio in 1991. As the Annual Report that year noted: "Plans include co-ventures between programming units and the Group, and the use of the stations as laboratories for new projects."

But as the nineties rolled on, Paramount further increased its commitment to television. In November 1993, the company announced intentions to start a Fox-like television network by 1995. In other words, Paramount would offer programming such as the *Star Trek* series to a network of affiliated stations for one or two nights each week. With its strong base in syndicated programming and station relationships, the move seemed a logical extension of Paramount's diversified activities. Yet some commentators still doubted the viability of another advertising-based TV network for the US market. (More discussion of relations with television follows at the end of this chapter.)

Paramount distributes its television shows and motion pictures (as well as some independent companies' products) to the home video market and participates directly in the cable industry as co-owner of the USA Network (with MCA), a basic cable network in the USA with an audience reach of nearly 58 million US households. Paramount's 1991 annual report explains:

Actively exploring new programming concepts worldwide, USA Network is on the cutting edge of an expanding industry. With cable compression technology promising greater channel capacity, USA is breaking away from the conventional approach of targeting specialized niche markets. The network appeals to an audience traditionally served by broadcast television – a strategy that has propelled it to the top spot overall as the most-watched advertiser-supported cable network in the country.

Paramount is also an investment partner (with MCA) in TVN Entertainment, a ten-channel pay-per-view service targeting the growing direct broadcast satellite (DBS), or backyard dish, market.

The company owns motion picture theaters in 12 countries, through Famous Players (481 screens), Cinamerica (464 screens, jointly owned with Time Warner), and United Cinemas International (339 screens, jointly owned with MCA).

The entertainment division also includes the Madison Square Garden (MSG), meaning that Paramount owns sports teams such as the New York Knicks and New York Rangers, as well as the Miss Universe, Miss USA and Miss Teen USA pageants. A new 5,600 seat Paramount Theater at the Garden offers concerts and family shows. But the MSG operation also involves the largest regional cable television sports network (the Madison Square Garden Network), which carries the Knicks', the Rangers' and the New York Yankees' games, and sports video marketing operations. Paramount recently purchased another company which promotes auto thrill shows (SRO/Pace Motor Sports).

Other parts of the entertainment division administer and license more than 70,000 music copyrights through Famous Music subsidiary, sell advertising time in TV programs produced and distributed by Paramount through jointly owned Premier Advertiser Sales (with MCA), and produce television commercials via Paramount Images and cable programming via Wilshire Court Productions.

Paramount's various publishing concerns have expanded to include products and services in a wide range of areas, from educational and consumer publishing, to business information products, computer-based learning systems and audio books. Paramount's publishing is mostly clustered under Simon & Schuster, the largest educational publisher in the USA, including imprints such as Prentice Hall, Silver Burdett & Ginn, Allyn & Bacon, Computer Curriculum Corporation and Pocket Books. The following description of consumer publishing activities alone indicates the extent of the company's publishing activities:

Consumer publishing operations encompass hardcover and trade paperback books for all ages (Simon & Schuster, Prentice Hall General Reference, Pocket Books Hardcover, Poseidon Press, Touchstone, Fireside,

Table 4.4 Paramount Communications Revenues Summary, 1991

	Revenues ($m)	% of revenues
Motion pictures and television features	1,176.9	49
Television	593.4	25
Station and network	184.6	8
Other	17.5	1
Theaters, sports and other entertainment	407.8	17

Source: Paramount Communications Inc. Annual Report, 1991.

Linden Press, Silver Burdett Press, Simon & Schuster Books for Young Readers, Little Simon, Green Tiger and Messner); mass market paperback books (Pocket Books, Pocket Star Books, Washington Square Press, Archway and Minstrel); travel information (imprints include American Express, Baedeker, Frommer's, H. M. Gousha, Insight, Mobil and The Real Guides); general reference and consumer information (imprints include Arco, Betty Crocker, Burpee, J. K. Lasser, Monarch Notes, Webster's New World Dictionaries); and audiocassette publishing (Sound Ideas, Audio Works). The Group also distributes books of other publishers.

At the end of 1991, the company reported 70 best sellers and 13 number one titles during the year. Clearly, Paramount does not depend solely on motion pictures, as indicated by the revenues summary in table 4.4. By 1987, the company received over $1 billion in revenues from home video and television series alone.[6]

Another indication was Paramount's bid to take over Time Inc. at the same time that Warner was negotiating with Time. Although Paramount moved to block the combination in the courts, Warner was eventually successful, as will be discussed shortly. Paramount's President Brandon Tartikoff summed up his company's future at the end of 1991: "As Paramount Pictures begins its 80th year, it is positioned to prosper from changes in the marketplace and in technology." One of the changes included Tartikoff's resignation shortly after this statement. However, his prophetic words rang true in the waning months of 1993 as Paramount became the focus of a struggle between two other media groups for further dominance in the media/entertainment field. One group was led by Viacom International – owner of MTV, VH-1, and Nickelodeon cable networks, Showtime and The Movie Channel pay-cable channels, five TV stations, 14 radio stations and cable systems reaching 1.1 million subscribers. Backing Viacom was Blockbuster Entertainment Corp., a video retail chain, and Nynex Corp., a regional telephone company, as well as investment bank Smith Barney Shearson and several of the country's largest commercial banks, including the Bank of New York.

The second group was headed by the QVC Group, a $1 billion cable shopping channel operator, headed by Barry Diller, former head of Paramount. Key cable industry allies included Liberty Media Inc. (owned by Telecommunications Inc. (TCI), the largest cable operator in the USA) and Comcast Corp. Additional support came from Cox Enterprises Inc. and Advance Publications Inc., owner of Conde Nast magazines and Random House books. In addition, six banks agreed to lend $500 million to assist QVC, and also QVC's investment banker, Allen & Co., offered support for the takeover.[7]

Both groups emphasized the role that Paramount would play in supplying programming for the future "electronic highways" that cable and/or telephone companies foresee delivering infinite volumes of news, information and entertainment to American homes. (For more discussion, see chapter 5.)

But the struggle over Paramount also revealed some interesting features about the relationship between Hollywood and communications technologies in the 1990s. The bids to merge or take over Paramount were obviously backed by financial institutions, representing their support and enthusiasm for such "information age" mergers. It also indicates that Hollywood companies have become even more pivotal in the exploitation of new communications technologies and the expansion of entertainment/information markets. And, finally, no matter who controls Paramount, it is clear that these new technologies, as well as the companies and industries that control them, are becoming increasingly more intertwined.

Time Warner Inc.

One of the surviving Hollywood majors, Warner Brothers, operated under the roof of the diversified conglomerate Warner Communications Inc. from the late 1960s through the end of the 1980s. On January 10, 1990, Time Inc. acquired the stock of Warner Communications Inc. to form one of the largest communications companies in the world. Despite an increase of $10.8 billion long-term debt, the arrangement was defended in Time Warner's 1989 Annual Report as follows:

> In the Eighties we witnessed the most profound political and economic changes since the end of the Second World War. As these changes un-

folded, Time Inc. and Warner Communications Inc. came independently to the same fundamental conclusion: globalization was rapidly evolving from a prophecy to a fact of life. No serious competitor could hope for any long-term success unless, building on a secure home base, it achieved a major presence in all of the world's important markets.

With this goal in mind, Time and Warner began discussions on joint ventures. The more we talked – and the more we learned about each other – the more obvious it became that the most significant and exciting possibility was a synthesis that would lift us to a position neither could achieve alone.

In a season of history when technology has combined with political and social change to open vast new markets, we are a company equipped to reap the greatest benefits.[8]

Time Warner created a huge international conglomerate with assets of nearly $25 billion and revenues of $7.6 billion. The new corporation's diversified activities include the publication of magazines and books, the operation of cable television systems, the production and distribution of motion pictures, television programming, videocassettes, compact discs, tapes, and vinyl records, pay-television and cable programming, and the ownership and administration of music copyrights, theaters and theme parks.

Magazines produced and distributed by Time Warner take over 20 percent of all advertising dollars placed in consumer magazines (see table 4.5 for a list of its publishing operations). In addition to distribution services, the company implemented a program entitled Target Select, which customizes and personalizes magazine advertisements through the use of computer-controlled selective binding and ink-jet printing. Thus, advertisements can be directed not just at specific target groups, but at individual subscribers.

In February 1990 Time launched *Entertainment Weekly*, which "provides reviews and reports on events in television, movies, video, music and books." Interestingly, those are business endeavors to which Time Warner is heavily committed.

Time Warner participates in the book industry through the ownership of Little, Brown & Co., Warner Books, Time–Life Books, Book-of-the-Month Club, and the Children's Book-of-the-Month Club. Warner Publisher Services distributes 400 magazines and books for 90 other publishers. In addition, the company publishes more than 60 regularly issued comic magazines, such as *Superman, Batman, Wonder Woman, Teen Titans* and *Justice League International*, as well as story collections sold as books, under its subsidiary, DC Comics.

Time Warner distributes music under a wide range of labels (see

Table 4.5 Publishing subsidiaries and magazines produced/distributed by Time
Warner

Magazines		Publishing Companies
Time	*Baby Talk*	*Southern Progress*
Fortune	*Ready for Baby*	*Whittle Communication*
Life	*Baby on the Way*	*American Family Publishers*
Sports Illustrated	*Baby on the Way Basics*	*Time Distribution Services*
Money	*Martha Stewart Living*	*Publishers Express*
People	*Sunset*	
Sports Illustrated for Kids	*Health*	
Entertainment Weekly	*Hippocrates*	
Southern Living	*Asiaweek*	
Progressive Farmer	*Yazhou Zhoukan*	
Southern Accents	*President*	
Cooking Light	*Dancyu*	
Travel South	*Elle Japon*	
Parenting	*Who*	
Parenting's Summer Fun	*Vibe*	

Source: Time Warner Inc. Annual Report and Form 10K, 1992.

table 4.6), and claims to be the largest record company in the world.
(Foreign sales represent more than half of total revenues.)

The combination of Time and Warner concentrated 25 of the top 100
US cable systems within one company. Through complete ownership of
Warner Cable Communications Inc., and 82 percent ownership of
American Television and Communications Corp. (ATC), Time Warner
became the second largest cable operator in the USA, with systems in
35 states. In 1989, the company's cable systems passed 10.43 million
homes and included 6.14 million basic subscribers. The company is vertically integrated in the cable business and owns cable programming
channels as well as cable systems. The oldest and largest pay-television
service in the USA, HBO, is owned by Time Warner, as well as Cinemax
and The Comedy Channel. The company owns 45 percent of Movietime
and 16 percent of Black Entertainment Television.

Time Warner operates in the field of filmed entertainment via Warner
Bros Inc. and its subsidiaries, plus Lorimar Telepictures Corp. (purchased
in January 1989 by Warner Communication). In the early 1990s, Warner
also distributed Disney and Touchstone pictures in foreign theatrical
markets, and theatrical products for Sony/Columbia Pictures to basic
cable in the USA.

Table 4.6 Time Warner Record Labels, 1992

Warner Bros. Records	Atlantic Recording Group	Elektra Entertainment	Warner Music International
Warner Bros.	Atlantic	Elektra	WEA
Reprise	EastWest America	Asylum	East West
Sire	Interscope	Nonesuch	Teldec
Giant	Third Stone	Mute	CGD
Warner Nashville	Rhino	Chameleon	Carrere
Tommy Boy	A*Vision	Hollywood (distrib.)	Erato
Owest	Select		MMG
Def American			WEA Latino
Capricorn			PWL
Maverick			ZTT
Paisley Park			rooArt
Music for Little People			DRO
			Anxious

Source: Time Warner Inc. Annual Report 1992, p. 33.

Television programming is produced by both Warner Bros and Lorimar, and together they claim to represent the largest supplier of original network programming in the USA. During the 1989–90 television year, the two companies produced 16 prime-time network series, one mini-series, and six made-for-television movies, as well as supplying first-run syndicated programming.

At the end of December 1989, Time Warner reported that Warner Bros' contracts "for the licensing of feature films, cartoon programs, syndicated series, mini-series and made-for-television movies to pay television and over-the-air broadcast television that will be recorded as revenue in 1990 and beyond amounted to approximately $977 million."[9] Time Warner's home video subsidiary is Warner Home Video Inc., which has a library of over 1,800 titles available on videocassette.

Warner Bros also owns the Licensing Corporation of America (LCA), which "acts as an agent in the licensing of rights to names, photographs, likenesses, logos and similar representations or endorsements, for individuals, organizations, fictional characters and entities." Thus LCA manages copyrights and trademarks for characters ranging from Bugs Bunny to television heroes such as J. R. (of *Dallas*) or Murphy Brown. Of course, LCA was involved in the merchandising campaign for *Batman*, a Warner Bros release.

Table 4.7   Time Warner Inc. revenues by business segment

	Revenues ($m)	%
Publishing	328	23
Music	585	24
Entertainment		
Filmed Entertainment	410	26
Programming-HBO	215	11
Cable	977	16

Source: Time Warner Inc. Annual Report 1992, p. 1.

Time Warner owns a 50 percent interest in Cinamerica Theaters (with Paramount), which includes operation of the Mann, Festival and Trans-Lux theater chains. The company owns and operates theaters in the UK, Germany, Denmark, Australia, and the Soviet Union.

Following the theme park trend of other majors, Time Warner also operates "Warner Bros Roadshow Movie World" in Australia, as well as Time Warner's 60 percent interest in Six Flags theme parks in the USA.

The revenue received from these diversified activities is presented in table 4.7, again illustrating that the production of motion pictures, or even filmed entertainment, is only one of many other activities for Time Warner, but also pointing to the broad-based media concerns represented in this one company.

The Walt Disney Company

It has been said before: the company that Walt built is no Mickey Mouse affair. While Time Warner has been criticized for its lack of synergy,[10] the Walt Disney Company is possibly the most synergistic of the Hollywood majors. The company that began as an independent production company producing cartoons distributed by others has moved into the ranks of the majors, gleaning nearly $7.5 billion in revenues in 1992, and proclaiming the 1990s as "The Disney Decade."

Since a major reshuffling of owners and managers in 1984, the Disney empire has extended its tentacles more widely and more tenaciously.[11] And, as with most of the Hollywood majors, the company's expansion has not depended solely on motion pictures, but on a wide array of business activities in which the new management team (calling itself "Team Disney") has aggressively exploited the Disney name and its characters. The company is organized as three major business segments, and within these divisions is a plethora of profitable projects.

Filmed entertainment   During takeover discussions in the early 1980s, the value of the Disney film library was estimated to be $400 million, but the same reports observed that if exploited more aggressively, the library could be worth even more. Team Disney has been aggressive, to say the least. Disney films were rescued from the vaults and released on videocassette, resulting in quick cash for the new management team.[12] The company continues to exploit its film library, carefully releasing already amortized products in new forms, and promoting them through their other business activities.[13]

But new products have been developed, as well. The new management team embraced the formula initiated by the old guard,[14] releasing some of its strongest box-office hits on the Touchstone label – untainted by the family-oriented, PG-rated Disney name. In addition, a new label (Hollywood Pictures) was introduced in 1990, expanding Disney's presence at the box office. An example is the claim made by the company that during the weekend of 3–5 August 1990, 7,400 theaters – 30 percent of theaters in the USA and Canada – were showing a Disney, Touchstone or Hollywood Pictures film. Another indication of Disney's success in the late eighties in its feature film activities is the number of years the company has led the Hollywood majors in the division of film rentals (see table 4.1 again). In 1993, Disney again expanded its box office clout by acquiring the successful independent distribution company, Miramax.

Financing for films often came from Silver Screen Limited Partnerships, which raised nearly $1 billion for Disney films.[15] More recently, Disney arranged a financing vehicle called Touchwood Pacific Partners I, with a group of Japanese investors, providing a total of $600 million for film production up until 1992. Disney sometimes works with partners, although the company typically wants control of everything they touch. In 1990, the studio had agreements to distribute a number of films with Cinergi Productions, Interscope Communications and Nomura Babcock & Brown.[16]

If there was one weakness in the Disney empire, it seemed to be finding successful formulas for prime-time network television fare. While *The Golden Girls* was a tremendous success, the company held only part interest in the series. Disney continued looking for other hits, but basically failed with such shows as *Lenny* and *The Fanelli Boys*. Finally, the company hit the mark with *Dinosaurs* and *Home Improvement*, both of which have been successful enough to reach syndication.

Team Disney has fared much better with syndicated programming, with 18 hours of first-run programming on syndicated television each week by the fall of 1990. While the popular network show, *The Golden Girls,* was an instant success in syndication, the company also offered *Live with Regis and Kathie Lee, The Challengers* (a game show) and *Siskel & Ebert*. The most successful syndicated programming, however, was The Disney Afternoon – a package of animated shows offered to independent TV stations, forming a two-hour block of Disney programming. The Fox network was an important buyer of The Disney Afternoon, but 350 other stations around the country also carried the programs.

Disney also has its own pay-cable operation. While the Disney Channel carries non-Disney shows, a major share of its programming is new or revived Disney fare. When Team Disney took over in the mid-80s, the Disney Channel was the most expensive of the new pay channels, charging more than $4 for each subscriber. Despite a $75 million deal in 1984 with the Cablevision system,[17] the company felt the channel could attract more subscribers. So, policy was changed, subscription rates slashed and lower prices offered to hotel chains.[18] By 1990 the channel attracted over 5 million subscribers.

The Disney Channel represents the synergistic policy of the company, as explained by Ron Grover in *The Disney Touch*:

> By late 1988, the Disney Channel was ... achieving [Michael] Eisner's goal of cross-promotion for other company ventures. Kids watching Winnie the Pooh or Mickey Mouse cartoons became a target market for Disney toys. Showing episodes of *The Mickey Mouse Club*, which had been filmed at the Disney-MGM Studios Theme Park, enticed 14-year-olds into pressuring their parents to take them to Orlando. When *Who Framed Roger Rabbit?* was aired on the channel, specials on EPCOT Center were also run, along with anniversary shows celebrating the parks.[19]

Through its Buena Vista Home Video label, Disney/Touchstone films as well as other products are distributed on videocassette. Disney has expanded internationally, with gross revenues increasing four-fold from 1986 to 1990, with branches in 45 countries.

Disney also has joined the ranks of broadcasters, as an owner of KCAL-TV (formerly KHJ-TV) in Los Angeles. An interesting move for the Disney company, which has usually stayed out of the arena of news and information production, was the introduction of an innovative three-hour prime-time news format. Of course, the station carried Disney's syndicated programs and The Disney Afternoon.

Theme parks and resorts   Disney's theme parks and resorts represent a sizable investment and a hefty share of the revenues for the company. The original Disneyland is located on a 320-acre site in Anaheim, California, although the company plans to expand the facility. Other California activities include the Disneyland Hotel (adjacent to the park), and the Hotel Queen Mary in Long Beach. In 1992, Disney followed up on their successful film *The Mighty Ducks* by purchasing the rights to a new expansion hockey team in Southern California, to be called . . . The Mighty Ducks.

Disney owns around 29,000 acres of land southeast of Orlando, Florida, where the Walt Disney World Destination Resort is located. At the beginning of 1990, the complex included the Magic Kingdom, Epcot Center, the Disney-MGM Studios Theme Park, eight hotels, a night-time entertainment complex (Pleasure Island), shopping village (Disney Village Marketplace), conference center, campground (Fort Wilderness), golf courses, water parks and other recreational facilities. The park's facilities attracted more serious visitors as well as tourists, as Walt Disney World represented the second most popular destination for corporate meetings.[20]

Tokyo Disneyland, which opened in April 1983, is built on a 600-acre landfill site in Tokyo Bay. The park has been a tremendous success, nearly equaling attendance at the original Disneyland. But the Disney company only collects 10 percent of the admission charges, 5 percent of food and merchandise sales, and 10 percent of corporate sponsorships, as the park is owned by the Oriental Land Company. Still, by 1984 the park was generating $40 million for Disney.[21]

In 1987, Disney announced plans to move into Europe. Euro Disney seemed a natural: the popularity of Mickey Mouse and other Disney characters in Europe is legendary, indicated by the fact that 25 percent of all Disney merchandise is claimed to be sold to the Continent.[22] While there was some competition as to where the complex would be located, France finally succeeded in attracting the company to a location 20 miles east of Paris. The French government had to make big promises, however: 5,000 acres of land at "rock-bottom price," millions spent on upgrading and improving the highway system and suburban rail line, and reduced interest rates on $1 billion in loans.[23] The actual agreement with the French government was much more complex, but essentially, as Grover notes, "was an impressive deal for Disney. For less than $200 million in equity and other expenses, the company had bought nearly half of a venture that was worth $3 billion." Others simply called it "a Cinderella story of business."[24]

Euro Disney finally opened in April 1992 with the usual Disney fanfare. However, the park reported a loss of $87.7 million during its first year, prompting a major debt restructuring which eventually cost Disney around $750 million, and increased the company's financial commitment to the park. Some analysts observed that the source of Euro Disney's financial problems had less to do with public sentiment than the Disney company's "abrasive and aggressive management style in planning, building and financing the resort." Despite the problems plaguing the park, by 1994 Euro Disney ranked as Europe's biggest paid tourist attraction.[25]

The war of the studio tours   The tale of the opening of the Disney–MGM Studios Theme Park provides some insight into Disney's mode of operation. Rather than go it alone, the company approached MGM with the idea of a joint project. In June 1985, Disney executives negotiated a 20-year agreement, with an accelerating yearly fee to MGM (starting at $100,000 and not exceeding $1 million) for the use of MGM's logo and films (with a few exceptions). The deal represented a real coup for Disney, while MGM executives were roundly criticized by owner Kirk Kerkorian. "In the end, Disney all but walked away with Leo the Lion's mane."[26]

But the controversies were not over. MCA (parent company of Universal) charged that Disney had impeded progress on their Florida theme park. While MCA claimed their idea came first, there was a race to finish the parks. But Disney had a few advantages. The company's holdings in Florida are governed by the Reedy Creek Improvement District, an independent quasi-government organization awarded to Disney by the Florida assembly. In other words, Disney projects did not need the typical regulatory reviews or licenses. Commenting on Disney's behavior, Sid Sheinberg, MCA president, said, "Disney's ability to decimate you by acting in a predatory way is chilling. Do you really want a little mouse to become one large, ravenous rat?"[27]

Disney–MGM opened in May 1990 at a cost of over $500 million. Promotional festivities included a General Motors (GM) commercial during the 1988 Academy Awards, featuring a GM car in front of the new park. GM paid the $500,000 bill for the advertisement. On the other hand, MCA's opening the next month included numerous publicized problems and the dubbing, "Universal's Swamp of Dreams." Disney had (for the moment) won the War of the Studio Tours.[28]

Disney's land   With the expansion of Disney's theme park activities, the company became heavily involved in real estate and hotel management. In addition to the existing parks and hotel complexes, there are plans for another Euro Disney park, for expanding the Disney–MGM Studios park, for a second theme park in Southern California and Tokyo, and for extensive hotel expansion to include 16,300 rooms.

Guiding this development are two of the company's many subsidiaries: Walt Disney Imagineering and Disney Development Company. The Imagineering unit provides design, engineering and new planning for the Disney magic at parks and other facilities, while the Development Company's staff are the master planners of real estate transactions and other projects. Despite all the planning and research, though, the company often has found itself in trouble. Environmental problems and resistance from the communities surrounding Disney playgrounds have emerged, often prompted by the company's fetish for controlling every aspect of areas in which they operate, from wildlife and water supply to transportation facilities and phone services.

While Team Disney attempts to downplay these conflicts, the company is not shy about the synergistic emphasis within its real estate empire. As noted in its Form 10K filed with the Securities and Exchange Commission (SEC) in 1990: "the Company believes its theme parks and resorts benefit substantially from the Company's reputation in the entertainment industry for excellent quality and from synergy with activities in other business segments of the Company."

Consumer products Disney's third division is Consumer Products, which "licenses the name of Walt Disney, its characters, its visual and literary properties, and its songs and music to various consumer manufacturers, retailers and publishers throughout the world." But this description does not adequately describe the deliberate and coordinated proliferation of Disney products and characters worldwide.

While Disney's merchandising activities are legendary, the new management team has emphasized the exploitation of "old" Disney characters, as well as new ones, which are featured in the company's other business activities, as well as in Disney Stores, mail order catalogs, and through hundreds of licensing arrangements with other companies. (Disney's merchandising empire will be discussed in more detail in chapter 8.)

News Corporation/Twentieth Century Fox

The News Corporation is well on the way to becoming the most versatile and skilled media company in the world.
The News Corporation Ltd, 1990 Annual Report

Table 4.8 News Corporation Ltd income and revenues, 1992 (percentages by segments)

	Operating income (%)	Revenues (%)
USA	55	64
UK and Europe	24	19
Australia and Pacific Basin	21	17
Filmed entertainment	8	24
Television	16	12
Newspapers	37	29
Magazines/inserts	24	16
Books	13	14
Other	2	5

Source: News Corporation Limited Annual Report, 1992, p. H7.

Twentieth Century Fox, the company started by William Fox which has maintained its position as one of the corporate pillars of Hollywood since the 1920s, was purchased by Rupert Murdoch's News Corporation in 1985.[29]

Murdoch's empire is said to be valued at around $11 billion, although the exact numbers seem obscured by some tricky and loose accounting procedures.[30] Nevertheless, the company claims to be the largest English-language newspaper publisher in the world, with a paid weekly circulation of over 15.5 million. But Murdoch's activities go far beyond newspapers. A complement of media concerns includes magazines, books, and newsprint manufacturing, as well as television, film, video and satellite distribution of entertainment and information, in addition to a variety of other companies sprinkled throughout the Murdoch empire. Total assets for the company grew from $6.4 billion to $19.7 billion in the six years ending in 1992, although reaching over $26 billion in 1990.[31]

While the News Corporation is incorporated in Australia, the company seems to live up to its own billing as "A Global Media Company." Its holdings are literally spread all over the globe (see table 4.8). In Australia and the Pacific Basin, the company owns or has a controlling interest in over 130 regional and city newspapers, nine magazines, a book publishing company, and commercial printing companies, as well as paper mills, a record company, travel companies, and an airline.

In the United Kingdom and Europe, the News Corporation owns key newspapers, such as *The Times*, *The Sunday Times*, *The Sun*, and *News of the World*, as well as 11 magazines and book publishing, commercial printing and other companies. One half of Sky Television and Sky Radio in the UK are controlled by the corporation, as well. Murdoch moved into continental European broadcasting during 1992 with a 40 percent interest in Antena 3 in Spain. A more important arrangement was made with Canal Plus in France, linking the "dominant suppliers of subscription television in Europe." Through their control of programming and encryption, the companies are well set to dominate the future development of digital compression and multiplexing in Europe.[32]

The News Corporation still receives over 50 percent of its revenues from the USA, where it has owned four newspapers, ten magazines, a book publisher (Harper Collins, the second largest English language book publisher in the world), commercial printing and a coupon insert division. Interestingly, the News Corporation's US publications have included entertainment-oriented magazines, such as *Premiere*, *Soap Opera Digest*, *Soap Opera Weekly*, and *TV Guide*, which works nicely with the company's extensive holdings in television and filmed entertainment

Control of Twentieth Century Fox Film Corporation would be enough to qualify the company as a major player in entertainment, as this includes Fox Film, Twentieth Television Corporation, CBS/Fox Inc. (a major video distribution company), and Deluxe Laboratories.[33] But the Fox entertainment empire has aggressively moved into the television arena through ownership of seven television stations in major US cities, as well as making television history with the Fox Broadcasting Company, or the Fox Network. By offering programming especially popular with younger audiences to a network of 117 affiliates, but also drawing on the strengths of the film studio, the Fox Network has been successful in challenging the three major networks' domination.[34]

Interestingly, this would seem to align Fox with the broadcasting industry as much as the film industry, and present problems with its ownership of television programming under the FCC's Financial Syndication rules (see end of chapter for further discussion.) However, the company has successfully argued that it is still not a *real* network, even though the number of prime-time hours it offers each week continues to grow. Fox will look even more like a regular network when it offers its own network news magazine (which was scheduled to begin in summer 1993) through Fox News Service in Washington.

Perhaps it is not too surprising that the Fox network has received some favorable treatment in Washington. The 1987 News Corporation Annual Report explained that Thomas R. Herwitz, Vice-President for Corporate and Legal Affairs for Fox Television Stations Inc., tells the Fox story to Congress. The 30-year-old lawyer regularly screens Fox motion pictures in the nation's capital for about 50 Congressmen, their wives and staffers. "We make sure members of Congress and other government officials know what we're doing. . . . These are popular social events, particularly at premier times, and our discussions with them allow them to know what's on our minds and us to learn what's on theirs. Lawmakers want to understand our business better – after all, they face questions in every session of Congress relating to television and movies.[35]

The News Corporation is expanding in other new technological arenas. The company recently purchased (with TCI Cable) Reiss Media Enterprises, active in pay-per-view and other international media enterprises. Reiss owns Request TV, which plans to offer a 40–50 channel pay-per-view system by 1994. (See chapter 5 for more on pay-per-view.)

In 1992 News Corporation announced the formation of two technology divisions. News Electronic Data (headquartered in the USA) will provide electronic versions of News Corporation's worldwide databases compatible with the digital electronic world, while the News Technology Group brings together the company's previously independent activities engaged in developing new media technologies, including Etak Inc., the world's leading provider of electronic road maps.

In addition, the UK-based News Datacom produces technologies dealing with media access control and encryption. An example is the "smart card" system for Sky Television (three million cards were produced for Sky and other customers during 1992).

As to how these diverse activities relate, Murdoch explains:

> Our underlying philosophy is that all media are one. The principles and skills involved in discovering and fostering creative talent – no matter the format, be it newspapers, television, magazines, films or books – are transferable.
>
> We believe that our future is to be the pre-eminent supplier of first rate creative and editorial product. The more we think about our businesses, and the more we look at the whole communications industry in all its facets, the more we define ourselves as a global supplier of what is now called "software." For us, the hardware developments that attract so much attention are secondary to our real business.
>
> Nevertheless, News Corporation is acutely conscious of the interaction between software and hardware, between technology and editorial opportunity.[36]

Murdoch's expansion into the world of television is explained more bluntly elsewhere: "Anyone who owns a media company would be foolish not to pay attention to the electronic side." Yet, the media tycoon was encountering a few problems with his TV ambitions in 1993. As a *Business Week* article observed: "Key executives have bolted, the film studio is saddled with flops, and flat ratings plague Fox TV."[37] While Fox's film and TV operations have contributed handsomely to the News Corporation coffers, they must continue to do so if Murdoch is to accomplish his future plans for cable channels in the USA and other countries, as well as expansion of his satellite-delivered broadcast television.

Sony/Columbia

The theme of synergy boldly emerged with the purchase of Columbia by the Sony Corporation. The Japanese electronics transnational formally became the owner of Columbia Pictures Entertainment Inc. on November 1, 1989. The price was $3.4 billion – the highest amount ever paid by a Japanese concern for a US company.[38] At the same time, the company also purchased the Guber–Peters Entertainment Company for approximately $200 million.[39] (Guber and Peters produced a number of profitable films, including *Batman*, *Rain Man*, and *Tango and Cash*.) Sony had previously purchased CBS Records, giving them a strong base in the manufacture of cultural products, as well as audio/video hardware. Another winner in the deal appeared to be investment banker Herbert A. Allen, who held 2.7 percent of Columbia's stock, worth around $88 million.[40]

As explained in Sony's 1990 Annual Report, the company is

> one of the world's leading manufacturers of audio and video equipment, televisions, displays, semiconductors, computers and such information-related products as micro floppydisk systems. Keenly aware of the inter-related nature of software and hardware, Sony is also bolstering its presence in the audio and image-based software markets through the CBS Records group and the newly acquired Columbia Pictures Entertainment, Inc.[41]

It seemed clear that Sony's motivation was the integration of hardware and software. Stung by the videocassette recorder "format wars" (see chapter 6), the Japanese hardware company moved to expand its interests in software. "Sony did not want to be caught without a market for its hardware again, so it purchased Columbia."[42] The attraction of rapidly expanding foreign markets for audio/video products also played a big role in explanations of Sony's move.

The purchase of Columbia and CBS Records made Sony a "powerful, vertically integrated, international empire," not unlike other media giants such as Rupert Murdoch's News Corporation.[43] Even though Murdoch, an Australian, had owned Twentieth Century Fox studios for several years, the takeover of an American movie studio by a Japanese company caused a good deal of controversy. *Tokyo Business Today* observed: "At issue is the scale of Japanese acquisitions in the US and the symbolic, even cultural, status of some of the properties involved."[44]

Sony became the owner of Columbia's library of over 2,700 movies and 23,000 TV series episodes. Columbia also owns TriStar Pictures, with major hits such as *Look Who's Talking*, *Steel Magnolias*, *Ghostbusters II*, and *When Harry Met Sally*. Each averaged over $100 million annually in the USA alone. (For more on TriStar, see chapter 5.) At the end of 1990, Columbia became the international distributor for Orion Pictures.

In addition, Columbia is active in television production, where it sometimes uses ideas from its successful films. Examples: *Baby Talk*, take-off of *Look Who's Talking*. The company also distributes the two "most popular game shows in the world": *Wheel of Fortune* and *Jeopardy!* The two shows have weekly audiences of over 40 million viewers in the USA and appear in foreign versions in over 100 countries. While Sony's film/television activities accounted for only 3.2 percent of the company's net sales in 1990, the hardware–software link is still emphasized by the company. The following announcement by the company is an example:

> Completing its initial Sega CD line-up, Sony Imagesoft has adapted two classic 16-bit titles for the Sega CD. *Hook* combines real scenes from the movie, twelve levels of intense play, never-before-seen computer graphics of Hook's ship, and selections from the film soundtrack. . . . Sony Imagesoft Inc., a subsidiary of Sony Electronic Publishing Co., develops, manufactures, distributes and markets interactive software products for the video game market, using the worldwide technological and entertainment resources of Sony.[45]

(For more discussion of video games, see chapter 8.)

The same philosophy has worked with Sony's record business, as CBS Records handles the software and Sony produces a wide array of audio equipment and production. The record division contributes 15.8 percent of the company's net sales, which includes the production of music videos by CBS Music Video Enterprises. The company also operates several direct marketing clubs under the Columbia House division, including its Compact Disc Club and Video Club, and in 1990 agreed to work with Time Warner to create a joint venture in direct marketing of music and home video products worldwide.

Sony reported assets of over $39 billion in 1993, while net sales were over $34 billion. Since its purchase of Columbia, Sony has invested vast quantities of capital in the enterprise. (One estimate in 1991 claimed the total investment was close to $6.5 billion.) However, Sony appears to be fully committed to their new software ventures, and have announced that they will devote the next ten years to a melding of their old and new lines of business.

Matsushita/MCA/Universal

If Sony's purchase of Columbia started waves of anxiety about the foreign takeover of American culture, then the sale of MCA/Universal to Matsushita in January 1990 prompted near-panic in the national press. Not only the new owners, but also the amount paid for the studio ($6.9 billion) attracted immediate attention, as studio executives and Wall Street experts were probed and prodded in interviews about the consequences of Japanese ownership of a substantial portion of the US entertainment industry. (Interestingly, Lew Wasserman, Chairman of MCA, was one of the interviewees defending the "merger." With 12 percent ownership of MCA's stock, he would come away with at least $800 million if he chose to retire.[46])

MCA was certainly a plum for Matsushita. The company had a fine record of box office hits (such as the *Back to the Future*, etc.) and successful television series (including *Murder, She Wrote*, *Major Dad*, etc.), as well as half ownership of the USA Network and full ownership of WWOR-TV. Of course, the company also is active in home video and merchandising, including Winterland concessions which licenses everything from recording stars (such as Madonna, Bruce Springsteen, and New Kids on the Block) to Major League Baseball, the National Football League, Hard Rock Cafe and Greenpeace. MCA operates a retail store chain, Spencer Gifts, which included 437 stores in 1990. The company is also involved in book publishing through GP Putnam's Sons, the Berkeley Publishing Group, and the Putnam & Grosset Group.

And, similar to Disney, MCA's Recreation Services division operates Universal Studios Hollywood, Universal Studios Florida and plans a European Universal Studios as well. Prior to the Matsushita purchase, the company managed the lodging, food and services for Yosemite National Park, but gave up such activities because of the concern over a foreign company operating services at a National Park.

Table 4.9 Matsushita Corporation Sales, 1990

	(Value billion yen)	% total sales
Video equipment	1,039	17
TV receivers	495	8
Audio equipment	561	9
Home appliances	802	13
Commercial/industrial equipment	1,375	23
Electronic components	781	13
Batteries/kitchen products	312	5
Other	574	10

Source: SEC Form 20F, 31 March 1990.

Another division of MCA is involved with the company's real estate, which includes extensive property in Universal City, the location of the Universal Studios, the Sheraton-Universal hotel, office buildings and a Cineplex Odeon complex.

But what about the company that bought MCA? Matsushita Electric Industrial Co. Ltd is the largest manufacturer of consumer electronic products in Japan and one of the largest in the world. The company was founded in 1918 by Konosuke Matsushita to manufacture electronic equipment for household use. Only recently has Matsushita expanded to non-consumer markets, such as information and communication equipment, semiconductors, etc. (see table 4.9).

With assets of ¥7,851 billion and sales over ¥6,000 billion in 1990, Matsushita led the world in the production of VCRS and related products, such as home video cameras and camcorders. The company also produces professional video equipment, especially for high definition television, and a wide variety of audio equipment. These products are sold under various names: Panasonic, National, Technics, Quasar, Victor or JVC.

However, the fastest growing activity of the conglomerate by 1990 was the manufacture and sale of communication and industrial equipment, such as office automation equipment (fax machines, word processors, personal computers), copiers, teleconferencing systems, telephone equipment, broadcast equipment, etc. The company also produces everything from refrigerators and irons to electronic pencil sharpeners and batteries.

Matsushita owns 117 companies in 38 countries outside Japan, depending on sales outside the country for 44 percent of net sales in 1990.

Increasingly, the company has shifted production, as well, to overseas locations.

The Second Tier – MGM/UA Communications

MGM/UA seems to be the only example of the old studio guard losing its grip. The MGM and UA alliance (MGM/UA Entertainment Co.) was formed in 1981, when MGM's owner Kirk Kerkorian took over United Artists. Since then, it has been a complicated saga of unusual buy-outs and aborted deals.

Kerkorian sold the company to Ted Turner in 1986, but several months later bought it back – that is, minus the film library and the studio real estate. Kerkorian also increased his share to 80 percent and reacquired the UA films.[47]

Since then, the company has been nearly sold on several other occasions, including to Quintex and Turner Broadcasting (again). In 1990, Giancarlo Paretti (Pathe Communications Co.) bought the company for $1.3 billion, backed by Credit Lyonnais Bank Nederland.[48] The bank also chipped in $145 million in April 1991, saving the company from bankruptcy. Apparently Paretti drained MGM/UA by shifting millions to his other investments. However, early in 1992 Paretti was forced to give up control of the company to the bank. Paretti, already in trouble for tax evasion in Italy (and in jail there at the time), was accused of breaching a corporate governance agreement.[49] Credit Lyonnais renamed the company Metro-Goldwyn-Mayer and is still attempting to get the legendary studio back on its feet.

MGM has certainly suffered from all of this dubious deal-making, sinking to a second-level distribution company in the Hollywood ranks. Yet, the corporation still holds valuable assets, with several hit films and successful TV series during the decade, plus various rights to many classic MGM and UA films. Thus, one report in early 1992 concluded: "Despite myriad layers of tarnish, the MGM logo still burns brightly around the world – a miracle of staying power."[50]

Illusions of Grandeur? Orion Pictures

Orion Pictures Corporation provides an example of the difficulties of playing with the big boys. Described as "a director's studio that took chances," Orion survived pretty well for nearly ten years, releasing some of the most acclaimed pictures of the decade.[51] The company represented an aspiring major, formed by experienced film executives out of Filmways Pictures in 1982, who stuck primarily to the entertainment business. The company produced and distributed motion pictures and television productions to the usual outlets (theaters, television, home video, cable), and sometimes even picked up foreign films through its Orion Classics label. By 1987, the company ranked fourth in overall film rentals, receiving 10 percent of the pot. (See table 4.1 again.)

While it seemed that Orion was progressing nicely, a few of its films in 1990 and 1991 failed to cover costs in domestic theatrical release or the home video market, as Hollywood films are sometimes wont to do. Their next batch of films (*Cadillac Man*, *RoboCop 2*, *Navy Seals*, *State of Grace*, *Mermaids*, *Dances with Wolves* and *The Silence of the Lambs*), however, promised big box office bucks. It took significant amounts of cash for the especially costly production costs and advertising/print expenses for these films, but the company generally managed to cover them. While several of these films were great successes,[52] Orion had dug itself a deep hole and didn't have the deep pockets to get out. Their troubles were aggravated as well by their recent expansion into television production. With the credit lines exhausted and cash reserves drained, the company filed under Chapter 11 of the Bankruptcy Act, with debts of over $1 billion in December 1991.

Within a year of filing bankruptcy, the exodus began. Despite incentive programs (sanctioned by the bankruptcy proceedings) offering "stay" and "transition" bonuses, key executives left. The number of total employees was reduced from 420 in February 1992 to 150 in August 1992. And with "key men" leaving, some of Orion's deals for pay cable and video distribution fell apart, as well.[53]

The company's attempts to survive included encouraging takeover bids from several companies, including New Line and Republic. Ultimately, John Kluge – claimed to be America's fifth richest person – came to the rescue and became Orion's dominant stockholder with 50.1 percent, as well as guaranteeing the company's debt. Orion emerged from bankrupcy in October 1992.

However, it was a new Orion. No film or television production. And at the beginning of 1993, only about 20 employees were left.[54] Orion still controlled some valuable properties – over 750 previously released theatrical and television motion pictures, television series and other television programs, including the valuable rights to sequels to successes such as *RoboCop*, plus ten unreleased, star-studded films. However, the company's survival was not guaranteed by these assets alone. The difficulties were described by the company itself in its 1992 report to the SEC, providing further insight into current industry relations and some of the problems involved in competing with the Big Boys:

> the Company will need to compete with many other motion picture distributors, including the "majors", many of which are larger and have substantially greater resources, film libraries and histories of obtaining film properties, as well as production capabilities and significantly broader access to distribution opportunities. Many of the Company's competitors have substantially greater assets and resources, and, unlike the Company, will not be restricted to non-recourse debt financing to acquire product. By reason of their resources, these competitors may have access to programming that would not generally be available to the Company and may also have the ability to market programming more extensively than the Company.
>
> Distributors of theatrical motion pictures compete with one another for access to desirable motion picture screens, especially during the summer, holiday and other peak movie-going seasons, and several of the Company's competitors in the theatrical motion picture distribution business have become affiliated with owners of chains of motion picture theaters. The success of all the Company's theatrical motion pictures and television programming is heavily dependent upon public taste, which is both unpredictable and susceptible to change without warning.[55]

Although Orion was attempting to get back into the game with a separate production unit in early 1993, it was still questionable whether or not the company could ever gain its past stature, much less challenge the larger, more well-endowed and more diversified industry giants.

Big Boy Issues

Takeovers from afar   The foreign takeovers of Columbia, TriStar and Universal prompted speculation and controversy in the USA. In October 1991, a California congressman proposed a bill that would limit foreign ownership of entertainment companies and national landmarks. Representative Leon E. Panetta (D-Monterey) called the foreign takeovers an "ominous trend," explaining that "it is increasingly apparent that our cultural industries, particularly the entertainment and motion picture industries, are in danger of being dominated by foreign owners. This phenomenon is not healthy for America, nor would it be accepted by any other nation."[56] Others in Washington seemed to agree. Panetta's bill would prohibit companies outside the USA from controlling more than half of the businesses devoted to such fields as motion picture and television production. Meanwhile, *Newsweek* reported that 43 percent of the American people also felt it would be bad for the USA.[57]

As predicted, the Japanese companies settled on a policy of local management, rather than on their typical centralized decision-making style in other industries. Some attention was directed toward some meddling with the script of Universal's film, *Mr Baseball*, including the elimination of certain jokes and the expansion of some Japanese characters' roles.[58] However, both companies seem to have acknowledged that Hollywood knows how to make films that sell, so the Japanese owners seemed to be willing to let those who know the business call the shots.[59] Meanwhile, there has been further discussion of whether or not the hardware–software link was really as valuable as anticipated by Sony and Matsushita.[60]

The syndication battle   For many years, the Hollywood majors have supplied the bulk of television programming in the USA. Since 1970, the majors have been favored by FCC regulations preventing ABC, CBS and NBC from owning the programs telecast on their networks; the majors have thus benefitted from the lucrative syndication markets. The controversial Financial Syndication rules have proven advantageous to the Hollywood community, but the networks argue that the market has changed considerably since the rule was adopted. For example, since 1970, the three networks' share of the prime-time audience has slipped from more than 90 percent to about 65 percent.[61]

While the Fin-Syn rules will not go down without a fierce battle involving political clout and lobbying expertise, the issue is complicated by some of the Hollywood majors' interests in television. Following the model of the Fox network, both Paramount and Time Warner plan to form TV networks during the next few years. Both companies intend to draw on their extensive supplies of syndicated programming, but will need to enlist the assistance of other companies to attract the number of TV stations necessary to form a successful network. Another possibility is that one of the majors may combine with an already existing network, forming an even more formidable media giant and clearly outdating the "TV" or "film" industry designations.

But for now, the Fin-Syn struggle is essentially a "Battle of the Gorillas," as large corporate entities bump heads over who will control more profits. At any one time, one group may prevail, but the profits will still flow as long as the syndicated programming market prevails.

Furthermore, it seems unlikely that programming will change very much, no matter who controls syndication rights. As a *New York Times* report points out: "The dispute has little direct impact on what viewers see on television, but the financial stakes are substantial. At the beginning of the 1990s, the syndication market was estimated at $3 billion or more."[62]

Why the Big Boys are Big

This chapter has focused on the corporate context in which the Hollywood majors exist. Obviously, they are still part of *diversified* conglomerates, no longer depending on movies as their only source of income, but involved in a wide range of cultural production, from audiovisual products, to publishing enterprises, to theme park operations.

The majors claim to encounter intense competition in the film industry, as well as in these other activities. At least in film production/ distribution, a number of companies have attempted to compete in recent years, but with great difficulty. Orion represents only the latest example. While a few smaller distribution companies managed to carve out niches for their products,[63] *Variety's* film rental breakdown for 1992 gives information on "several extinct operations, from the so-called "instant majors" of a generation ago (National General, Cinerama) to the more recent casualties of merger, reorganization, and fiscal pipe-smoking (DEG, Lorimar, Embassy, Allied Artists)" – a haunting reminder of the risks involved in playing with the big boys.[64] (The problems of independent producers have been a common theme over the last decade, and will be discussed in more detail in later chapters.)

Clearly, the corporations described in this chapter are not omnipotent, as indicated by the case of MGM/UA. As with other corporate entities, the majors are susceptible to economic ups and downs, recessions, depressions, and other problems. The Hollywood companies, in particular, have continually encountered criticism for escalating production costs, inefficient and unstable management, and luxurious habits and lifestyles. Concerns also have been expressed over the drawbacks of companies actually becoming too big.[65]

Nevertheless, there still seem to be clear advantages to large, strong, diversified companies. The ability to influence the political process to their advantage is one area that already has been well documented.[66] The following chapters will document how the Hollywood majors have been able to influence and take advantage of an economic and political climate which has created new market configurations, as well as to exploit new technological development.

5

The Wired Nation and the Electronic Superhighway: Cable Television, Pay Cable, Pay-Per-View and Beyond

Cable technology has existed in the USA since the late 1940s, when early attempts to boost signals and import distant signals led to Community Antenna TV systems throughout the country. Meanwhile, experiments were conducted with subscription or pay television, and, as we have already discussed in chapter 2, Hollywood was involved in both the initiation of and opposition to some of these early efforts. Thanks to a good deal of opposition, pay systems folded, as did Hollywood's immediate interest in cable.

The service languished as merely an enhancement of over-the-air channels until 1975, when pay-cable channels started offering recent feature films and sporting events using satellite distribution to cable systems around the country. Since then the US cable business has become an extremely lucrative venture, as well as representing the commercially oriented, concentrated and integrated nature of an advanced capitalist media system. But cable also represents an important market for Hollywood product – for instance, over $175 million is received yearly just for retransmission of Hollywood films broadcast on over-the-air stations carried on cable. It also seems that cable would have been a logical extension of the business of Hollywood companies.

Setting the Scene: The Ups and Downs of Communication Policy

It is necessary to look briefly at the political context within which cable (and some of the other new communication) technologies were introduced, specifically considering the components of US communication policy which have influenced the development of these new systems during the last few decades.

Regulatory questions pertaining to cable began to emerge around 1959, as the FCC investigated the effect of distant signal importing on local broadcast markets. At this point, the FCC found no reason to regulate emerging cable systems. However, when microwave technology was introduced, the FCC found that local broadcasters could be economically injured and placed cable under its jurisdiction in the Carter Mountain case. Meanwhile, cable was growing, but rather slowly. By 1975, only 13 percent of US households subscribed.

By the 1980s, the prevailing political and economic climate in the country supported marketplace solutions for a wide variety of social problems. Hollywood provided Washington not only with a President supportive of such ideals, but with a new rhetoric for an intensified marketplace mentality. For instance, Mark Fowler, as Chairman of the FCC, referred to regulation as "a kind of evil empire" and to himself as Luke Skywalker.

But deregulation did not start with Fowler or even the Reagan administration. Several Congressional and FCC investigations laid the foundation for "unregulating" communications.[1] In most of these studies, several arguments were made supporting policy changes. Basically, spectrum scarcity was no longer seen as a problem, thanks to new technologies. In addition, there was general agreement that competition in telecommunications would further the traditional FCC goals of diversity and technological development. A competitive marketplace was accepted as the best means to promote consumer welfare because of the "efficient allocation of resources." As one study noted, "Competition in the economic marketplace and in the marketplace of ideas, then, is to be vigorously encouraged." And, if competitive marketplaces led to diversity and technological dynamism, there was little need for regulation.

But how to assess competition in the marketplace of ideas? In most studies, the method was the same as in other markets: some type of quantitative measurement, either concentration ratios or simple counting techniques. What was counted? Conduits. It was assumed that there is a competitive marketplace for programming or content if there is a sufficient number of distribution outlets or conduits. So, regardless of content, conduits were to be counted. For instance, one market may have only ten media outlets or conduits, including radio and TV stations, cable channels, and distribution of VCRs per capita. Another local market may have over 100 conduits.

Further, conduits were to be counted that are available to consumers, not those actually used or consumed. In other words, as long as enough outlets or conduits are offered for consumption, a competitive market is said to exist. But, conduits are counted only in local markets, as it is argued that national markets need not be measured for concentration, thus need not be regulated by ownership limitations.

From only a brief look at Hollywood in the nineties, it seems that there may be some problem in measuring competition this way. Most studies conclude that there is considerable concentration at the national level, in the production and distribution of entertainment programming. Can it be assumed, therefore, that a local market will be competitive, given the heavy dependence on program acquisition from national sources by local network-affiliated broadcast stations as well as by cable channels and video retail outlets?

There also are problems where the notion of diversity is concerned. Counting those conduits available to consumers does not measure the quality or range of programming and information presented on these channels. The approach used in the studies arguing for deregulation is consistent with a welfare economics model, where a distinction is made between access and content diversity. In other words, most attention is given to determining diversity of access. The argument that citizens should be exposed to a variety of political and cultural ideas is ignored in the usual economic welfare calculus, as explained by two media economists:

> While this perspective undoubtedly has some merit, there is no objective way to quantify those benefits and so we will ignore the social externality aspects of content diversity . . . any standard devised to permit welfare evaluations of this type of externality must of necessity embody personal value judgments on the relative merits of various types of programming . . . In addition, we suspect that a video industry that meets reasonable standards for access diversity and effectively provides programming in response to a wide range of tastes will also perform adequately when the social benefits of content diversity are considered.[2]

Another disturbing aspect of these government studies and economists' reports is the shift to referring to the public as consumers in a marketplace, relegating the notion of the public interest to broadcasting history textbooks.

A seldom noted point in these reports is that new services require additional and on-going investments by the public. What about those unable to invest or participate in the marketplace for information and entertainment products – the disenfranchised of the marketplace of ideas

– the information poor, or in the case of cultural products, the entertainment poor. This is consistent with the redefinition of the concept of access, which takes on a specific meaning in these discussions: a company or advertiser's access to consumers, rather than the public's access to information and entertainment.

So, the on-going deregulation of communications has been based on this type of analysis. It has contributed to the recent popularity and takeovers of various communications corporations, as well as the lack of control over marketplace prices by the government. But it also explains some of the reasons why companies have been allowed to develop the latest technologies, as we shall see in the following chapters, to give us "more of the same."

We will return to the regulatory background of cable, with attempts to re-regulate the industry in 1992, after describing the evolution of cable, pay cable and pay-per-view in the USA since the 1960s.

Old Wine in New Bottles: Pay Cable Catches On

While the FCC finally authorized pay cable in 1968, cable and pay cable's dramatic growth was in the late seventies when the government loosened restrictions, and computers and satellites were used to offer previously unavailable, exclusive programming on pay channels linked with cable systems. The move by a company called Home Box Office (HBO) in 1975 to offer relatively new, uncut Hollywood movies and special sporting events, distributed by satellite to cable systems around the country, was an important development that boosted cable's perceived value to viewers, and thus initiated the cabling of the country. While the idea behind pay cable was not new – prompting some to describe it as "old wine in new bottles"[3] – the time was right.

A typical early description of the promises of cable gives an idea of the appeal of the new medium: "For a monthly fee, pay-television can bring ballet, Shakespeare, boxing, opera, lectures and movies into any home."[4] However, as a cable TV operator noted at the beginning of the eighties, "Films have always been the No. 1 attraction."[5]

During the emergence of pay channels, theater owners actively resisted the new technology, urging distributors not to rent to HBO and fighting cable in Congress through their task force called the Committee to Protect the Public from Paying for What It Now Gets Free.[6]

However, the rest of the film industry seemed to ignore cable for a while, concentrating on keeping their films in theaters for several years before offering them to other outlets. Hollywood found support in 1970 when the FCC applied its restrictive rules for over-the-air pay services to pay cable, thus severely limiting the type of programming that could be shown on the new channels. The philosophy behind the rules was to protect broadcast programming (or "free" television) from being siphoned off to various forms of pay television.

In 1975, however, the Commission issued further rules for pay cable, which included complicated provisions for pay-cable programming. For instance, from 1975 until 1977 (when the courts overturned the ruling), pay TV companies were restricted from showing movies less than two or more than ten years old. But this type of restriction was lifted from pay cable in 1977 and its growth was dramatic.[7]

It was not until HBO "revolutionized" the cable industry that Hollywood woke to the realization that pay services were becoming increasingly more profitable, and, most often, profits were being made using Hollywood products. By May 1974, there were 45 pay-cable channels with a total of 67,000 subscribers. But HBO became the leader of the pack.

HBO and the Cable Boom

HBO and Hollywood had the symbiotic relationship of mutual parasites who loathed each other but couldn't survive without each other. To use an old Texas expression, they were like two strange dogs on their first meeting, circling and sniffing, sniffing and circling. Each one had no greater pleasure than lifting his leg on the other.

George Mair, *Inside HBO*

A cable service offering movies and sports was envisioned around 1971 by Chuck Nolan, the head of a small cable company owned by Time Inc. By the next year, HBO started licensing films from distributors and arranging for the coverage of major sporting events. Subscribers paid an extra amount (around $8–10 per month) above the basic fee and local cable systems paid HBO a proportion of the charge (usually $3–5).

In September 1975, HBO became the first cable service to shift from microwave to satellite delivery of its programming. RCA's SATCOM I satellite delivered 12 hours of HBO programming each day via two separate transponders. The move was successful, thanks to the change in FCC regulations that allowed smaller and less expensive dishes. (In 1979, even further deregulation allowed even further reduction in prices.) Thus, HBO could provide programs simultaneously to the entire nation of cable systems.

Among the problems encountered in the seventies by Time's new subsidiary, as well as other pay channels, was getting new movies. In his book on HBO, George Mair points out that a pay-cable channel like HBO has 8,760 hours a year to fill. But the studios had a nasty habit of keeping their films in theaters for several years, as well as adhering to those nasty FCC regulations. This explains, of course, the repetition of movies on the pay channels, especially in the early years. As noted by Jack Curry of the *New York Daily News*, "Show me a Home Box Office patron, and I'll show you someone who has seen *The Great Santini* 15 times."[8]

Most of those opposed to pay television, such as the movie studios, theater owners, and broadcast networks, seemed not to understand anything about the new technology and its implications. Or, if they did understand it, they did not care, because they apparently did not think Home Box Office could make it work financially.

Despite the problems and the opposition, HBO did become successful – very successful. "It's a channel that gives you everything you ever wanted in home movie entertainment," exclaimed an industry observer.[9] One of the factors in HBO's success, in Mair's opinion, at least, was the "stupidity of its competitors."[10] However, it also might be noted that HBO was able to sustain its "pioneer" efforts thanks to the capital backing provided by its parent company, Time Inc., and its bankers. For instance, in 1976 HBO acquired Telemation Program Services, a company that distributed programming to systems without ground stations. (Telemation was renamed HBO Program Services in 1980.)[11]

Mair describes the life cycle of HBO: from 1973 to 1977, trying to stay alive; from 1978 to 1982, hauling in big profits; from 1983 to 1987, fighting off competition and diversifying beyond cable systems.[12] His chronology is useful in framing HBO's development and on-going relationship with Hollywood.

HBO presents By 1981, HBO wanted its own production company. The company was paying substantial license fees which contributed to film production costs, yet was receiving no profits from any other markets. HBO President Frank Biondi explained that the company wanted to participate "in the whole stream of revenues in return for the healthy percentage of film cost we pay."[13]

So Time Inc. reorganized its Video Group to become a broad entertainment and information programming company, which would include foreign cable, home video, and theatrical exhibition. Thus, during the Hollywood wars (discussed in the next section), HBO (and the other pay channels) relied more on their own programming. For instance, in February 1983 HBO ran only 28 Hollywood movies, The Movie Channel only 35, and Showtime 48.[14]

HBO also started developing "pre-buys" – putting money into an independent producer's hands before shooting to get exclusive pay-TV rights to a film. *The First Deadly Sin* and *The Legend of the Lone Ranger* were examples of pre-buy deals. Although the films were not successful, their budgets were only about $3.5 million. Other HBO pre-buys included *Sophie's Choice, High Road to China, Daniel, First Blood, The King of Comedy* and *The Pope of Greenwich Village*.[15]

Needless to say, the pre-buy strategy outraged movie studios. To add insult to injury, HBO created Silver Screen Partners (with E. F. Hutton), a film financing arrangement which generated $100 million to produce 12 features.[16]

Hollywood at war with HBO   As HBO grew to become the dominant force in pay cable, the Hollywood majors' resentment grew as well. Primarily, the film companies complained about the ability of HBO to name its own price for films. Of course, the price was usually not as much as the Hollywood majors felt they should be receiving, or, in their own words, their "fair share." By 1982, when other movie channels were paying 45–50 cents per subscriber for a feature film, HBO paid a flat rate of about 30 cents.[17]

Some cable systems also resented HBO and began dealing directly with the studios instead of relying on HBO as middleman. (Examples included Times–Mirror Co. and Spotlight.) HBO responded by running exclusive films. The studios, however, started resisting HBO's demands for exclusivity, as well as insisting on selling their films on a per-subscriber basis.[18]

So waged the war between HBO and Hollywood. An industry observer at the time noted, "Like most business conflicts, the battle between HBO and Hollywood is simply over money – in this case, billions of dollars."[19] Finally, Hollywood settled on three strategies in its assaults on HBO, as follows.

1   It initiated legal actions. The Motion Picture Association of America (MPAA) threatened in 1978 to file monopoly charges against HBO, and a Department of Justice investigation started in 1979.[20]

2   It withheld films. While this strategy may have been satisfying to the studio executives for a while, cable revenues still represented additional profits for the film companies.

3   It started competing with pay channels. As cable was becoming an extremely lucrative venture, the studios finally became eager to jump into the business. Universal and Paramount were said to be "salivating to get a piece of the cable business."[21] Viacom, one of the lesser studios mostly involved with television production, had created Showtime in 1976, while Warner Communications had tried to get into the business years earlier, with a system in the mid-Atlantic area called Gridtronic.[22] Warner eventually joined with American Express to start The Movie Channel in 1979, as well as Nickelodeon (1979), and MTV (1981). (These moves worked especially well with Warner's and Viacom's roles as cable system operators. In other words, these pay channels would be seen on these companies' cable systems. See further discussion later in this chapter.) Disney launched its own pay channel in 1983, while United Artists, Columbia Pictures and Madison Square Garden (owned by Gulf + Western, which also owned Paramount Pictures) formed the basic cable channel USA Network in 1980.

Premiere   The most audacious effort to get into pay cable and to undermine HBO was the Premiere Channel. On April 21, 1980, Twentieth Century Fox, Universal, Paramount, Columbia and Getty Oil signed an agreement to form the Premiere channel, apparently as a direct assault on HBO.[23] Getty (at the time, majority owner of the popular cable sports channel, ESPN) was to supply most of the capital and satellite distribution facilities, while the studios supplied the films. Though the venture was promoted as a boost for competition, especially for independent productions, the group proposed not to sell films to any competing pay-cable service for nine months after the films were aired on Premiere. They further agreed that the license fees for their films paid by Premiere would be decided collectively. While such policies seemed obviously anti-competitive, some suspected that the strategy was to attack HBO and earn profits, while the Justice Department dealt with the legalities.[24]

And, sure enough, Premiere was challenged by the Justice Department, in a suit which pointed out that the four movie companies provided 34 percent of HBO's films and 44 percent of the films licensed to Showtime.[25] The suit also claimed that the Premiere agreement would amount to price fixing and an illegal boycott, and sought not only an injunction blocking the venture, but a preliminary injunction to prevent any plans for the opening of the channel on January 1, 1981. The studios countered by pointing to the "real monopolist" – HBO – which, at the time, was actually under investigation itself in the Justice Department's pay-television investigation.

The case was heard in the NY Federal District by Judge Gerard Goettel, who issued a preliminary injunction preventing Premiere from starting operations. Despite HBO's domination of pay cable, Judge Goettel thought potential subscribers had many services to choose from, and even praised HBO's "pioneering skill." In his opinion, "The popularity of [pay-TV] has grown so rapidly that it is not impossible that, by the end of the century, it will be the prime method of viewing motion pictures. This case is about who will reap the enormous revenues available from this enterprise."[26]

The film companies did not push the case (it seemed clear they would have lost), and folded the Premiere project. Ultimately, the endeavor cost the partners $20 million, including $5 million in legal fees. During this period (1980–1), the four studios had boycotted pay services by holding back movies to release on Premiere. However, The Movie Channel had run through its backlog of movies, and was desperate for films after the court case. Thus, lucrative deals were made with Universal and Paramount.

Meanwhile, apparently out of anger over the Premiere case, Twentieth released 9 to 5 to home video ten weeks after theatrical release – the earliest that any major movie had gone to the home video market. It seemed a clear signal that pay cable was going to be different, as the studios sought to boost home video as a way to hurt pay cable, and more particularly, HBO. The pay-cable world in 1982 was changing, and HBO faced increasingly tough competition.

The Showtime/Movie Channel merger Yet another attempt was made by the studios to collectively challenge HBO's dominance. In November 1982, Paramount, Universal, Warner and American Express announced plans to become joint owners of The Movie Channel (already owned by Warner and American Express). Two months later, Viacom joined the group, which then proposed to merge The Movie Channel and Showtime (owned by Viacom). The four film companies would own 22.58 percent of the new pay channel, while American Express would own 9.68 percent.[27]

Again, the antitrust implications seemed obvious: the three majors involved received nearly 50 percent of total revenues from theatrical rentals and nearly the same from pay-cable license fees. The newly created pay channel would command about 30 percent of the pay-cable market, and thus become an oligopoly with HBO, which then held 60 percent of the market.

The partners again argued that the merger would promote competition and challenge HBO's control. Yet, again, the Antitrust Division did not buy it. In June 1983, the partners were told that the merger would be challenged in court. Two other plans were submitted, until finally the two channels were merged under a partnership involving Viacom, Warner and American Express. And even though Paramount and Universal were kept out of the deal, the new alliance still increased horizontal integration in an already concentrated pay-cable market. By 1987, Time and Viacom controlled 83.6 percent of the market in a neat little oligopoly.[28]

Nevertheless, the failure of the Showtime/TMC merger and the Premiere proposal meant that collaborative efforts by the film industry in the world of pay cable seemed doomed. The industry retreated to other strategies, especially trying to formulate favorable deals with existing pay channels, as discussed below.

The bickering between the studios and HBO subsided, as they managed a somewhat strained relationship. Yet even through the "war," there had been various alliances or forms of cooperation. And, although the studios held back their films during a few tense periods, they still sold their movies to HBO. Despite the claims that it was difficult for HBO to get Hollywood films on an exclusive basis, Columbia even agreed to sell its films exclusively to HBO for a five-year period in 1981 – the beginning of a new policy of exclusive arrangements between pay services and the studios.[29] As Mair observed, "in spite of bickering and contradictions, Hollywood and HBO have always needed each other."[30] The same might be said generally for the cable industry and Hollywood.

TriStar A classic example illustrating this cooperation was the formation of TriStar – an alliance which also involved a broadcasting company.

On November 30, 1982, CBS, HBO and Columbia met to discuss a business plan originally called Nova. By December, the alliance announced the formation of the "first major studio in 40 years." Each company would contribute $200 million, plus $200 million from six banks led by the First Bank of Boston. Six to ten films were to be produced each year, with an average budget of $12 million. The number would be increased eventually to 12–15 per year, with *The Natural* as the first picture to be produced. The arrangement would work nicely: Columbia was to distribute to theaters, HBO to cable, and CBS to network TV. All the participants were interested eventually in developing a pay-per-view system for cable.[31]

While initially the National Association of Theater Owners (NATO) were up in arms about the proposal, they eventually withdrew their opposition and TriStar Pictures started limited operations in March 1983, releasing its first picture, not *The Natural*, but *The Evil Men Do*.[32]

Even though the Premiere proposal had been rejected by the Justice Department, on September 14, 1983, William F. Baxter, Assistant Attorney General, Antitrust Division, announced approval of the joint venture and licensing agreement between members of TriStar. He explained: "the agreements under scrutiny here involve only a single pay-TV programmer, HBO, and only one of the six major distributors, Columbia. The nature of the financial arrangement does not encourage Columbia to collude with its production or distribution competitors."[33]

Though TriStar was up and running, it did not initially win any races. At the end of 1983, the company reported an initial loss of $3.8 million.[34] By November 1984, the company received 4.9 percent of the domestic box office and ranked seventh among the major distributors. Around the same time, the salaries of TriStar's top executives were released: President Gary Hendler received an annual salary of $1 million, with past bonuses of $350,000, $240,000, and $150,000, while Chairman Victor Kaufman was paid an annual salary of $400,000, plus bonuses of at least $200,000.[35] Indeed, the business was paying off for at least some of the participants.

Gradually the company began to make money, selling home video rights to its releases, as well as distributing the top box office film of the year in 1984, *Ghostbusters*. But despite the success, CBS was forced sell its 29 percent share in a restructuring plan, partially due to Ted Turner's attempted takeover of the network.[36] Late in 1985, Columbia began negotiations with HBO to become the principal TriStar shareholder after the CBS sellout. Finally in 1989, TriStar became a subsidiary of Columbia, contributing nicely to the studio's profits with films such as *Look Who's Talking* and *Total Recall*.

Thus, the cooperative efforts of three competing companies led to the creation of a new, successful film company, in the midst of what was generally acclaimed to be a hostile, competitive period in the entertainment industry.

The Latest Period: Cable and Hollywood Co-exist

Despite claims to the contrary, Hollywood was involved with cable in various ways from its beginning. However, the studios either pursued dead-end technology or inappropriate strategies, or used their typical monopolistic style. As cable television evolved, the studios mostly withdrew to their own concerns, only to find others moving in during key periods of cable/pay cable's development in the mid-1970s.

Again, the industry reacted to others' success with moaning, resentment and hostility. But, cable and pay cable were here to stay, and indeed offered film distributors additional markets for their product via basic and pay channels and pay-per-view services, as well as over-the-air stations carried on cable systems. By the 1990s, the film industry was intimately involved with cable, pay cable and pay-per-view – if not in terms of ownership, then in a customer relationship. To get a better sense of the latest period for Hollywood and cable, an overview of the US cable system may be helpful.

The US Cable System in the Nineties

Cable operators and MSOs   Cable systems in the USA are operated almost always by private companies granted franchises by municipalities. These companies typically have a monopoly in a specific location – in 1991, only 50 cities had competing cable companies.[37] In 1992, there were 11,314 operating systems serving 30,579 communities.[38] While this may seem to be a relatively high number of systems, it also indicates the considerable concentration which characterizes the cable industry.

Most systems are operated by Multiple System Operators (MSOs), companies that own many cable systems and consequently serve large numbers of subscribers. The level of concentration in this sector of the cable industry is indicated in table 5.1. By 1991, Telecommunications Inc. (TCI) and American Television and Communications (ATC) served 24 percent of all basic subscribers, with TCI serving one out of every four subscribers.[39] Since then, Time Warner has acquired all the stock in ATC and combined ATC with Warner Cable to create Time Warner Cable, which served over 6.3 million subscribers in 1992 (see table 5.1). By the end of 1992, Time Warner's Annual Report stated that their systems served over 7.1 million subscribers.

The other trend in the cable industry is the integration of cable systems, cable channels and program producers (typically, Hollywood studios). The primary example is Time Warner; it is the second largest cable operator in the USA, but Time Warner is also the owner of pay channels (HBO, Cinemax, etc.), and several major production companies. (More discussion of integration will follow in later sections.)

Plate 2 High-Tech Dishes Giant satellite dishes are mounted outside a local cable system's headquarters, receiving signals from national and regional cable and pay-cable channels and superstations and sending them via cable to local homes. While there are over 11,300 cable systems in the USA, only a minuscule number of communities have competing cable operations. Multiple Systems Operators (MSOs), in particular, TCI and Time Warner Cable, own the vast majority of US cable systems. *Photograph by Carlos R. Calderon*

Costs and revenues The initial costs of setting up a cable system may be considered relatively high, as laying cable runs at around $10,000 per mile in rural areas, $100,000 in urban centers, and $300,000 per mile for underground installations. Yet, there are few other expenses. Cable systems initiate very little programming, and only about one half originate any programming, with the average time per week at around 23 hours. Equipment costs are extremely low, compared to other programming sources.[40] Other expenses include fees paid to basic channels and pay services according to the number of subscribers on each system. (Example: the USA Network receives 13 cents a month for each cable subscriber.[41]) These programming fees have increased over the last few years.

While these expenses are claimed to be high, there are big payoffs for such investments. From the mid-seventies, revenues for the cable business grew steadily, although annual revenue growth slowed during the

Table 5.1 Top cable MSOs in the USA, 1992

Company	Basic service subscribers
1 Telecommunications Inc.	9,516,244
2 Time Warner Cable Group/ATC	6,316,081
3 United Artists Entertainment	2,896,605
4 Continental Cablevision Inc.	2,800,000
5 Comcast Cable Communications	2,764,500
6 Cox Cable Communications	1,643,604
7 Storer Communications Cable Division	1,619,000
8 Cablevision Systems Corporation	1,614,376
9 Jones Intercable	1,600,000
10 Times Mirror Cable Television	1,118,000
11 Cablevision Industries Inc.	1,090,000
12 Viacom Cable	1,058,000
13 Adelphia Communications	1,030,570
14 Sammons Communications Inc.	920,000
15 Century Communications Corporation	884,000
16 Prime Cable	694,626
17 Maclean Hunter Cable TV	674,247
18 TeleCable Corporation	640,000
19 Scripps Howard Cable	634,800
20 Falcon Cable TV	606,220
21 KBLCOM Inc.	558,850
22 Cencom Cable Associates Inc.	550,000
23 Tele-Media Corporations	500,000
24 MultiVision	477,200
25 Post-Newsweek Cable Inc.	443,674
26 Lenfest Group	437,336
27 TCA Cable TV Inc.	420,000
28 NewChannels Corporation	378,000
29 Colony Communications	316,999
30 Palmer Communications	190,000

Source: *Broadcasting & Cable Market Place 1992*, New Providence, New Jersey: R. R. Bowker, 1992, p. F100.

end of the decade, from 38 percent in 1980 to 13 percent in 1990 (see table 5.2). By 1990, total revenues reached nearly $21.4 billion, including basic and pay-cable subscriptions. Cable operators still keep a large percentage of subscriptions (as much as 80 percent), while the remainder is paid to the program supplier.

But operators also profit from miscellaneous revenues, such as the

Table 5.2 US cable systems' revenues and capital investment, 1989–91 (in $m)

	1989	1990	1991
Basic cable revenues	9,300	10,575	15,300
Pay-cable revenues	4,751	4,828	5,080
Other revenues[a]	4,830	5,990	6,650
Total revenues	18,881	21,393	23,360
Total capital investment	1,825	2,000	1,400

[a] includes advertising, installation, converter rentals, pay-per-view, expanded basic service, and other revenues.
Source: *Standard & Poor's Industry Surveys*, "Media," 7 February 1991, p. M29.

sale of advertising, installation, converter and remote control rentals, pay-per-view, fees from shopping channels, expanded basic service, and other services.[42] Advertising is the fastest growing source of miscellane ous revenues, seen by many as cable's "next frontier."[43] By 1987, cable advertising sales were reported to be "eat[ing] a hole in local broadcast revenues," as low-budget cable spots attracted local and regional advertisers at 1,400 cable systems.[44] By the beginning of the decade, 21 percent of all systems accepted advertising on their local origination channels. Even though these local channels derived little advertising revenue overall (less than 5 percent) through the 1980s,[45] some systems were receiving over $30 million annually from local ad sales by the early 1990s.[46] As a whole, advertising was expected to provide cable systems with $2.8 billion in revenues in 1991.[47]

Subscribers and rates   At the beginning of the 1990s, 95 percent of US television homes had access to cable. The cable penetration rate, however, or the actual percentage of homes which subscribed to cable, was only 60.3 percent in 1991. The number of homes actually receiving cable was yet another percentage – obviously unknown – as some homes received the service via unauthorized means or by pirating.

While the average 24-hour audience share for basic cable was 19 percent in 1985–6, that share had increased to 34.5 percent between October 1990 and January 1991, sending the major over-the-air networks into a tizzy as their share of the audience dwindled to around 65 percent.[48]

Average fees charged to subscribers have varied with each system over the years and have been influenced by government regulation. But with cable deregulation measures in 1984, it is safe to say that most cable rates generally increased. By 1991, the average monthly basic rate was $18.[49] According to the General Accounting Office (GAO), basic rates have increased by 61 percent since deregulation.[50] The GAO further observed that between December 1986 and October 1988, cable rates climbed at twice the rate of inflation. Another study recently cited these above-average increases in cable rates as one of the non-market prices affecting inflation.[51]

The rapid increase in cable rates was one of the primary forces behind the move to re-regulate cable through the Cable Act of 1992 (see end of this chapter for more details). But in anticipation of re-regulation, the cable companies started other schemes to glean even more revenues. The process of tiering – adding separate tiers of basic cable channels at different rates, or "unbundling" the channels that basic cable offers – became common again in the late eighties. Tiering enhances cable companies' revenues, while offering subscribers a "confusion of menu choices and pricing schemes."[52] Such actions prompted claims that cable companies were simply offering "the perception of choice," while increasing subscription fees.[53]

Basic cable

Basic channels are those that cable systems offer for a basic monthly fee. (Cable operators are required to carry at least 20 channels.) They include a range of cable channels (sometimes referred to as networks), plus superstations, such as WTBS, WGN, and WOR, as well as home shopping channels, such as the Home Shopping Networks I and II, the QVC Network, and JC Penney TV. (See table 5.3 for a list of top basic channels.) While the cable boom in the seventies was related to pay-cable's menu of movies and special events, basic channels (such as ESPN and CNN) also offered viewers services not available on over-the-air channels. Channels such as Discovery and Arts & Entertainment present a range of documentaries and informational programming, while CNN features 24-hour-a-day news coverage.

In addition to news, sporting events and weather reports, some cable channels expanded their involvement in original programming. For instance, TNT and USA offer made-for-cable movies and specials. Also, attempts were made to produce original programs which might appeal to smaller audiences, such as the cultural programming offered by CBS

Table 5.3 Top basic cable networks, 1991

Cable network	Subscribers	Ownership
ESPN	57,200,000	Capital Cities/ABC
CNN	56,702,000	Turner Broadcasting[a]
WTBS	55,515,000	Turner Broadcasting[a]
USA Network	54,100,000	Paramount; MCA.
Discovery Channel	53,200,000	TCI (35%); Cox Cable (24.5%); Newhouse (24.5%); United Cable (14%); management 1%.
Nickelodeon	53,200,000	Viacom
Nick at Nite	53,200,000	Viacom
MTV	52,900,000	Viacom
C-Span	52,100,000	Cable operator supported
Nashville Network	51,911,000	Gaylord Broadcasting
Family Channel	51,695,000	International Family Entertainment
Lifetime	51,284,000	Capital Cities/ABC (33%); Viacom (33%), Hearst (33%).
TNT	51,152,000	Turner Broadcasting[a]
Arts & Entertainment	49,600,000	Capital Cities/ABC (38.1%); Hearst (38.1%); NBC (23.6%).
Weather Channel	47,176,000	Landmark Communications
Headline News	44,708,000	Turner Broadcasting[a]
VH-1	38,700,000	Viacom
QVC Network	37,000,000	Comcast (27.7%); TCI (26.3%); Time Warner (11%)
FNN	35,400,000	Infotech (46%)
WGN-TV	32,600,000	Tribune Broadcasting
Black Entertainment Television	29,400,000	Bob Johnson (52%); TCI (32%); HBO (16%).
American Movie Classics	29,000,000	Rainbow Programming[b] (50%); TCI (50%).

[a] Turner Broadcasting: Turner (60.7%), TCI (9.85%), and Time Warner (8.25%).
[b] Rainbow Programming: Cablevision Systems (25%) and NBC (25%).
Source: *Broadcasting Yearbook 1991*, Washington, D.C.: Broadcasting Publications, 1991, p. D-3.

Cable and ARTS in the early 1980s (although both of these services ultimately failed).[54] But a good deal of cable's programming is recycled from other sources. In other words, cable offers yet another outlet for programming which has already been seen either in theaters, on video, or via over-the-air television.

Basic cable can be quite lucrative if a toehold can be established in the cable spectrum. An example is the USA Network, which received total revenues of $267 million in 1990. Just under 38 percent of this amount was from subscribers' monthly bills, while advertisers supplied the bulk of USA's revenues.[55]

The USA Network is not unusual, in that cable programming is increasingly surrounded by advertising messages. Despite early promotion touting advertising-free content, more and more cable channels rely heavily on advertising for increased revenues – including channels which could be considered *only* advertising, e.g. home shopping. By 1986, almost $1 billion was received annually from local and national advertising revenue. By the end of the eighties, there were over 70 advertising-supported cable networks.[56] Some of these channels experienced dramatic increases in advertising revenues, as cable continued to eat away at the traditional broadcast networks' hold on a mass audience. The Discovery Channel's revenues increased nearly 60 percent in 1990, while the USA Network's gross advertising revenues were $197 million, a 40 percent increase from the previous year.[57] Meanwhile, MTV generated $269 million from advertising in 1990, while ESPN brought in $260 million.[58]

Home shopping networks offer "pure" advertising, exemplified by the Home Shopping Network (HSN), which was carried on 1,644 cable systems and 24 television stations in 1992, claiming over 5.5 million customers, 4 million of which made four or more purchases each year. By mid-1993, home shopping networks also included the QVC Network, NBC Direct, America's Value Network (AVN), Cable Value Network, Consumer Discount Network, Shop Television Network, Telshop, and Video Shopping Mall. Several other department stores also were planning their own channels, including Nordstrom and R. H. Macy & Co. Meanwhile, in 1991 the Home Shopping Network started 24-hour programming consisting principally of "infomercials" – commercial time of two to thirty minutes disguised as programs. Home shopping visionaries predicted video shopping malls (with detailed consumer information on products), targeted advertising, devices to issue coupons with items purchased, and advertisements that consumers specifically pay to watch.[59]

At the same time, there are considerable problems in introducing new basic channels. An example was the Courtroom TV Network, which experienced typical problems for a new cable service – low subscriber count and virtually no advertising. However, the channel ultimately may succeed because it is a joint venture of Time Warner, Cablevision Systems Corporation and NBC, and its base is "made up of a chunk of cable systems owned by TCI, Time Warner and Cablevision Systems."[60] These corporate ties proved helpful to Turner Broadcasting System's

TNT channel when it was introduced. TNT could rely on the systems owned by Turner's part owners, TCI and Time Warner, to carry the channel.[61]

Other new channels opened or promised for the early nineties were typically owned by well-established cable veterans, and very often opened as part of the tiering trend. These included the Cartoon Channel (Turner), the Sci-Fi Channel (USA Network), Romance Classics (American Movie Classics), the Game Show Channel (United Video and Sony), and the Game Channel (International Family Entertainment).[62] Another problem confronted by these channels was the lack of space on most cable systems. However, the new technical possibilities to expand channel capacity (see end of chapter) promised an end to such difficulties.

Meanwhile, in early 1993 the FCC was deciding the fate of several new cable networks. The list (as described in *Daily Variety*) included a wide range of interests:

- Worship, a religious network put together by Bud Paxson, former head of the Home Shopping Network;
- Americana TV, a service grounded in country/bluegrass music;
- The Military Channel, which will focus on news, docus and movies related to the armed services;
- RecoveryNet: The Wellness Channel, which will promote services for former addicts;
- Ole TV, a Spanish-language net;
- Prime Plus, a sports-news operation tied to all-sports Prime Network;
- New Culture Network, which will tap into the vast storehouse of foreign films and independently produced American movies;
- R&B TV, a music-video net.[63]

Also the How-To Channel, the Cowboy Channel and a Golden American Network aimed at seniors were announced around the same time. But cable-system operators seemed unwilling to add any of these new channels, waiting to see how Washington was to enforce new cable regulations. (See end of this chapter.)

Pay Cable

Cable systems arrange to carry pay services through contracts (usually from three to five years in length) which specify fees paid by the operator plus other provisions. Typically, the cable operator keeps 50 percent of

Table 5.4 Top pay-cable channels

Pay Channel	Subscribers	Ownership
HBO	17,300,000	Time Warner
Showtime	7,400,000	Viacom
Cinemax	6,400,000	Time Warner
Disney Channel	5,665,000	Walt Disney Co.
Bravo	5,000,000	Rainbow Programming
The Movie Channel	2,800,000	Viacom
Playboy	350,000	Playboy Enterprises

Source: *Broadcasting Yearbook 1991*, Washington, D.C.: Broadcasting Publications, 1991, p. D-4.

pay revenues, while the remainder goes to the program supplier.[64] While the operator chooses which pay services to carry, there may be specific incentives and/or restrictions which favor the system carrying only one service, rather than two competing services. Indeed, there is some evidence that systems affiliated with MSOs owning pay services typically carry the parent company's pay channel.[65]

Pay channels can be found on 9,000 systems, reaching over 51 million subscribers.[66] Pay cable penetration has increased slowly, from 25.9 percent in 1984 to 29.4 percent in 1989.[67] The average monthly rate for typical pay-cable services was $9 in 1990, while revenues for pay cable amounted to $4.8 billion in 1990.[68]

Early studies indicated that the main reason subscribers wanted pay cable (or even cable) was to view uncut, relatively recent movies.[69] Thus, it is not surprising that the mainstay of pay-channel programming in the USA is Hollywood films; and this is often touted as the basis of cable's diverse programming (the motto of Cinemax: "More Movies, More Choice").

This proliferation of films on pay cable is more understandable when considering that ready-made Hollywood movies still represent extremely economical programming. (Arrangements will be discussed in the next section.) It also is not too surprising that pay-cable channels are connected in some way to the film and television production community, despite the presumed separation between the "film", "television" and "cable" industries.

Despite the slight decline in pay subscribers in the late 1980s due to home video and the emphasis by operators on basic cable, pay cable is still a lucrative endeavor dominated by only a few companies.[70] Table 5.4 lists the top pay-cable channels, and also illustrates the dominance of HBO, as well as the oligopoly of Time Warner and Viacom. These companies also have developed various strategies to boost subscriptions, as well as to create the illusion of more competition.[71] For instance, HBO and Showtime split their services into two or more channels (a process called multiplexing), but offered no new programming on the new channels.

Programming

Cable programming comes from a wide array of sources, including original productions for cable and sports presentations. However, as noted previously, feature films and television programs are overly abundant on pay, as well as basic, channels. And this type of recycled programming is supplied by a relatively small number of companies, most often connected in one way or another to the Hollywood majors.

The sale of feature films to pay cable represents a lucrative activity for these companies, as these outlets offer additional revenue for a feature film. However, there has been more than a little friction between the Hollywood majors and the cable community. A closer look at this relationship may be useful in understanding the interaction and integration between these supposedly separate industries.

Feature films   Pay-cable release of major motion pictures usually follows home video release. Basic cable channels typically purchase feature films after independent broadcast stations (or the syndicated market), although in the late 1980s film distributors started by-passing the syndicated market by sometimes selling first to basic cable.[72]

Typically, Hollywood studios sell films to pay services under long-term contracts (one year, in the case of HBO and Cinemax), for a fee plus a specific amount per household.[73] Often the fee is between $6 and $8 million per film, but sometimes license fees are connected to a film's box office performance.[74]

Film distributors typically receive over 45 percent of the box office receipts from theaters, but complain about getting much less from pay cable. Nevertheless, in one year, HBO and Cinemax alone may run over 550 films.[75] One estimate in 1983 claimed that HBO spent over $300 million on film license fees.[76] Thus, film companies generate a good income from selling their films to pay cable. In 1984, it was estimated that the film business received $600 million from the pay-cable market.

Around the same time, pay-cable revenues were said to contribute about $3 million to an average Hollywood film's revenues.[77]

Since the failure of the studios' collective efforts to capture their own pay channel in the early 1980s, they have increasingly arranged exclusive deals for film packages. The efforts to obtain exclusive contracts has enhanced the competition between major pay services – that is, HBO/Cinemax versus Showtime/TMC. But the competition also has meant arrangements which tie the pay services to specific studios. An example is the output deal in which Showtime agreed to license all of Paramount's films during a five-year period in December 1983. While Showtime could refuse some films under certain conditions, Paramount reserved the right to sell films to other pay services, such as STV and regional pay services. The deal was said to involve Showtime in paying between $600 and $700 million for 75 Paramount features over the five-year period.[78] After similar deals with other film companies (Cannon, Atlantic, DeLaurentiis, and Touchstone), Showtime was said to have committed about $1 billion for exclusive movie rights.[79]

Meanwhile, HBO countered by signing non-exclusive deals for films, thus preventing Showtime's stranglehold over product, but also in order to acquire films for lower prices (exclusive deals are more expensive than non-exclusive). Nevertheless, while HBO promoted the virtues of non-exclusivity, HBO's deals still involved long-term contracts with major studios. The first was with MCA in March 1984, and included access to Universal's films from 1983 to 1988.[80] Another was with Twentieth Century Fox and involved recent and "classic" films from the studios vaults, as well as arrangements for co-financing films made for pay TV and Fox distribution of HBO's productions in theaters. HBO also arranged non-exclusive deals with Warner Brothers (with an "exclusivity under certain circumstances" provision) and Orion Pictures.[81]

HBO's non-exclusive deals also made Showtime's policy of exclusivity problematic, as those companies who had sold non-exclusively to HBO could not offer Showtime exclusive arrangements. Thus, HBO's deals became de facto exclusive. The battle raged on at the end of the eighties with Showtime flaunting its exclusivity policy in advertisements, and HBO arguing that it was "self-destructive" for the industry.[82]

Another trend affecting pay cable has been the proliferation of Hollywood blockbusters. It still takes big bucks to get the big films on pay cable. One example from the early nineties was *Terminator 2*, which Showtime reportedly pre-paid $9 million to run on its channel.[83] (Such deals also often include an arrangement for the production company to shoot footage for a "Making of . . ." feature which will later run on the pay-cable channel to promote the film.)

But there are other consequences of exclusive arrangements, long-term contracts, and blockbuster prices. As a researcher noted in 1987, "Showtime's exclusivity policy and the current array of licensing agreements probably will prevent the emergence of a successful competing service since all major studios appear to be aligned with one of the two dominant services ... which have a suffocating oligopoly within pay cable."[84]

Sure enough, at the beginning of the 90's, there were no new pay cable services, and Time and Viacom still held their "suffocating oligopoly."

Broadcast programming Film distribution companies also receive royalties from films seen on over-the-air broadcast stations which are carried on cable systems, in a sense receiving double payment for the same screening of a film (i.e. for the sale of the film to the TV station and again from the cable system that carries that station).

Early complaints from copyright holders and broadcasters claimed that cable systems importing signals "disrupted the system of exclusivity by which such programming had traditionally been marketed – a system in which broadcasters bought exclusive geographical rights to air motion pictures, TV series, etc. based on so many showings over a specific time. In other words, cable operators did not pay copyright royalties for retransmission of broadcasting signals while broadcasters did."[85] Thus, lower income was received from broadcasters, in addition to lower income from revenues not collected from cable operators. This conflict erupted as part of the copyright revision hearings in 1965, as "Congress basically sought to impose copyright liability for programming contained in retransmitted local and imported signals."[86] Meanwhile, in United Artists Television Inc. v. Fortnightly Corp., the District Court found that cable retransmission of broadcast signals constituted a "multiple performance" and thus infringed copyrights.[87]

Sensing that they may be liable for full copyright liability, the cable industry offered the idea of a compulsory license, or the establishment of a "reasonable" royalty fee by statute, as a compromise during the Senate hearings in 1966.[88] Copyright holders were adamantly opposed to any such compromise. Meanwhile, the cable section of the House bill was deleted before it passed in 1967.

Copyright revision for cable stalled, further complicated by a Supreme Court decision which found that cable retransmission of broadcasts did not constitute a "performance," and the cable system was similar to a viewer rather than a broadcaster. Though the decision seemed contradictory and thus questionable in light of the future growth of cable television, Ron Bettig points out that "the decision to maintain the status quo (no copyright liability for cable) appears ultimately as an attempt by the Court to force Congress into settling the matter in a comprehensive way."[89]

This still left a "stalemate produced by the contradictory actions of legislative, judicial and administrative institutions and the uncompromising stances of the industry sectors."[90] However, after $5 million in research funds dedicated to cable by the policy-planning network (FCC studies, think tanks, etc.), the Copyright Royalty Tribunal was established by the Copyright Act in 1976 to administer jukebox and cable royalties.[91] As noted previously, the payments for films shown on cable by 1993 provided over $175 million each year to the major Hollywood distribution companies.[92]

Pay-Per-View

The possibility of viewers paying for individual programs or special events has been around for a while. As we have seen, subscription television (STV), in one form or another, is the oldest of the pay-TV approaches, in existence for the last 40 years. Coinciding with the cable boom in the late seventies, several companies operated STV stations using over-the-air scrambled signals, a service which had been authorized by the FCC in 1968. By 1984, STV attracted 1.7 million subscribers. But it faced stiff competition from pay cable, as well as rising operating costs, subscriber complaints, and piracy problems. Only a few STV stations were in operation in the early 1990s.[93]

Ultimately, STV could not compete with the growing cable systems, which increasingly offered another form of pay-TV – pay-per-view. Over one quarter of cable systems in the USA are addressable, allowing customers to order specific programs or events for an extra fee beyond their monthly basic or pay-cable charges. By 1991, the addressable universe consisted of 15 million homes, and pay-per-view services had garnered revenues of over $400 million in the previous year.

Several pay-per-view services started in late 1985, including Viewer's Choice, offered by The Movie Channel/Showtime, and Request TV, started by former Showtime President, Jeffrey Reiss[94] (see table 5.5). Movies available on Viewer's Choice were to be offered at the same time as videocassette release. Meanwhile, The Exchange was an arrangement providing for pay-per-view exhibition of motion pictures from Twentieth Century Fox and most of the other majors.[95]

Table 5.5 Pay-per-view services, 1991

Service	Subscribers	Ownership
Viewer's Choice I	8,000,000	ATC, Cox, TeleCable, Warner Bros (10% each)
Viewer's Choice II	2,433,000	(same)
Request I	7,500,000	Reiss Media Enterprises (50%); Group W (50%)
Request II	3,500,000	(same)
Playboy at Night	4,000,000	Playboy Enterprises
Spice	3,000,000	Graft PPV
Drive-In Cinema	1,200,000	Graft PPV
Cable Video Store	1,000,000	Graft PPV

Source: *Broadcasting Yearbook 1991*, Washington, D.C.: Broadcasting Publications, 1991, p. D-4.

While some pay-cable companies have been viewed by the majors as formidable obstacles to the control of an important distribution outlet, Hollywood has been more excited about (read: has anticipated better returns from) pay-per-view. The film companies especially like pay-per-view's potential of bringing in as much as $40 million in one night for a blockbuster film. An example was *Star Wars* on pay-per-view, which attracted 1.5 million customers at $8 each.[96]

For the studios, pay-per-view represents an "unbundled" method of pricing, as opposed to the "bundled" pricing of pay cable. In other words, it allows more direct pricing of a given film or supply of films. As David Waterman has observed, "[it] permits the same kind of self-selection of high value consumers for individual movies as the theater turnstile does."[97]

While feature films have played a key role on pay-per-view, there has been heavy competition from home video. Cable operators have been reluctant to add the addressable feature to systems as long as home video first receives feature films. Consequently, sporting events are currently more prevalent on pay-per-view.

Concentration and Integration: Working Together

Concentration and integration are well established in the US cable industry. Concentration is especially strong in cable-system operations,

Table 5.6 Cable integration exemplified

	Time Warner	Viacom
Program producers	Warner Bros Lorimar Prod. (Geffen)	Viacom Entertainment Viacom Productions Viacom Pictures
Cable channels	HBO Cinemax The Comedy Channel	Showtime The Movie Channel Nickelodeon Lifetime MTV VH-1
Cable systems	ATC Warner	Viacom Cable

as well as in pay cable and program suppliers. And there is considerable integration between cable-system operations, basic and pay-cable channels, and program suppliers. Because of these integrated activities, it is increasingly more and more difficult to distinguish between cable, television and film industries, although the industries and the government still insist on these distinctions.

Industry lines have been blurred considerably since the formation of Time Warner. HBO, once the "nemesis" of Hollywood, is now part of a company which incorporates one of the Hollywood majors. Warner Brothers and Lorimar actively produce programming which appears on HBO, Cinemax and the Comedy Channel, which are carried on 25 of the top 100 cable systems, owned by Time Warner Cable.

Viacom also presents similar vertical integration: it combines television and film production with running cable channels such as Showtime, The Movie Channel, Lifetime, MTV, VH1, and Nickelodeon, and also represents the 12th largest MSO in the USA (see table 5.6).

Integration of programming services makes it possible for cable operators to withhold programming from rival cable companies or new outlets. An example: planning ended in June 1991 for Sky Cable, a direct broadcast satellite (DBS) venture of Murdoch's News Corporation, General Motors, NBC and Cablevision, because of fears about program access.[98] The same problem may face telephone companies if and when they enter the cable business (see next section).

Déjà Vu All Over Again:
1992 Cable Re-regulation

From the mid-seventies onwards a profitable cable system was established in the USA. At the beginning of the nineties, however, technological and regulatory developments forecast changes in the more or less wired nation. Final sections of this chapter will focus on these technological and regulatory changes, the merging of cable and telephone activities, and the policy context in which these changes are taking place.

While numerous bills were proposed during the late eighties to curb the cable industry's excesses, such attempts failed because of the enthusiastic unregulators and stiff opposition from the well-organized cable industry. But by 1992, the excessive rate increases had taken their toll and even the well-endowed cable lobbyists could not save the day. The Cable Television Consumer Protection Act, introduced by Representative Edward J. Markey (D Mass.), was an attempt to curb the escalating rates of basic cable TV service and give cities back the authority to regulate cable TV that was taken away with the 1984 Cable Act.[99]

The bill attracted its supporters (broadcasters and consumer groups, such as the Consumer Federation of America (CFA), the US Conference of Mayors, and the National League of Cities) and its opponents (the cable industry and the Hollywood majors). The movie industry focused its opposition on the retransmission provisions, arguing that studios were being left out of royalties payments that would be made for the use of films seen on local over-the-air stations.

During the heated debates, the CFA played up the fact that MPAA president Jack Valenti had admitted at a 1988 Congressional hearing that cable rates had jumped dramatically following deregulation. They also pointed out that the film industry had switched its position once Time and Warner Communications had become one company. Valenti claimed, however, that the film industry would have supported re-regulation with provisions for payment to studios for local retransmission.[100]

Re-regulation proponents countered by pointing out that the studios were already appropriately compensated when programming was bought by local broadcasters and networks, in that these payments accounted for cable homes. In fact, "[t]he attempt by the film studios to obtain further monies by inclusion in retransmission fees amounted to an effort to receive double payments, reregulation proponents charged."[101]

The cable industry claimed that the retransmission provision would add more than $1 billion to cable companies' annual expenses, which meant that subscriber fees would have to increase or such programming would not be offered. Re-regulators pointed out that the retransmission fees would be only half that amount and that cable companies could offer local broadcasters other kinds of compensation, such as channel positions or advertising time.

Eventually the bill passed both the House and Senate, surviving a veto by President Bush with a Congressional override (the only one during Bush's presidency). The support for re-regulation seemed so strong that another bill would probably have followed a successful veto.

An *Entertainment Law and Finance* article adequately summarizes the otherwise confusing legislation:

> The 1992 Cable Act bars local governments from handing out exclusive cable franchises and requires the regulation of the basic tier of cable service, including public access, educational and government channels and local over-the-air signals. "Reasonable" fees for these services are to be established by taking into account cable subscriber rates in cities where cable companies face some form of competition (which could result in a 20 percent reduction in cable subscriber fees in re-regulated communities). Under this procedure, the FCC would also be able to determine fees for cable converter boxes and other equipment used for basic cable service. The FCC rates would affect about 95 percent of the cable companies now in business. For the next tier of cable service, such as the USA Network, ESPN and CNN, the FCC would handle the rates issue by fielding consumer complaints. Rates for premium channels like HBO and Showtime won't be affected by the new law.[102]

At the beginning of 1993, the effect of the legislation seemed unclear and depended on how vigorously the new "Clinton FCC" chose to enforce the law. The FCC was to establish rules by April 1993. In addition, the cable industry challenged the must-carry provisions in Federal Court (similar rulings had been found unconstitutional twice before).[103]

The new cable re-regulation package was certainly not popular with the cable industry and many in the film industry. But it was even criticized by some re-regulatory proponents, who said the legislation lacked strong enforcement measures and avoided dealing with new competitive technologies such as wireless cable. Representative Markey admitted that the re-regulation package might only be an interim measure. In light of the technological developments that were sweeping the industry around the same time, it was not surprising that the re-regulation move was to be seen as only temporary.

A Quantum Leap: The 500-Channel Universe

More channels for the queens While cable systems offered a larger number of channels than previously available via over-the-air broadcasting, even more cable channels could be offered with digital technology developed in the early 1990s. Various types of compression technologies were developed to squeeze more information onto copper or coaxial cable wires, or fiber-optic lines. For instance, digital compression uses various computerized techniques to squeeze three to ten programs into a single cable channel. The advantage to cable systems was clearly stated by a representative of ATC: "People will pay more money for more channels."[104]

The first major test of compression technology was introduced in December 1991, when, using fiber-optic transmission lines and digital compression, Time Warner's New York City Cable Group offered their 150-channel system called Quantum to a limited number of households in Queens. Around the same time, the average cable system offered 35 channels, often without pay-per-view or other information services.[105] Time Warner promised that their system would eventually be made available to 10,000 homes in the affluent Queens neighborhoods of Whitestone and Bellerose, as well as nine other areas.[106]

Quantum offered two Cinemax channels and three different HBO channels, as well as its own Nostalgia Channel (with *The New Art Linkletter Show*), a NASA channel (with launch-to-landing coverage of space missions), four home shopping channels, news from Sweden, Malaysia and Turkey on SCOLA, and 57 (although some reports cited 55) channels reserved for pay-per-view movies around the clock (in other words, a choice of 17 movies, offered every half-hour) for $3.95. "These 55 channels are what we call bringing a video store into your home," said Richard Aurelio, the president of the New York group. "It's a virtual video-on-demand service."[107] Thus, the Quantum system followed the same pattern set by cable systems of the past and featured a strong diet of movie fare.

Time Warner was reported to be spending $150 to $200 per subscriber for Quantum upgrades. At the same time, customers were not paying any more for the same services, but receiving more channels, although most were pay services. While some of the Queens families received the service free for a year, in exchange for submitting to interviews from the press, the system cost other subscribers around $43 a month (including three premium channels).[108]

While press reports were typically glowing, it was difficult to avoid calling attention to the vast amount of time and programming consumed by such a system. For instance, a *Washington Post* reporter described the viewing habits of one of the Quantum system families:

> Alas, they are unable to make full use of their cathode-ray cornucopia. By the time everyone drives home from the family business, Brooklyn Fan and Blower Sales Co., and eats dinner, there are only four hours a day to devote to televiewing. Jerome and Richard watch a lot of sports, and everyone watched the William Kennedy Smith trial on Court TV, but no one shops via the tube or uses the channels programming in Greek, Hindi, Korean, Cantonese or Mandarin.
>
> The Nashville Network? "Never," Norma says. The Prayer Channel ("reverent contact with God throughout the day")? "Never." Mind Extension University, through which viewers can earn college degrees? "We all have degrees already," Richard says. Norma turned to Nostalgia once – it features Big Bands and Art Linkletter – but she can't remember what was on. The major change, really, is in movie viewing. The service the family previously used already allowed them to order movies using their remote control, but Quantum offers a greater variety, including six "hits" (*Terminator 2* and *Hudson Hawk*, for instance) that start every half-hour.[109]

"This is the world of tomorrow," said Larry Gerbrandt, senior Vice-President of Paul Kagan Associates, the California-based media consultants. While it would take the rest of the country a few years to catch up, another analyst concluded that "the cable deluge is coming."

The deluge: 500 channels   By the end of 1992, 150 channels sounded downright old-fashioned. In December TCI announced a 500-channel system that would utilize digital compression techniques, expanding five channels to 50. Eventually, 10:1 compression could allow even TCI's smallest, 36-channel systems to upgrade to 360 channels. But the "500-channel universe" became the buzz phrase of the industry.[110]

While other companies had made similar moves, the TCI vision was said to represent "the first major application of digital compression technology in the TV universe."[111] TCI would purchase up to one million set-top digital compression terminals from General Instrument using AT&T's compression technology. Experimentation in homes with the first order of boxes would determine the pace of further expansion in TCI's universe of more than 9 million subscribers.

The promises sounded familiar: "We're creating a new platform for the distribution and deployment of new programming and information ideas for the industry," explained TCI's John Malone. "Our ultimate goal here is to give our customers control of their TV service. That means giving them hundreds and hundreds of options, letting them control what they want to see and what they pay for."[112]

Eventually TCI plans to deliver hundreds of additional channels and data services, many of them interactive. Although a variety of marketing concepts are to be tested, Malone noted that a large number of channels will be programmed with pay-per-view movies and programs. Malone also noted that "services targeting special interest groups like gays and ethnic minorities are likely to spring up."

Meanwhile, the previously cited Quantum family – with a paltry 150 channels at their disposal – responded to the possibility of 350 or 450 additional channels:

> "Six hundred?" Jerome gasps. "It's just ridiculous. What could be on 600 stations? Six hundred, Norma! You couldn't even comprehend the thought. It would take you a day just to scan the channels."[113]

Cable Telephony

> Build the system and the consumers will come.
> Alfred Sikes, FCC Chairman, in *Hollywood Reporter*, 1992

Meanwhile, another more potentially revolutionary move was afoot. For years, the telephone industry has eyed the lucrative cable business, but has been prevented by court order and government restrictions from entering the field. Towards the end of the 1980s, however, the stage was set for what promised to be the most far-reaching changes in home entertainment and information services for the 21st century. The courts and the FCC started lifting prohibitions on telephone company entry into cable television.

Unleashing the telcos During the summer of 1990, Judge Harold Greene lifted the ban on phone companies providing cable and data services in areas where they operate. Then, in October 1991, prompted by Chairman Alfred Sikes, the FCC issued a statement supporting telephone companies' entry into a wide range of computer data and communications services, including cable television.[114] Although the commission would still prohibit the companies from controlling program content, support was given for them to participate with other companies (such as Hollywood studios or TV networks) to provide a cable service without franchises from local governments in areas where they already provide a phone service.[115] While the support was not unanimous (Commissioner James Quello stated that full entry of telcos into cable would result in "the greatest monopoly known to man"), the proposal was supported with the now-expected promises of "more information and entertainment to more people from more sources," and "greatly enhance[d] competition." Meanwhile, Commissioner Ervin Duggan asked, "Does this proposal reflect actual demand for new services or is it driven by mere desire?" while consumer advocate Ralph Nader accused the FCC of "retarding the democratic control of the electronic media."[116]

Video dial tone On July 16, 1992, the FCC approved video dial tone, allowing phone companies to send video signals, linking telephone lines with televisions.[117] Under the new rules, local telephone companies could make available to multiple video programmers and service providers a basic platform that delivers video programming and related services under common carrier regulation. In other words, telephone companies would have to provide access to video dial tone services on a nondiscriminatory basis.

Other provisions allowed the telephone companies to provide enhanced services related to video programming, if they offered sufficient access for other video programmers. For example, telephone companies would be allowed to offer video gateways or menus, VCR-like services such as program pre-selection and storage, billing and collection for the programmers, and the sale of video equipment and inside wiring.

Certain financial relationships between telephone companies and video programmers would also be possible. Without rising above 5 percent ownership, a telephone company's business dealings with programmers could include debtor/creditor relationships, interconnection agreements, joint ventures of various diverse structures and consultant/client arrangements.

The promises? As explained by the FCC's Common Carrier chief, Cheryl Tritt:

First, we must acknowledge one of video dial tone's most striking benefits: choice. We are setting in motion the creation of a diversity of choices in the telecommunications marketplace that will someday meet any consumer's needs.

Second, there is the potential for empowering consumers in a way only dreamed about before. For them, video dial tone can radically change the nature of viewing from a passive activity to one permitting the viewer to become the programmer. . . .

Third, video dial tone represents the initial lowering of another artificial barrier – between cable TV and telephone companies – that opens the public network's horizons to new and innovative possibilities. . . .

What this Order really represents is a broader, more vibrant form of competition – the "network of networks" that Chairman Sikes has written and spoken about for years.[118]

But Tritt was not the only one to repeat the promises: Commissioner Sherrie Marshall explained that in its vote, the FCC reaffirmed its commitment to competition in the multibillion-dollar communications industry: "We are endorsing a host of new opportunities for American consumers and economic growth."[119] The FCC's ruling further stated the new competition would drive down prices in the video marketplace and improve service. "Competition should encourage new investment in our telecommunications infrastructure as well as create more diversity in the viewing opportunities now available to the American public . . . This decision can hardly be viewed as a death knell for the vibrant US cable industry."[120]

Other visions included people "roaming through remote electronic libraries that offer texts, data and video. Rural hospitals would be able to transmit and receive detailed, complex images from medical tests. Universities and businesses would be better able to exchange large volumes of computer data at high speed."[121]

Telco's cable ownership and unbinding cable While these actions opened the door for telephone companies to participate in video transmission, other moves were made to allow telephone companies to directly own cable companies. While the Cable Act of 1984 generally prohibited phone companies from owning cable systems,[122] bills introduced in both the Senate and the House during the early 1990s would permit such telephone/cable combinations.[123] The legislation, which won the cautious endorsement of the White House at the time, was intended to encourage the phone companies to invest in advanced technologies, arguing that such investments are crucial if America is to meet the future global challenge in high technology.[124]

Meanwhile, Bell Atlantic filed a suit in December 1992 challenging the restrictions on telephone companies pertaining to the ownership of video programming, arguing that it would be a violation of their First Amendment rights.[125]

Around the same time, cable operators received permission from the FCC to develop a new "wireless" telephone service. The technology involves compressed fiber-optic wiring with the potential to supply hundreds of programming channels to the home, as well as interactive communications, movies and musical releases on demand, and digital information services.[126]

Cable versus telco   These developments have been described in terms of industrial conflict and struggle. But the battle between the cable industry and the phone companies should not be seen as a David and Goliath saga. Both industries have established virtual monopolies and are profitable enterprises.

Certainly the phone companies tend to outweigh their cable foe in many ways. Cable service is subscribed to in about 60 percent of US households, while telephones are in 95 percent of all homes. The telephone industry represents more sizable assets of $193 billion, four times that of the cable industry. For example, the revenues of just one phone company (such as GTE which had sales of $19.6 billion in 1991) almost equals that of the entire cable industry ($20 billion the same year).[127] But both industries are immensely profitable and see the others' business as a way to finance the new technologies that will make them even richer. Phone companies need to move from copper wire (which can carry voice and data, but only limited video transmissions) to optical fiber, which has massive capacity to carry not only video, but two-way services, such as interactive video. The cable companies also want to upgrade their coaxial cables, which have more capacity than copper wire, but are still limited compared to fiber-optical wiring. In 1991 the USA had 6.8 million miles of fiber, 90 percent used for telephone applications and 10 percent for cable television and data communications.[128]

Cable has some advantages, however. Although phone operators had about a ten-year head start in deploying fiber-optic wire, in the early 1990s cable systems were laying fiber about three times as fast and could catch up in a few years. Cable also has skills dealing with the entertainment world, having struggled for years to develop amicable relationships with program producers and sometimes moved into program production themselves.

The telephone company has been the monopoly that legislators and regulators have most often picked on;

But the mood in Washington has shifted. Traditionally, the telephone company was the utility that the public loves to hate. Cable now appears to hold that distinction, thanks to growing public resentment over the rapid rise in cable rates – up 78% since 1985. . . . The phone companies appear to be cashing in on the anti-cable sentiment.[129]

The cable industry, as well as others, points out that the phone companies will compete unfairly using the large quantity of ratepayer funds to underwrite new enterprises.[130] The phone companies counter by referring to the federal regulations which prohibit this activity. Yet, there are numerous examples of misconduct by the telephone giants, which exemplify the difficulties (or lack of will?) of FCC regulation.[131]

Telephone representatives, however, argue that they are better prepared and able to provide the wide variety of interactive technologies that will be part of the electronic superhighway, as it has become known, into people's homes. "That requires expertise in switched, or two-way, service, a craft practically invented by the phone companies."[132] But video dial tone represents "the last link in their ultimate high-tech fantasy: the Integrated Services Digital Network." While several of the US phone companies are developing ISDN software to become the primary conduit for virtually all communications services, they have been hampered by the withholding of regulatory approval for increasing telephone rates to cover installation costs.[133]

Another thorny question is the telephone companies' ownership of video programming. While some feel that telephone entry into cable service would provide healthy competition to the cable monopoly, there is real concern over the telephone companies' control of programming.[134]

Monopolists Expand: The Experiments

But no sooner have the battle lines been drawn, than supposed competitors have started to cooperate again. As the cable and telephone companies have been unleashed from their regulatory chains, they have moved quickly, sometimes alone, but often together, to plan for the new electronic superhighway.

In May 1992, AT&T announced that it will provide the technology and equipment (transmission equipment and the set-top boxes) to deliver an improved pay-per-view service and "video-on-demand" to consumers' television sets. Working with the regional phone company US West and TCI, the plan includes compression technology that would substantially increase the channel capacity of existing cable television systems and the ability to request a movie at any time from a large list.

The technology is based on a technique that AT&T developed for HDTV in partnership with the Zenith Electronics Corporation, and involves editing out more than 96 percent of the information in a signal which is carried at 120 million bits a second. The process varies the amount of information delivered, depending on how complex the visual context is. For most movies, with many static scenes, as few as 1.5 million bits a second would work, although more fast-paced activities, such as a football game, could require as many as 8 million bits.

The AT&T system also would work with Comstream Corporation, to deliver television signals via satellite and News Datacom, a subsidiary of Murdoch's News Corporation, which would provide techniques for processing customer preferences. The system at first would send programming to the head end of cable television systems and was to be available in 1993.

But the company also said it was exploring partnerships that would deliver the programming directly to consumers' homes, and ultimately would offer "an end-to-end program-delivery system that would increase the channel capacity of today's cable systems by 3 to 13 times."[135]

IBM also was reported to be working on a similar home-entertainment and information system, and had sought partnership with a number of different companies, including TCI, Time Warner, Disney and Paramount.[136]

Meanwhile, Bellcore, the research arm of the regional Bell companies, and Northern Telecom Ltd's Bell-Northern Research announced a new video-on-demand set-up for all seven of its Bell owners. The systems would include "information warehouses" storing thousands of films on 8 mm tapes or in computers. The films would be translated into a digital format by supercomputers and compressed to travel over copper telephone wires.[137] While the system is probably more suited to large-scale use than others, it was not to be available until sometime in 1994.[138] While no specific alliances were announced, the project referred to the involvement of film companies or rental chains (such as Blockbuster Video) as possibilities for such warehouses. TV networks could also send live programming over the system, as well as making TV programs available on demand.[139] A similar scenario involved cable companies offering a version of video-on-demand, sending movies to individual homes where they would be stored on set-top disc drives.

Another $5.4 million experiment involved Bell Atlantic sending video over "twisted pair," the old-fashioned copper wiring still used for most local phone services, instead of waiting for high-tech fiber-optic lines.

The basic technique, called Asymmetric Digital Subscriber Line, was developed by Bellcore, and sends video signals at super-high speeds to a box in the home where the signals are amplified. Bell Atlantic planned to introduce the service in six states during 1994, and hoped to offer between 30 and 100 videos to each home. Additional titles would be added, as well as video material for education, home banking, and shopping.[140]

Meanwhile, GTE Corporation was conducting a long-running trial of video-on-demand via fiber in Cerritos, California. In other telco–cable partnerships, US West was working with TCI to introduce a new video system in the Denver area, while Nynex Corporation and Liberty Cable announced plans to offer 200 channels of video-on-demand in 1993 to a group of Manhattan apartment buildings using microwave technology, fiber-optic cables and video switching facilities.[141]

In a move that startled many in the two industries, Southwestern Bell (which provides telephone service in the Southwest) announced in February 1992 that it would buy two cable systems in the Washington area from Hauser Communications Inc. for $650 million in cash and stock. While not yet allowed to purchase cable systems in their own operating areas, telephone companies were permitted to do so in other markets.[142]

And finally, Time Warner announced in early 1993 that by the end of the year, the company's Orlando, Florida, cable system would feature a full-service network, including video-on-demand, interactive games and shopping, as well as a long-distance telephone service to 4,000 Orlando homes.[143]

But the quintessential move representing the linking of telephone and cable was the announcement of merger plans between TCI and Bell Atlantic in October 1993. Although the plan was later abandoned, the merger would have created a $44 billion monster, dominant in both the telephone and cable industries and poised perfectly to pave the path for the much-touted electronic superhighway. While some observers announced that it was "the perfect information-age marriage," the proposed merger represented a blatant example of increasing concentration in the communications sector, as well as further blurring of industrial lines.

Hollywood and the superhighway The prospect of more cable or video channels ultimately involves the question of programming, and thus Hollywood's role in the 500-channel universe or the new electronic superhighway. In announcing their Orlando system, Time Warner's chairman addressed this question directly: "This is a challenge to the creative community. We have a dedicated path to every home."[144]

Another executive echoed these remarks: "This represents a massive increase in outlets for the production community. Thankfully, the United States has the most sophisticated video production and distribution system in the world, because they're going to be faced with quite a challenge filling all these channels!"[145] Meanwhile, a report in *Time* magazine concluded:

> Producers of computer software, books, video games and Hollywood movies – as well as the hardware companies that make computer chips, high-definition television screens and VCRs – are investing heavily in products to supply the dominant pipeline into the home. It is a market that is expected to ring up nearly $1 trillion in revenues by the year 2000, accounting for 14% of the U.S. economy. Bringing advanced fiber-optic wires into every home in the U.S. could eventually cost anywhere from $150 billion to $500 billion. Whoever controls these wires will not only have a say in what the TV of the future will look like but will also have a grip on the lifeline of those leading-edge industries whose fortunes are tied to the network.[146]

But what role will Hollywood play in the television of the future? It remains to be seen, however some of the cable companies introducing (or resisting) these innovations are already entertainment producers, such as Time Warner.

Some of the existing experimental systems, such as Quantum in Queens, may show us a glimpse of the future, where heavy doses of commercial films and TV programming serve as the mainstay of these new expanded systems. The proposed 500-channel universes, video dial tone systems, and video-on-demand, while offering a myriad of other services, still often base the appeal of their vision on Hollywood films, albeit provided in more convenient, and even sometimes manipulable, forms.

Many agree that video-on-demand would be welcomed by the Hollywood majors. Indeed, the MPAA's statements in the FCC's Video Dial Tone decisions basically supported the entry of the telephone companies into the cable business.[147] And, given the history of Hollywood's interaction with cable, it is not surprising to find the majors anticipating a "better deal" (i.e. larger revenues) than they have been able to negotiate thus far with cable companies (or, for that matter, with the video rental system, as we shall see in chapter 6).

More predictable is the struggle over the control of software, which will make the FCC's decision regarding financial syndication even more important. As one media analyst explained:

All of the blue sky talk about new technology is going to be played out over the next several years. Software will emerge the winner – anyone with the capacity to produce or supply not just entertainment, but information, data, and services of all kinds. Now the real fighting begins. These events are going to pull the trigger on fin-syn. There are now bigger software issues to be considered. The big question driving so much of what happens in the future is who controls the software.[148]

While the telephone companies previously were reported to have had limited contact with Hollywood companies, the FCC's Video Dial Tone decision prompted announcements and rumors of a wide range of alliances and partnerships.[149] From these clues, it is possible to predict that Hollywood will be playing an important role as the electronic superhighway emerges during the next decade.

The Electronic Superhighway and Public Leadership

While some leadership seems crucial to protect the public's interest in these developments, it remains to be seen if and when it will be forthcoming. The Clinton–Gore campaign stressed high-tech development and investment, including the construction of a fiber-optic infrastructure by the year 2015. Clinton's "telecom-savvy VP," Albert Gore, was given the role of "coordinating Clinton's vision of technology as a pivotal force in the US economy," while watching over the work of technology-oriented agencies within the government, including the Commerce and Defense departments as well as the FCC.

Before the inauguration, one Clinton adviser explained: "A Clinton administration is more likely to take discreet government action – whether it be regulatory or funding legislation – that would promote the development of technology and at the same time protect consumers. This is a departure from the Bush administration, which worships at the altar of free markets." The same adviser also noted that along with Clinton's belief in telecommunications as an economic necessity, "he is also concerned that consumers don't get stuck with the enormous costs that are part of this new era."[150]

But Congressional movers and shakers, on both sides of the issue, may beat the White House to the punch. As the Clinton administration took over, numerous bills were still pending dealing with the various impending changes in the telecommunications system.[151] In addition, the

Bell Atlantic suit promised to settle the question of phone companies entering the video business before the Administration or Congress devised a more moderate compromise. As *Broadcasting* magazine pointed out:

> Telecommunications technologies invariably advance too fast for Washington policy makers to react in time. Advances in fiber optics, digital processing and signal compression have blurred the lines between traditional telephone service, cellular telephone and the upcoming personal communications services, cable TV and other industries to the point that some critics say the "telephony" section of the 1934 Communications Act should be torn up and rewritten. Bell Atlantic and cable MSO Telecommunications Inc. have announced plans to speed up installation of these technologies. With the next series of technical advancements, the administration and Congress may lose all control of the situation.[152]

Others have pointed to the lack of public debate over important questions relating to the high costs of these new systems, as well as privacy issues. One computer advocate who was asked about the promises of an electronic highway noted:

> A problem with the visions of the future has been that they are technologically glamorous but not always well thought through. People talk a lot about the need for fiber to the home and a national broadband network. While I have no doubt that is ultimately where we'll end up, how we ought to get there and what we ought to be doing with it has gotten astonishingly little discussion.[153]

Again, the technology – as controlled and developed by the corporate sector – may ultimately determine the next step towards an "information age."

The Promises of Cable

The promotion of cable has encompassed a wide range of promises, including a "television of abundance" envisioned by the Sloan Commission in 1970,[154] and the more recent visions of an electronic superhighway. Interestingly, both of these visions, separated by over 20 years, include many of the same components: more diverse programming, educational channels, interactive systems and a wide variety of information services.

Some of the early promises of cable have been fulfilled. Government channels, such as C-Span and local government channels, have given those who care to watch some insight into the legislative process at national, state and local levels. Some educational channels have been added to the cable menu, but certainly not to the extent imagined by early cable enthusiasts. There has even been the glimpse of truly public communications through public access channels, included by cable systems around the country, at first because of an FCC mandate, and sometimes sustained through agreements between cable companies and municipalities. However, without regulatory support or local pressure, cable franchises have either closed or severely limited public access activities.[155]

Indeed, cable has offered us far more channels and increasingly more narrow programming selections than the previous over-the-air system. It has been argued that these changes have contributed to the fragmentation of the previously mass audience, as individual viewers no longer share the same viewing experiences.

But it might be noted as well that *entertainment* has been the primary emphasis and main attraction of the cable boom in the USA. It dominates cable fare, and no doubt will probably continue to dominate programming into the distant future, whether offered via telephone or cable companies' systems. While some cable channels offer news and information, a large percentage of cable programming is made up of films and television reruns. Pay channels, especially, have developed some new programming, but cable channels still often serve merely as conduits for recycled entertainment programming, i.e. yet another outlet to gain profits from the same initial product.

In a survey of the programming on the 150-channel Queens system, journalist Peter Marks offered his reactions to the new system. Marks reported that he had gained "[a] renewed respect for the awesome blandness of TV and the endless ingenuity of the television industry to get us to watch way more TV than can possibly be good for us." (He also concluded that "in the age of cable, old TV stars are like space junk, still in orbit long after their usefulness has ended.")[156] Marks' observations were echoed by many others in responding to the expansion of the cable universe. Another forecast of the future was: "500 channels and nothing on!"[157]

Again, a new technological innovation potentially promising enlightenment and diversity has evolved as part of the further commodification of our communication and information environment. Cable has in many ways taught the American public/consumers an important "information age" lesson – thou must pay directly for entertainment and information products – thus clearly exemplifying Vincent Mosco's notion of the information society as a pay-per society.[158] It is likely that future information/entertainment systems, in whatever form they emerge, will be accepted as pay-per systems quite "naturally."

While the cable industry was unregulated, cable access grew dramatically to reach nearly 90 percent of US homes. Cable companies combined advertising revenues with subscriber fees to profit handsomely, even during a recession when local broadcasters and national networks suffered and competitive technologies, such as satellite broadcasting, developed slower than predicted. While broadcasting was once called "a license to make money," cable might be referred to as "a franchise to make even more money."

Meanwhile, the companies which own most of the systems are connected to large communications conglomerates, thus increasing concentration of the media and information system. Ironically, then, as channels, and supposedly program choices, have expanded, *control* over those choices has narrowed, and promises to continue to do so into the future.

Finally, while Hollywood has struggled with cable, it has been mostly over the price to be paid for programming. As we have seen in this chapter, some of the majors participate actively in the cable business, as owners of systems as well as of program channels, thus complicating the industrial divisions often assumed in public debates. In general, Hollywood has played a key role in the establishment of cable as basically an entertainment medium and benefits from yet another delivery system which recycles and promotes its products as part of an overall marketing process. While it is difficult to predict future developments, it seems likely that the new delivery systems contemplated by the cable and telephone industries will rely on Hollywood's products, in addition to serving as further profit centers for the Big Boys of the entertainment industry.

6

Talkin' 'Bout a Revolution: Home Video

Home video has had a revolutionary effect on the entertainment habits of the nation.

1991 International Television and Video Almanac

Videocassettes are the new opiate of the people.

G. D. and O. H. Ganley, *Global Political Fallout:
The VCR's First Decade*

By the beginning of the 1990s, home video machines were in over 70 percent of the television homes in the USA. Over 30,000 video stores, devoted primarily to the rental or sale of videocassettes, dotted the urban and rural landscape, while video sales or rentals were common features in a wide variety of businesses, from bookstores, record shops and large department stores, to small grocery stores and gas stations. The video industry claimed that 300 million tapes were rented from video stores each month, and three times as many people rented videos as attended motion picture theaters.[1]

This "video revolution" has been accompanied by its own assortment of promises, both for the industry and the public. Consumers are said to have more control over the time and location of viewing a wider range of entertainment and information. They can even create their own entertainment using home video cameras and recorders. A. M. Rubin and C. R. Bantz conclude simply that "VCR technology allows the audience more choice, participation and control."[2]

In terms of the entertainment business, independent film and video makers have been offered new, less expensive outlets for the distribution of their products. And new video distribution activities and rental outlets have provided new sources of entrepreneurial activity. Thus, video was another opportunity for competition in the entertainment industry.

Hollywood again has projected a schizophrenic attitude towards this new technological innovation. On the one hand, the popularity of home video has been a competitive threat, not only to the film industry (especially the exhibition sector), but also to broadcasting, cable and other leisure time activities. In 1990, consumers spent $14.9 billion renting or buying videocassettes, outpacing theatrical box office revenues by nearly $10 billion.

On the other hand, home video has become yet another market for Hollywood films, and an extremely lucrative one. Out of total home video revenues of $11.3 billion for 1989, $4.1 billion went to the suppliers of video programming – mostly the Hollywood majors.[3] By 1992 an estimated 35–40 percent of distributors' total revenues for new films were derived from worldwide video distribution.[4]

If home video represented simply another outlet for motion pictures, why did Hollywood panic and Jack Valenti depict video as the biggest threat facing the film industry?[5] Why did Hollywood companies spend millions of dollars challenging viewers' right to record video signals in their home? And then, only a few years later, why were the same people embracing home video as though they couldn't live without it, with Valenti exclaiming, "If ever there was a union of interests, it is electronics and movie-making"?[6]

And what about those promises offered by home video technology – is there really more diversity, independence, and competition?

To answer these questions, it is necessary to look more closely at the growth and structure of this new branch of the entertainment and information business.

The Evolution of Home Video Technology

The history of video technology is part of the history of television, as efforts to record television signals began as early as television itself. These developments break roughly into three chronological stages: (1) video recording-mostly professional; (2) consumer video – pre-Betamax; and (3) VCRs/videodiscs – after Betamax.

Video recording From the beginning of television, a variety of techniques have been proposed for recording television images and sound. By the end of the 1920s, three different processes had been suggested.

One of the earliest efforts was by John L. Baird in England, who was experimenting with recording television signals on phonograph records during the 1920s. Baird called his recording device a "phonoscope," but did not pursue the process.[7]

Meanwhile, Boris Rtcheouloff filed a patent in England in January 1927 for a process recording television signals on magnetic material, based on the concept of magnetic recording developed by Valdemar Poulsen, the Danish physicist who had invented magnetic recording around 1894.[8] However, it is not clear that Rtcheouloff's device was ever built.

Around the same time, Ralph Vinton Lyon Hartley and Herbert Eugene Ives, inventors at AT&T, suggested a method of recording televised images on film.[9] The process was later called the intermediate film method and was further developed during experiments in Germany, England and the USA during the 1930s. The first actual television film recordings are said to have been produced in 1933 in Germany. The intermediate film process remained the only viable system of recording television images until the 1950s.[10]

During World War II, the US military became interested in television film recording and experimented with airborne television equipment, such as "Project Ring" and the "Block" systems, used to record images sent from aircraft and guided missiles. After the war, the Navy initiated a series of experiments, which generated the first postwar black-and-white television recordings in 1946.[11]

Hollywood also became involved in electronic recording methods, as Paramount experimented with large-screen television, using the intermediate film method around 1948–9, and Twentieth Century Fox planned to use the Swiss Teleidoscope system for theater television. In fact, several of the majors (unsuccessfully) petitioned the FCC for specific frequencies for theater television.[12] (For more discussion, see chapter 2.)

Although radio personnel apparently had been suspicious of taped programming, television broadcasters were extremely interested in television recording processes, especially in the USA where time-delayed broadcasts and program distribution were special problems. A national audience for programming and advertising could be built if the same show could be seen during the same time slots around the country.[13]

Although many systems were proposed, broadcasters came to rely on the kinescope process, which employed a special 16 mm or 35 mm film camera mounted in a large box aimed at a high-quality monochrome video monitor, called a kinescope. Early "quick kines" could be processed in less than three hours, although a good deal of work was necessary to perfect the technology.[14] Later kinescope processes were fairly reliable, although not very good quality and quite expensive because of the amount of film used. By 1954, television facilities in the USA used more raw film for kines than all the Hollywood film studios combined.[15]

The next advance in recording technology would solve that problem. The use of magnetic tape not only was less expensive, but more flexible and technically superior to previous methods. The principles of magnetic recording had basically been solved by Poulsen by the end of the 19th century. The task in the 1950s, therefore, was to apply them to video.

Four companies (RCA, the BBC, Ampex Corporation and Bing Crosby Enterprises) were involved in developing magnetic video recording, each one with slightly different interests in television broadcasting. However, the first prototype machine was demonstrated at Bing Crosby's studios in Los Angeles, in November 1951. Crosby had worked with audio taping and was especially keen on using similar production techniques for television. A $1 million contract from the US government for developing recorders for military use was another motivation for the Crosby company's experiments.[16]

The first recorders were longitudinal machines, similar to audio recorders, which operated at extremely high speeds and used relatively large reels of tape. A portable recording system using a helical scanning system had been patented in Germany in 1953, but proved too expensive and impractical (tape could only be used once, for instance).[17] In 1952, the BBC started working on a longitudinal system called the Vision Electronic Recording Apparatus, or VERA, using a 5 foot reel for taping a half-hour program.[18]

Meanwhile at RCA David Sarnoff personally encouraged his engineers to improve the video taping system, and it might have been expected that RCA would take the lead in this technology.[19] Indeed, an RCA tape machine (recording in both mono and color) was demonstrated in 1953. But the tape speed was 30 feet per second, and the reels held only about 3–4 minutes of programming.[20]

Despite RCA's experience and resources (including funds from the Defense Department), a small company in Redwood City, California, developed the first practical video recorder in the USA. Ampex had experience with audio magnetic recording and had the capital to devote to developing video recording.

Ampex Corporation's engineers incorporated transverse scanning and FM (frequency modulation) recording to produce a broadcast-quality recorder, which recorded more slowly and on longer reels than previous machines. In April 1956, Ampex introduced a quad system, or quadruplex recorder, including four recording heads on a rotating drum, using 2 inch wide magnetic re-usable tape. It was "the most sensational demonstration of magnetic recording equipment thus far" and was in use at CBS's Hollywood studios by November 1956.[21]

By 1957 RCA and Ampex had agreed to share patents through a cross-licensing agreement, and both were producing color video tape recorder (VTR) equipment. However, Ampex took the lead and became the dominant force in video taping equipment markets around the world through the late 1960s.[22]

Although VTRs were first intended to be used for network programming time delays, the system actually meant the death of live television. Recorded programming became the norm, and networks and stations replaced their expensive kinescope equipment with video recorders.

Meanwhile, Japanese companies were working on similar technology, but more specifically aimed at the consumer market. In July 1960, Ampex agreed to work with Sony, one of the leaders in consumer electronics.[23] Ampex was to concentrate on professional equipment for the broadcast market, and Sony would focus on the consumer market. By 1966, their partnership was over, and they competed against each other for industrial and educational customers.[24]

Consumer video: pre-Betamax   Home video systems became a possibility with the introduction of the helical-scan format which many electronic companies were working on in the late 1950s. While a transverse scanning system includes tape heads mounted on a drum that rotates at a right angle to the tape movement, helical-scan (or slant-track scan) systems involve fewer playback heads (one or two), which are mounted on a drum that rotates in the same direction as the tape, which is wrapped around the drum in a helical manner. The helical-scan systems typically produce lower quality images than quadruplex machines (because the tape travels slower). However, the new systems were less complex and less expensive and included a number of other features, such as slow motion and still framing – characteristics making them more suitable for non-professional use or consumer video systems.

Sony is often attributed with the first "home video" system; many other systems, however, were aimed at the consumer market before the introduction of Sony's Betamax.

(1)   Ampex: the American company apparently produced several "home entertainment systems" based on their video tape recording devices in the early 1960s. An example was the Signature V, advertised in the 1963

Neiman–Marcus Christmas catalog for $30,000, featuring a VTR, black-and-white camera, music center and television receivers.

(2)   EVR (CBS): in the early 1960s Peter Goldmark, President of CBS Labs, presented his idea for Electronic Video Recording (EVR) to CBS. Although CBS at first was uninterested, Goldmark turned to the government and received research funds (although apparently not officially) from the US Air Force. EVR was perceived to be useful for weapons training. By 1964, EVR also was supported by CBS.

A prototype machine presented in 1967 used one-hour black-and-white cartridge with film, but was able only to play back and not to record. Despite this drawback, a public demonstration in March 1970 impressed its audience and attracted a great deal of attention. EVR was promoted as the "video long-playing record of the future" and the "greatest revolution in communications since the book." CBS created an international consortium (called EVR Partnership) to sell players and cartridges, and Motorola was to produce players selling at $800 each. And one of the Hollywood film majors (Twentieth Century Fox) even agreed to license some of their films.

However, EVR never actually reached the marketplace. Numerous problems plagued its production, including difficulties with generating masters for cartridges, high costs for cartridges, and, finally, competition from Sony's U-matic. EVR became economically untenable, and CBS abandoned the project after only a few hundred cartridges were produced, at a cost of $33 million.

(3)   Holotape (RCA): in 1969 RCA announced yet another video system, using lasers and holograms to record pictures on pieces of plastic film; they were then played back on television monitors. At first the device was called Holotape, then Selecta Vision, and it was to go into production in 1972; the machine was to sell for about $400, and half-hour programs for $10 each. When the effort failed, RCA reserved its favored Selecta Vision label for other systems.

(4)   Cartrivision: this was perhaps the most interesting of the pre-Betamax video systems. In 1972 Cartridge Television Inc. offered a video-cassette recorder, together with programs on half-inch tape. Although Cartrivision was started by non-Hollywood people, the company became popular with movie companies because of its recognition of the importance of programming. One movie company, Avco (which owned Avco-Embassy) even joined the endeavor.

But to obtain films from the studios, Cartrivision had to devise a unique system of distribution. The initial set of cassettes was packaged in black boxes and sold with the machine. Rental cassettes were packaged in special red boxes, with locking devices making them impossible to rewind. Only retailers could rewind them on special machines, equipped with counters. Thus, unofficial copying was prevented.

Cartrivisions were sold at Sears stores, with 111 black cassettes available for sale only (such titles as *Fishing with Gadabout Gaddis* and *Basic Crewel*), and 200 red cassettes (including films such as *Casablanca* and *Dr Strangelove*) available for rental only.

At first glance, it would seem that Cartrivision had it made, even anticipating future arrangements in the home video business:

> And yet, of all the systems conceived, announced, and demonstrated in the pre-Betamax years, Cartrivision was the only one of American manufacture to be submitted to the judgment of the marketplace, and after that judgment had been rendered, Cartrivision's promos could claim with reasonable fidelity to the truth that fully three years before Sony unleashed the home video revolution, another company – an American company – had been selling a product capable of doing everything a Betamax could do.[25]

However, the company ultimately had too many problems. The company and its product was not popular with the press, as it lacked the slick promotional campaigns of larger corporations. Its lack of marketing expertise made selling a low-quality machine, together with a television set, difficult. In addition, the no-rewind feature of the red cassettes was inconvenient and unpopular. And to add to these miseries, the first batch of tapes began disintegrating after being shipped.

Although Cartrivision seemed to appreciate the importance of programming, there were still difficulties with their system. As long as there were only a relatively few machines, distributors and retailers were unwilling to handle programming. And, without programs, the machine population would not grow.

Despite these nagging problems, the company continued to spend large sums of money, but received little in return. Avco eventually pulled out, after having spent $48 million on the project, and Cartrivision became merely a stepping stone in the history of home video.

(5)   Sony's video systems: meanwhile, Sony had devoted a great deal of its corporate resources to developing a consumer video system. Sony's half-inch CV-2000 (CV: consumer video) was introduced in 1965, and promoted as "the world's first home videocorder." The system used a

7 inch reel which could hold an hour of material. The first models included a TV set and cost around $1,000. The intention was clearly to record TV programs for later replay, as the more expensive model included a timer. (Cameras were also available.)

But there were plenty of drawbacks: it was a complex system, with tape on open reels, and only black-and-white. It became more popular for industrial and educational customers, thus Sony renamed it "commercial" instead of "consumer" video.

The solution for some of these problems was in the technology of videocassettes. Audiocassettes had been introduced in 1962, but it was not until 1971 that Sony solved the problem of videocassettes, and introduced the U-Matic. Utilizing three-quarter inch color tape, it was claimed to be the first videocassette recorder to reach the market. However, it was not very successful in the market for which it was originally intended. The machine and the cassette apparently were too big and too expensive (over $1,000 for the recorder and $30 each for half-hour cassettes). But, even though consumers did not go for the U-Matic, it was a great success in the educational, industrial, and professional markets. Indeed, the beginnings of electronic news gathering (ENG) have been traced to CBS News's use of the U-Matic and Ikegami video camera in 1974.[26]

Betamax (and VHS): the beginning of consumer home video   Most of the companies manufacturing video technology introduced consumer products in the late sixties and early seventies.[27] However, Sony claimed to offer the first successful home video machine. The Betamax system was introduced in 1975, using a narrow half-inch tape; but it recorded only one hour per tape, with blank tape priced at around $20. The first models cost around $2,295, and included a 19 inch Trinitron. The Betamax deck, however, went on sale in February 1976, priced at $1,295, and was an immediate success.[28]

The Betamax was promoted at first for time shifting, a term attributed to Sony head, Akio Morita, and referring to the process of recording programs from television and playing them back at a later time. The idea of time shifting in Sony's advertisements attracted the attention of consumers, as well as the movie industry, and prompted Universal's legal case against Sony (more later).

Meanwhile, Matsushita and other electronic companies in Japan had refused Sony's offer to produce a standardized machine. In 1976, Matsushita and JVC introduced a competing format – VHS (video home system), which developed as the primary competition to Sony's Betamax.

VHS was a smaller machine, with a different loading system, but offered a longer tape running time of two hours, later extended to four, then six hours.

Sony, JVC, and Matsushita struggled to recruit other electronic companies to their systems. By 1978, Zenith was distributing Betamaxes, but a number of other American companies had joined the "VHS family." Although VCRs carried the name General Electric, Magnavox, Curtis Mathes, Montgomery Ward, Sylvania, RCA, or Panasonic, the machines were made by Matsushita, which soon produced two-thirds of the world's home VCRs. Despite Beta's slight technical superiority, and even though Sony increased the length of their cassettes, lowered the price and added other improvements to the basic Betamax, by 1979 twice as many VHS systems were selling as Betamaxes.

Videodiscs   Meanwhile, several of the electronic manufacturing companies were developing videodiscs, which provided excellent quality playback, yet no recording capabilities.

RCA had been working on their CED (capacitance disc) player for years, but hesitated, trying to perfect a low-priced unit that would compete with videocassette players.

But RCA faced competition from Philips and MCA's Magna Vision, an optical scanning videodisc system, marketed in 1980 at $775 per unit, with the help of Magnavox and IBM. Meanwhile, MCA's Discovision used a laser beam to decipher a picture recorded on a plastic disc and played back on a TV monitor.

Of course, videodisc machines were especially interesting to movie companies as they could not record, thus, could not copy movies. MCA considered working with Sony to manufacture videodisc players (ironically, at same time suing Sony for copyright violation). And RCA had involved the Hollywood companies in its project, with programming agreements from Paramount, United Artists, Disney, and others committing about 1,000 titles.

Finally, in March 1981, RCA introduced their Selecta Vision Video-Disc player for around $400. Zenith, CBS and Matsushita also marketed the system. At this point, RCA expected to profit from the sale of discs, which could be sold for around $10–20 each, compared to $80 for tapes. But despite the superior technology and the lower costs (at one point, $200), disc players moved rather slowly in the market. By the end of 1983, RCA had only sold 500,000 players, and was reported to have lost between $400 million and $580 million on its videodisc project. In fact, RCA had sold more cassette players than disc players.[29]

Accepting defeat in April 1984, RCA blamed the problem on "the enormous growth in videocassette recorders, the rapid development of a rental market in videocassettes, and the loss of control over videodisc software." The popular use of video recorders for time shifting was another limitation. RCA described videodiscs as a "technological success but a commercial failure." As Robert Sobel concluded in his book on RCA, "Perhaps videodiscs would have been viable had they been introduced in the early 1970s, before the nation became hooked on the videocassette units."[30]

Format wars   While the VHS and Beta formats battled to become the industry standard during the eighties, NV Philips and Grundig introduced another technically superior machine. Video 2000 was based on Philips's audiocassette technology and incorporated a flexible video head, making better use of tape and thus producing a higher quality. The equipment was introduced in Europe in 1980. However, Philips had declared defeat by 1983, unable to compete with the Beta and VHS models of the Japanese companies. Philips was reported to have lost $55 million on the project, which again demonstrated the advantages of an early market lead.

Gradually other Beta-producing electronic companies added VHS and dropped Beta. By 1988, Beta's share of the US market was only 9.9 percent.[31] Around that time, Sony finally gave in and added a VHS to its line as well as producing a version of Beta compatible with VHS (ED Beta).[32] While there were various reasons given for Beta's decline, one was the release of Hollywood films on VHS format rather than Beta.[33]

But the decline of Beta in the USA also seemed tied to problems with Sony itself:

In the 1950s, Sony had managed to maintain a monopoly over the Japanese tape recorder business by vigorously asserting its patent rights. By the eighties consumer electronics had become such a fiercely competitive business and the products themselves had become so fantastically complicated that no company could produce state-of-the-art equipment by relying on its own R&D. The sharing and trading of patents had become essential and routine, and when a truly new product emerged, its discoverers knew that no matter how secure their legal position, if they tried to construct a patent barrier against would-be imitators, the people they gave the cold shoulder to today could be the people they needed a favor from tomorrow.[34]

Bells and whistles   As saturation point approached in the late 1980s, the electrical industry added further modifications to prompt consumers to buy more advanced recorders or additional equipment. Some did not make it, others were blocked before they reached the market.

New formats were introduced, including 8 mm, a smaller format video (by Sony and others), Super VHS, and 8 mm Hi-Band.[35] Meanwhile, compact disc video was introduced in June 1987. The system records on optical discs with small pits on the surface which carry digital audio or video information. A laser reads the disc and translates it into high-quality sound and pictures.[36]

Meanwhile, Panasonic introduced a video recorder that could be programmed via a phone, and Sony produced a Video Walkman. Additional features for machines included picture in picture (separate picture from different source) and channel scan (sampling channels). More "bells and whistles" would follow (often, at higher prices), in attempts to lure first-time buyers or potential two-VCR families.

Other devices were created to work with VCRs. TV Genies were wireless transmitters for VCRs, sending signals to other TV sets not connected to a VCR. The Genies, however, were declared illegal around 1986.[37] And a Portland, Oregon, company (Vidcraft-Portland) produced a contraption that was bound to upset advertisers: the Commercial Cutter automatically removes commercial breaks during taping.[38] While many other innovations tried to capitalize on the home video boom, a combination VCR/Popcorn Maker proposed by *Video Review* in 1986 had yet to appear by the beginning of the nineties.[39]

The most controversial video innovation might have been video recorders with two decks, which of course would allow easy copying of pre-recorded videos. Go-Video, a small Arizona company, developed a dual-deck recorder (VCR-2) around 1984 and approached NEC to produce the machine.[40] Meanwhile, a double-deck recorder was introduced by Sharp in the Middle East in early 1985. The film industry responded – strongly. Valenti called it a "two-headed dragon," an "amoeba run amok," and, finally, "the crudest blade of all."[41]

However, Sharp and other electronics firms, apparently under pressure from the MPAA, agreed among themselves – with the consent of the Electronic Industries Association of Japan (EIAJ) – not to produce or supply parts for dual-deck VCRs.[42] Go-Video actually filed an antitrust suit in June 1987 against 20 Japanese and Korean manufacturing companies, the EIAJ, and the MPAA, claiming that they were trying to block production of their machine. By March 1989, the company had collected $1.8 million in out-of-court settlements, their stock had taken dramatic leaps, and Samsung had agreed to produce the machine. Meanwhile, the MPAA had backed off when Go-Video agreed to include anti-copying devices with the machine.[43]

When the Go-Video machine finally was available (as GV-2000, priced at around $1,000), it was promoted as a device for editing; however, many found it less than adequate for the job.[44] Meanwhile, other recorders were introduced, such as Samsung's The Translator, permitting an 8 mm format to be turned into VHS, but also allowing copying.[45]

The Business of Home Video/Hardware

The revolutionary character of home video is most often supported by the rapid sales of the hardware itself. The proliferation of home video technology is measured in different ways, and several organizations and publications gather statistics, including Arbitron, Gallup, the Electrical Industry Association (EIA), and home viewer publications, such as *Video Marketing*. But these sources often report conflicting data.

The average cost of machines has dropped – from $830 in 1981, to around $200 by the end of the eighties.[46] Sales of machines increased gradually from 800,000 in 1980 to 2 million in 1982. By 1985, the boom had begun – from 25,000–30,000 machines were reportedly purchased daily,[47] with nearly 11.9 million VCRs sold during the year. During the next two years, over 13 million recorders were purchased.[48] Sales dropped slightly in 1987 to 11.7 million, and to about 10.5 million in 1988.[49] By the end of the eighties, sales were leveling off, but still reached nearly 12 million each year.[50]

One of the most popular measures of the video revolution, though, is the "video penetration" measure, which is the percentage of TV households to own video equipment. In 1983, only 7 percent of US homes owned either videocassette recorders or videodisc players.[51] By 1984, only 15–20 percent of US homes owned video equipment. However, during 1985 video penetration grew to 25–33 percent. In 1986, the EIA stats claimed 40 percent of the TV households owned home video equipment.[52] By mid-1988, 55–60 percent of households included VCRs, although Gallup said it was 65 percent.[53] And AC Nielsen Co. reported 62 percent TV homes with machines in late 1988.[54] (See table 6.1 for a profile of the US home video market from 1983 to 1992.)

VCR ownership also is reported demographically, by area, by city, by income, two-VCR families, etc. A sample report from one of the video trade publications in 1985 noted:

Table 6.1   Profile of US home video market

Year	Number of VCR households[a] (millions)	% of TV homes with VCRs	Videocassette sales (millions of units)	
			Prerecorded[b]	Blank[c]
1992	E70.0	E75.2	E350.0	380.0
1991	67.5	73.3	300.0	365.0
1990	65.4	70.2	240.0	338.0
1989	62.3	67.6	200.0	285.6
1988	56.2	62.2	135.0	296.9
1987	45.8	51.7	110.0	285.0
1986	32.5	37.2	84.0	280.0
1985	23.5	27.3	52.0	182.0
1984	15.0	17.6	22.0	109.0
1983	8.3	9.9	9.5	57.0

E-Estimated.
[a] At year-end.
[b] To US dealers, excluding adult and public domain material.
[c] To US consumer market.
Sources: Motion Picture Association of America, Electronics Industries Association, *Billboard* magazine and Standard & Poor estimates. Presented in *Standard & Poor's Industry Surveys*, 11 March 1993, p. L25.

Most surveys peg the current VCR owner as well-educated, between the ages of 25–50, with an income between $20–50,000. They are technologically savvy; they own stereos and computers. Half are women. They live in urban areas with about 25% each in four areas: the Northeast, the West, the South and the Central portion. 75% have VHS machines. They are heavy TV watchers and use the VCR to time shift.[55]

Some of the primary beneficiaries of this video explosion, of course, have been the electronics companies. By the mid-1980s, however, 95 percent of the VCRs sold in the USA, marketed under 86 brand names, were made by Japanese companies. By mid-1988, there were 50 different brands and more than 100 different models – but *all* made by Japanese companies, despite labels such as RCA, General Electric, JC Penney, Sears, and Curtis Mathes.[56] Japan's share of VCR imports to the US was 96 percent in 1986, but dropped to 87 percent in 1987, with South Korea's share growing to 11 percent from 3 percent. In 1987, 230,000 machines were produced in the USA, but by Japanese-owned companies.[57]

The Evolution of Home Video Software/VCR use

The growth of home video must be considered, however, in light of factors other than the availability of the hardware and assumed market demand. The perfection of home video technology at costs affordable to many households had been accomplished by the early 1980s – but for what use? Why would a consumer want to purchase a video recorder or playback machine?

Basically, there are at least three possible uses for video recording or playback equipment:

1   to *record* from other sources, especially off-the-air television programs, or *time-shifting*.
2   to *play back* pre-recorded video material.
3   to *produce* video tapes, or direct recording.

To Record and (Maybe) to Play Back

Early promotion of VCRs by manufacturers emphasized time shifting. So it may not be surprising that for the first few years, taping programs from television was the most popular use of home video technology.[58] However, the emphasis on taping programs off the air did not escape the attention of the Hollywood majors, some of the most important suppliers of television programming.

Universal v. Sony/Betamax case   The first major response to home video recording by the film industry was prompted by Sony's advertising campaign in September 1976 for Betamax as a way to time-shift television programming. Universal and Disney filed a lawsuit in November 1976, challenging the copyright law pertaining to fair use. At Universal's initiative, all the majors were asked to join, but only Disney agreed to be co-plaintiff.[59]

Disney's lawyer expressed the sentiments of both companies when he explained simply that "the videotape machine would be used to steal our property." However, the other studios, represented in the amicus curiae brief submitted by the MPAA, were less interested in the case. As Sid Sheinberg, head of Universal at the time, noted: "It's a constant problem in this industry that most people in high places are not worried about what might happen ten years down the road. They're worried about getting to the Polo Lounge."[60]

Although Sony suggested a royalty fee on machines and cassettes as a compromise, MCA was not listening. As Sony's US representative observed, "I don't think it was accidental that the company that took the lead in fighting the videocassette was the company that held all the patents on the videodisc."[61]

The trial started on January 30, 1979, and was tried by Judge Warren Ferguson, US District Court, Central District of California. The case received a great deal of public attention and revealed the film industry's attitude toward home video at the time, as well as serving as a test for the standards of fair use described in the new copyright legislation. More specifically, the 1976 law delineated fair use as:

1   the right to reproduce the work in copies;
2   the right to distribute those copies;
3   the right to prepare derivative works (such as translations and dramatizations) based upon copyrighted works;
4   the right to perform or display the work publicly.[62]

While interpretation of these rights was pivotal for the defendants, several other issues also were emphasized during the trial. First, it was argued that revenue would be lost from the sale of movies to network TV. In addition, television networks and stations would lose advertising revenue because viewers would not be watching at specific air times. Despite the claim that the studios (specifically, Universal, MCA, and Disney) had encouraged Sony's development of home videotape recorders, MPAA President, Jack Valenti, called the Betamax a "parasitical" device.

Finally, in October 1979, Judge Ferguson decided that the concept of fair use was applicable, as home taping was done in private homes, and the film companies had "voluntarily" transmitted their works over public airwaves: "Home-use recording from free television is not copyright infringement, and even if it were, the corporate defendants are not liable and an injunction is not appropriate."[63]

Although the hardware manufacturers breathed a sigh of relief, their triumph was short-lived, as the plaintiffs pursued the case to the US Court of Appeals, Ninth Circuit, which ruled on October 20, 1981, that home video recording *was* an infringement, and Sony was responsible. The response to the controversial decision was widespread and immediate, as cartoonists, editorialists, and comedians envisioned a "Video Police State."

According to James Lardner, "In the long history of its offenses, that much-maligned branch of government, the judiciary, had probably never issued a decision that attracted more abuse and less sympathy."[64]

The decision prompted several bills in Congress, introduced by Reps Parris, DeConcini, and Mathias. Meanwhile, the film industry – although pleased about the reversal – also responded to the widespread criticism by preparing an alternative to the home recording ban. A provision for royalties on VCRs and blank tapes was proposed as "a compromise which would preserve the interests of consumers and creators simultaneously."[65]

Thus, the battle raged on. In March 1982, Rep. Mathias added royalties for audiotaping as well as videotaping to his bill, as well as giving copyright owners the exclusive right to authorize rental of pre-recorded tapes – an issue which, as we shall see in the next section, was becoming increasingly more important as a video rental system emerged.

Meanwhile, Sony enlisted assistance from the Electronics Industry Association, forming the Home Recording Rights Coalition. They also found support from video dealers, who in addition to resisting tape royalties, wanted to fight the added rental provision.

The battle lines were drawn between the "Home Recorders" and the "Copyrightists," as numerous PR and lobbying firms were hired by both sides. Debates took place in the press, through direct mail campaigns, and on television talk shows. Charles Ferris (former FCC commissioner) was hired as a spokesman for the Home Recorders, and became the rival of Jack Valenti, spokesman for the Copyrightists, who called VCRs "millions of little tapeworms" eating away at the core of the American film industry.

A Home Taping bill was eventually introduced in the House and hearings were held in April 1982.[66] Much of the Congressional activity was placed on hold in June 1982 when the Supreme Court decided to hear the Betamax case. But as a landmark 27 amicus curiae briefs were filed with the Court, the hearings and debates continued. In 1983 *Variety* reported that the struggle was "reaching new heights of acrimony."

As Lardner observed:

> By the middle of 1983 the two lobbying coalitions had assembled between them a vast Washington brain trust which included two former cabinet-level officials; four former top advisers in the Carter White House; two former senators; five former representatives; two former chairmen of the Federal Communications Commission; two former White House economists; and two former chief counsels to the Senate Judiciary Committee. Hardly any issue facing the nation in recent memory had engaged the attention of a more formidable array of elder statesmanhood.[67]

On the other hand, there was a great deal of skepticism and derision of these activities. "It's corporate pigs versus corporate pigs," was one Congressional aide's assessment. "So you sort of watch it like a pig fight. All these people running around with five-hundred-dollar suits and three-dollar cigars. You walk into the hearing rooms and it's wall-to-wall pinstripes."[68]

Then, on January 17, 1984, the Supreme Court, with a vote of five to four, reversed the District Court's decision:

> One may search the Copyright Act in vain for any sign that the elected representatives of the millions of people who watch television every day have made it unlawful to copy a program for later viewing at home, or have enacted a flat prohibition against the sale of machines that make such copying possible.[69]

While the majors had lost their eight-year battle, they were, at the same time, busily jumping into the video market. Indeed, the arguments made during the Supreme Court case often referred to the majors' increasing profits from home video ($400 million in 1983). Another example of Hollywood's schizophrenic attitude towards video is offered by Lardner, who explains that Disney even made a deal with Sony to distribute its videocassettes before the case was settled. A Disney executive was said to soothe his worried Sony colleague by telling him, "Look, the people who are suing you are a different division of the company. If this makes economic sense for both of us, why should we let the lawsuit stand in our way?"[70]

So, viewers had "won" the right to tape at home. And despite the fears of the film and broadcast industry, and the claim that VCR owners were "independent entertainment seekers," early research by Mark Levy indicated that "most VCR households record and playback much the same programs which are watched and enjoyed by the mass audience."[71]

Levy further concluded that, for the short term, at least, the TV networks would be the principal beneficiaries, since the prime source for recordings was network-affiliated stations. Yet, Levy also hinted at long-term effects on broadcast audiences. Later research revealed that while viewers used VCRs for time shifting, the process was actually incomplete, as recordings were made, but often not replayed.[72] The important point, however, was that the popularity of VCRs at the time was related to the time-shifting convenience. This, again, partially explains the popularity of VCRs over videodisc players.

Levy's research also indicated that, at least for the first few years of home video growth, recording movies was the most frequent time-shifting/recording activity.[73] So it seems that the growth of home video also was related to the availability of films on TV, especially offered by pay-cable channels such as HBO.

With the popularity of time-shifting activities, the growth in blank tape sales also expanded rapidly: retail sales grew from around 24 million in 1982 to nearly 300 million in 1986.[74] One indication of the growth in tape sales was the announcement by Eastman Kodak that the traditional film supplier would enter the video tape business in 1984. The explanation? "We believe that our entry into the videotape field is properly timed to match these new business opportunities," stated a Kodak executive.[75]

Yet, by the time that the Universal/Sony case was settled, the time-shifting novelty was gradually wearing off. One study noted that by 1986, the primary reason most people gave for purchasing a VCR was to view rental movies.[76] According to another estimate, only 30 percent of VCR viewing by 1987 was watching tapes recorded from television or cable, and the majority of VCR activity centered on watching pre-recorded videos.[77] By mid-1988, it was reported that the average VCR owner spent only two-and-a-half hours recording tapes, but almost four hours playing tapes.[78]

Later indications were that there was probably less time shifting than reported, as consumers seemed to have some difficulty in actually programming their VCRs. A series of solutions was proposed and introduced, including easier programming procedures by manufacturers as well as various devices (such as bar codes) linked to television schedules. One popular system, accepted by many VCR manufacturers, was VCR Plus+, a device that automatically taped programs which were pre-assigned numbers listed in TV schedules.

Pre-recorded Videos: To Sell or to Rent?

The use of home video technology for pre-recorded tape playback had grown more slowly, as this activity depends to a great extent on the availability of such tapes. As home video machines became more popular in the late seventies, direct sales were emphasized, but at high prices. Only about one million cassettes sold annually. The most prevalent types of pre-recorded tapes available at first were pornography or X-rated films, often selling for $60–125 each. (Some were even as high as $300.)[80]

According to some reports, the earliest effort to distribute pre-recorded tapes of major motion pictures was by Andre Blay, an "industry outsider" who had formed Magnetic Video in Farmington Hills, Michigan, in 1969. Blay contacted the majors about obtaining rights to sell their films on video.

And, while some people at the studios were considering video distribution, none had made the move. At first, the studios' interest seemed related only to time shifting, and focussed on Universal's Betamax case. However, the ultimate concern was losing control over product, whether it was expressed as fear of time shifting, direct sales, or piracy. Consequently, the majors were hoping that the "right" video technology would prevail, in other words, videodiscs, which did not allow recording or copying. But, videodisc systems quickly lost ground to VCR systems; thus, the market was ripe for pre-recorded programs on videocassettes.

Apparently only Twentieth Century Fox was interested in Blay's proposal to buy the rights to films for sale on videotape. In 1977, Blay purchased the non-exclusive rights to 50 Fox films, which had already appeared on network TV. His agreement with Fox involved a $300,000 advance, plus a minimum of $500,000 a year against a royalty of $7.50 on each cassette sold. Blay chose (from a list offered by Fox) films such as *M*A*S*H*, *Patton*, and *Sound of Music*, and sold them to retailers for $37.50, or to individuals for $49.95 each through a direct-mail operation, called the Video Club of America.

> Fortuitously the Fox titles went on sale just as RCA and Sony were going head to head with their pre-Christmas ad campaign and just as a new competitiveness – spurred by the arrival of models that bore the Zenith, Sylvania, and Magnavox labels – brought prices under $1,000. As the number of VCRs grew, so did the demand for pre-recorded cassettes.[81]

By March 1978, Blay had sold 40,000 cassettes, to retailers and Video Club members. By the end of the year, he had sold 250,000 tapes, and started buying additional titles from independents (Avco Embassy, Viacom, etc.), as most of the majors were still reluctant to offer their films for sale.[82]

About the same time, a few enterprising individuals began to rent copies of movies purchased from companies like Magnetic. But the legal status of such activities seemed unclear. As companies began selling their films on tape, their contracts specifically prohibited rental. But, was it actually illegal to rent video copies of films after purchase?

One of the early pioneers in video rentals, George Atkinson, again an "industry outsider," received the following advice from his lawyer (according to Lardner): "You can't copy it, you can't publicly exhibit it – that's a violation of copyright. But yes, you can rent it, you can eat it, you can destroy it. You bought it. It's your property."[83]

The First Sale Doctrine, a provision of the Copyright Act of 1976, allows the legitimate buyer of a copyrighted work to dispose of the copy as he or she wishes.[84] In other words, after a cassette has been *sold* to a retailer, no further royalties can be claimed, and the copyright owner loses control of that copy.

While the studios philosophically supported a rental system as a more appropriate system of distributing their films on video, they certainly did not care for the First Sale Doctrine, and, thus, tried to prevent rentals via contractual restrictions, as well as pushing a direct sales rather than a rental market.

Nevertheless, video entrepreneurs, such as Atkinson, obtained copies and continued to rent, as well as starting others in the video business through franchises (Atkinson's franchises were called Video Stations). By the end of 1978, a rental system was emerging, despite the reluctance of the major distributors. As Lardner notes,

> Over the next few years the VCR and the pre-recorded videocassette set hearts on fire in entrepreneurial breasts all over the land. Americans from every imaginable walk of life cracked open their nest eggs, remortgaged their homes, and put the arm on their parents, siblings, and in-laws in order to become the proud proprietors of Video Castles, Connections, Corners, Hutches, Huts, Palaces, Patches, Places, Shacks, Sheds, Sources, Spots, and Stations. It was as if someone had hung a classified ad in the sky: "Retail Oppty. – Lo Cash/EZ Startup."[85]

While the majors still tried to prohibit rentals in their contracts, they eventually yielded to the popularity of rentals, and did not enforce the restrictions. They also started releasing more of their films on video.

Fox and Warner were the first of the majors to enter video distribution, but by 1981 all of the large Hollywood distributors had their own video divisions (even MCA, which had hesitated because of the Sony suit), or they combined with another company to distribute their films in video form (i.e. RCA/Columbia, CBS/Fox).[86]

However, the business was still expected to develop as direct sales, and so the film distributors priced their cassettes at $79.95. This would allow a royalty of about $10 – "a handsome return if multiplied by millions of individual purchasers, but a far less attractive one when multiplied by ten or fifteen thousand video store owners, each of them free to take a cassette which had cost, say, $50 wholesale, and rent it out a hundred times or more at $5 a shot."[87]

As the rental system emerged, the studios wanted more, arguing that they were not receiving their "creative share" when video store owners were not required to pay them a percentage of each rental transaction. Though they continued releasing films on video, they also initiated a series of challenges from 1980 to 1982 (called "the rental wars" by Lardner), in an attempt to get more of their share from rentals.

Several different proposals were offered by the studios around this time. In 1980, Disney proposed a two-track marketing system, featuring rental-only and sale-only cassettes. During 1981, the Warner Home Video Rental Plan was introduced, with leased cassettes on a weekly basis. In addition, Fox and MGM/CBS proposed different rental plans. And, in 1982, Warner's Dealer's Choice offered rental terms of four to six weeks, for A and B titles.

The distributors claimed that the retailers could actually make more money by agreeing to these schemes. But,

> [h]owever the studios explained the rationale behind their plans, it looked to the dealers as if the underlying purpose were to capture a bigger share of the take from each rental. They felt like colonists who had been through a few tough winters and were about to harvest a bumper crop only to learn that the mother country was going to raise their taxes.[88]

Thus, each plan was resisted by the retailers, who responded by forming two national organizations in 1982 at the Las Vegas Consumer Electronics Show. The Video Software Retailers Association (VSRA), the more militant group, even proposed a boycott. ("Let's pull their booth apart," "Rip their catalogs apart, and throw them in their faces.") The Video Software Dealers Association (VSDA) was more moderate, but still would not accept the studio's proposals. They pointed out that not only would they potentially lose money, they would also lose control over their business, and especially, their inventory, which provided the basis for bank loans, etc. "The reason people go into small business is to have some control," pointed out one dealer. "If you look at the history of Hollywood, it's been a history of trying to have disproportionate control – complete vertical control."[89]

By mid-1982, the new rental plans had been scrapped. One studio executive moaned, "We couldn't fight the tide," while others attributed the lack of cooperation by retailers to their immaturity. "Immature they might be. Ineffective they weren't. Their ability to mount a coordinated campaign of resistance from coast to coast was a source of amazement and annoyance to the studio people."[90]

As previously discussed, the majors turned to legislative efforts to change the First Sale Doctrine, especially after the Supreme Court's Betamax decision. Bills introduced during the 98th Congress received the majors' full attention, as they waged one of their typical Washington campaigns. Although well-paid and influential lobbyists called on legislators to help out their Hollywood friends, and a few powerful allies, including the White House, were enlisted, the "Home Recorders" ultimately were able to rally video dealers around the country and squash the legislation.[91]

Hollywood lobbyists also tried to get a royalty tax on rentals and sales of copyrighted movies, but failed. In 1986, the industry tried another tactic: pushing legislation that would require manufacturers to install anti-copying devices in all VCRs. As Jack Valenti explained in his testimony, "Unauthorized back-to-back copying is a malevolent threat to the creative future." As he went on to compare the practice to "a deadly virus," it appeared that creativity was not the only issue, and perhaps not even the most important one: "Every unauthorized copy made from a pre-recorded videocassette potentially displaces a sale or rental of a pre-recorded videocassette."[92] The virus continued, but the legislation failed.

During 1987–8 the introduction of pay-per-transaction (PPT) was another attempt by the majors to work around the First Sale Doctrine. Video copies of films were to be leased to retail outlets at prices much lower than outright sale, and a percentage of each transaction (50 percent) then paid to the supplier and distributor – "a revenue-sharing plan," noted *Variety*, "which splits the actual dollars consumers spend."[93] The plan also involved computer systems which recorded each transaction, and, of course, could be accessed by the suppliers. Orion was the first program supplier to offer all retail outlets PPT deals. But one of the largest retail chains, National Video, also pushed the program, claiming that it would solve the retailers' problem of depth of copy, or the number of copies of a specific title. Eventually pay-per-transaction was killed by the retailers' less than enthusiastic reaction (cries of "big brother" and "capitulation to Hollywood's dictates" were common), but also by the studios' reluctance to push a scheme that most retailers resisted. Although pay-per-transaction died a slower death than the previous schemes, the retailers had again resisted the dominating force of the Hollywood majors.

There have been other schemes to gain more control over the rental business. One system kept track of the number of times a cassette had been played through a built-in counter.[98] Thus, the supplier could charge the dealer per transaction, but also the dealer could charge consumers for the number of times the cassette was played. A few years later several companies, including Polaroid, developed cassettes that destroyed themselves after a specific number of plays, reminiscent of the self-destructing taped assignments in the *Mission Impossible* television series. Another version was a cassette that automatically erased after 25 plays.[95]

The Birth of the Video Industry

Meanwhile, rentals grew and direct sales diminished. According to a Nielsen report, the proportion of VCR owners who rented tapes for playback increased from 37 percent in 1984 to 45 percent in 1985.[96] In a 1985 Nielsen report, 74 percent of VCR owners had rented a pre-recorded cassette at least once, while 67 percent were active renters and rented at least once per month.[97] One study reported that 42.5 percent of VCR owners rented in 1987 and 44.3 percent in 1988.[94] (See figure 6.1 for *Video Store Magazine's* summary of rentals and sales.)

The home video business was growing, with a distinct industrial structure emerging. And the retail revenues doubled. And doubled again. In 1983, sales and rentals of videos totaled $1.06 billion. Revenues of $2.04 billion were reported in 1984, and $4.5 billion in 1985. By 1987, revenues were $7.46 billion, far exceeding theatrical box office receipts.[99]

In addition to their efforts to persuade Congress to change the First Sale Doctrine or provide another form of "relief" for the film industry, the majors gradually dropped their retail prices to encourage the sell-through market. In 1984, Paramount offered *Top Gun* (including a Pepsi commercial) for $26.95. By the end of 1987, nearly 3 million units had been sold, and according to *Variety*, ". . . re-established the viability of low-priced blockbuster films and made sure the industry's first major experiment with a commercial on a film cassette was a huge success."[100] In 1988, Nelson Entertainment went even further and launched a new sell-through product line at $14.98, the lowest price at that time for top films from a program supplier.[101]

Around the same time (1986), however, the video companies announced that they would increase their prices to wholesalers from $79.95 to $89.95 or $99.95, thus raising retailers' prices far beyond the standard $50.[102]

Figure 6.1   Video consumer spending estimates, 1985–92 ($ billions)

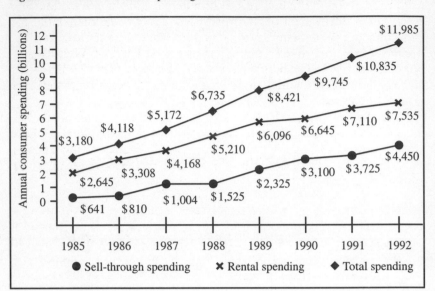

Source: Video Store Magazine, in *1993 International Television & Video Almanac,* New York: Quigley Publishing, 1993, p. 664.

So, the marketing of pre-recorded cassettes has gone through three phases:

1   1975–8: emphasis on sell-throughs at high prices;
2   1979–84: mostly rentals;
3   1985-present: mix of rentals and sell-throughs at lower prices.

Home video has proven to be an extremely lucrative business, attracting attention from the popular press and jealousy from other entertainment sectors. But this success cannot be attributed only to consumers' fascination with a new technology and the declining prices for VCRs. Home video has become popular in the USA because of the availability of software, or pre-recorded tapes, especially Hollywood movies, and the development of a popularly accepted distribution system (rentals). In other words, the home video market has become yet another profitable market for theatrical motion pictures.

Despite the early resistance, Hollywood has not only accepted home video but has embraced the new distribution outlet. Various observers have attributed this acceptance to the inability of the studios to challenge or lobby away the First Sale Doctrine, to successful box office receipts from 1988 through the end of the decade, and to the realization that home video distribution of films provided not only another outlet for their films but an extremely profitable one, with extremely low distribution expenses involved.[113] Thus, by 1988, the head of Walt Disney Studios, Jeffrey Katzenberg, was calling video retailers "Hollywood's ambassadors," and noting that video and theatrical distributors are not as much competitors as "synergistic allies."[104]

To further understand Hollywood's turn-about, as well as its involvement with this new distribution medium, we need to look more carefully at the business of home video. The following sections of this chapter will describe the production, distribution and retailing arrangements for motion pictures on video.

The Business of Home Video: Production

> Network rights . . . ad infinitum . . . video tapes . . . bubble chips, and all other methods of recording, known or unknown.
> Theatrical agent reading rights to victim, Ben Richards,
> in *The Running Man*

Despite claims that there is a wide diversity of videos available, most of the revenues received in the home video industry are from films which have been released first in theaters. Consequently, the rights to video release of films are valuable assets.

Video rights are arranged in at least two ways. First, video distribution can be negotiated after a film has been released in theaters. This has been the case for a large number of films produced before the video era, and early video retailers were anxious to stock such films. Since the video boom, though, the home video rights are typically arranged as part of the initial production/distribution deal. Thus, older films have become more problematic to release on video.[105]

The sale of video rights represents an important potential source of capital for film producers. As noted previously, Standard & Poor's estimate in 1992 was that a new Hollywood film receives 35–40 percent of its revenues from worldwide video release. However, some have claimed that the amount is even higher. *Video Marketing Newsletter* reported in 1986 that 45 percent of all revenue received by a film producer was from the video marketplace.[106] Meanwhile, independent producer Brad Drevey explained, "Home video accounts for 60 percent of our revenues."[107] Another producer noted early in 1989, "The economics of the industry have shifted so that no producer today makes a film without considering the video market – downside *or* upside."[108]

During the first years of home video, an independent producer could maintain control over video rights. But as the majors opened their own video distribution companies, it has become increasingly more difficult for independent producers to arrange distribution deals without including video income.[109] Studios reportedly get 80 percent of video revenues, 20 percent of which goes to negative cost and profits (if any).[110] For films previously made, i.e. from film libraries, video revenues are close to "pure profits," for the costs of making the films have been previously accounted for on a company's balance sheets.[111]

Keeping in mind that many major Hollywood films are produced and distributed by the same companies, we turn to the business of home video distribution.

The Business of Home Video: Distribution

To explain the home video distribution process, we must first identify the players. *Distributors* are middlemen or wholesalers, who buy products from manufacturers and sell to retailers. *Manufacturers* or *suppliers* are companies that own the video rights to titles. They produce videos and market them to wholesalers, distributors and large retailers. *Duplicators* make video copies for suppliers. And *retailers* are businesses that deal exclusively with consumers. Some large retailers may do wholesale business, too. (See figure 6.2 for video industry structure and distribution process.)

There may be some confusion over the term "distributor," or whether one is referring to *home video distributors* – wholesale companies buying from suppliers, selling to retailers – or to *film industry distributors* – companies that distribute and sometimes produce films for release in many markets, but called manufacturers or suppliers in the home video business. In this text, home video distributors will be referred to as wholesalers, and film industry distributors as suppliers or manufacturers.

Since the evolution of a rental system in the early 1980s, the structure of video distribution has operated in one of the following ways:

1 two-step process: suppliers (and duplicators) to wholesalers to retailers and other outlets;

Figure 6.2   Pre-recorded videocassette distribution process

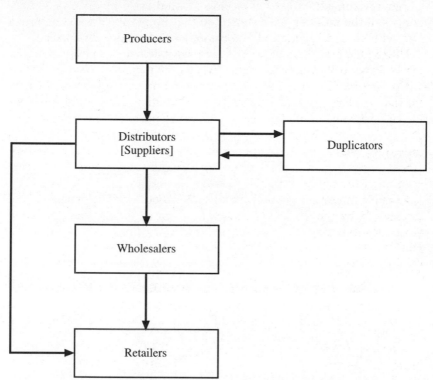

Source: David Waterman, "Prerecorded Home Video and the Distribution of Theatrical Feature Films," in Eli Noam, ed., *Video Media Competition: Regulation, Economics and Technology,* New York: Columbia University Press, 1985.

2 direct distribution: suppliers (and duplicators) directly to retailers and other outlets.

The two-step process dominated the business through the eighties, although suppliers continually considered the second method of direct distribution.[112] One of the compelling reasons was the typical breakdown of returns for each sector of the home video trade around 1984 (see table 6.2). Suppliers already received a relatively large share (28 percent) of revenues, which was claimed to be justified by costs of inventory, operating expenses, advertising and promotion.[113] However, by eliminating the wholesaler's 12 percent cut, suppliers claimed that they could make up some of the "lost" retail revenues denied them by

Table 6.2 Distribution of revenues by industry branch in pre-recorded
software sales, 1984

	Videocassettes @ $50 retail		Videodiscs @ $30 retail	
	%	$	%	$
Producer/copyright holder	12	5.80	12	3.48
Distributor [supplier]	28	14.20	21	6.42
Duplicator	18	9.00	25	7.50
Wholesaler	12	6.00	12	3.60
Retailer	30	15.00	30	9.00
	100%	$50.00	100%	$30.00

Source: David Waterman, "Prerecorded Home Video and the Distribution of
Theatrical Feature Films," in Eli Noam, ed., *Video Media Competition: Regulation,
Economics and Technology*, New York: Columbia University Press, 1985.

the First Sale Doctrine, and bring them closer to the percentage received from theatrical revenues. Wholesale representatives, of course,
pointed out that such a move would lead to the loss of the independent
wholesalers' "entrepreneurial spirit."[114]

The following sections look more closely at these different sectors of
the home video industry.

Program Suppliers/Manufacturers:
(Mostly) the Hollywood Majors

Program suppliers/manufacturers are companies with video rights to a
title. However, a large part of the business is dominated by companies
affiliated with, in joint ventures with, or subsidiaries of, the Hollywood
majors. In other words, the major video suppliers are the major Hollywood distributors.

Early in the short history of home video, the rights for a film's video
release were "up for grabs" and often pre-sold as a method of financing.
A title could be licensed to a sales agent or manufacturer for an
advance and a percentage of wholesale or retail revenues generated by
the product.[115]

Not too surprisingly, as revenue from home video sales and rentals increased, the fees for video release increased as well. In 1984, *Silkwood* set an early record, with video distribution rights selling for $1.5 million. Embassy then bought *Cotton Club* for $4.7 million, and *Prizzi's Honor* video rights went for $4.5 million.[116] For a while, the average price range remained around $3–4 million, although blockbusters were another story. For instance, (worldwide) distribution rights for *The Empire Strikes Back* were sold to CBS/Fox Video for $12 million. (*American Film* reported $14 million). But prices gradually increased for all new films. As examples, in 1987 *Willow* received $15 million from RCA/Columbia, while *Baron Munchausen* sold for about $8 million.[117]

As the market expanded, video rights to groups of films quickly became the norm. For instance, an early deal involved MGM/UA selling rights to Cannon for various films for $25–30 million. Meanwhile, Embassy Home Entertainment paid $10–15 million for over 100 titles, while Prism Entertainment bought 70 films for $1.5 million, and Twentieth Century Fox bought rights to Blackhawk Films.

As Austin Furst of Vestron explained in 1987, "Today, bidding for the rights to distribute theatrical films on videocassettes is like eight hungry men bidding on a TV dinner." His company made some tidy profits on films such as *Butterfly,* which grossed $2 million in video sales but had only cost Vestron $100,000 for the rights. A new company like Vestron could survive at first because there was little competition for these video rights. However, as more independent companies joined the business, the studios started their own subsidiaries for video distribution and the competition became tougher.[118]

The potential for enormous profits may seem possible from video release of a major motion picture, as customers pay over and over to rent the same cassette, and typical manufacturing costs for cassettes and discs run at around $7.50–$10.[119] However, as mentioned previously, the suppliers have been restricted in the USA by the First Sales Doctrine, limiting them to the amount gained from the initial sale of videocassettes or discs to wholesalers or retailers, or selling directly to consumers via mass merchants, etc.

Nevertheless, these sales tend to add up quite nicely. For instance, if a videocassette sells for $89.95 retail, a supplier may sell it to a wholesaler for around $56. The costs of the cassette itself, duplication, and marketing are deducted, leaving approximately $40 for the supplier.[120] If 200,000 units are sold in this manner, the company nets around $8 million. However, many big films easily sell over a million copies. In addition, the suppliers were raising prices for A-films at the beginning of the nineties, meaning higher prices paid by wholesalers. Before 1986, prices were generally $79.98. With the release of *Aliens* in 1986, the suppliers charged around $89.98. But by mid-1990, prices were hovering around $99.95.[121]

Another profit incentive for suppliers is the amount paid (or *not* paid) in royalties for video release. One anonymous agent told *Variety* in 1990 that "the studios collectively refuse to consider home video revenues as profit when calculating percentage payments to actors. Instead, all the studios put a 20 percent royalty from homevid into the profit pot." Some actors were trying to negotiate a percentage of video sales, pointing out that these revenues were often boosted by a star's name.[122]

Thus, the amount received from home video has contributed handsomely to the Hollywood majors' revenues. In 1980, only $20 million, or 1 percent of the industry's total revenues, were gleaned from home video sales. In 1983, that amount grew to $625 million, or 14 percent of total revenues.

By 1986, the president of CBS/Fox Video was admitting, "This industry is prone to obscene profits."[123] And the next year, program suppliers reportedly received 18 percent more, or $3.04 billion (41 percent) of the total home video revenues of $7.46 billion.[124] (Although another source reported that the Hollywood studios received nearly $1.5 billion from selling movies on videocassette the same year.[125]) By the end of the decade, however, the rental and sale of videocassettes was claimed to provide nearly 50 percent of the studios' total revenues, or $4.75 billion in 1991, and another $5.3 billion in 1992.[126]

In the early years, home video was described as a new competitive arena, attracting new players and companies. The National Association of Video Distributors listed 31 members in 1987.[127] A company like Vestron could survive quite well distributing films obtained relatively cheaply or "small" films. In 1986, Vestron Pictures announced that it would produce and distribute ten pictures per year, plus 18 low budget films at $2 million each.[128]

However, the field has since narrowed to a smaller number of key players. As the industry developed, fewer stores needed to buy new stock (or "library material") and consumers apparently became more interested in major hits; although it also is possible to argue that consumers' interests were fueled by distributors' and retailers' emphasis on hits. (See the following sections on wholesaling and retailing.) Consequently, a hits-oriented business favored the major studios, and many of the smaller companies (like Vestron) started having trouble.[129]

Top suppliers in 1988 included Paramount, CBS/Fox, Disney, Warner, RCA/Columbia, MCA, HBO, Vestron, MGM/UA, Orion Media Home Entertainment, International Video Entertainment, Lorimar, Nelson, New World, and Virgin Vision.[130] Warner Home Video reported

Figure 6.3   Supplier market share of rental-priced product, 1991 (in percentage of units sold)

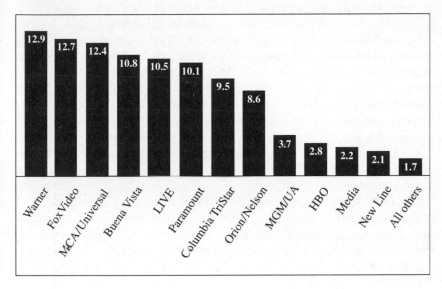

Source: *Video Store Magazine*, in *1993 International Television & Video Almanac*, New York: Quigley Publishing, 1993, p. 663.

worldwide revenues of $400 million in 1987.[131] By 1991, though, Warner received $680.6 million from the North American market alone.[132] Disney led all companies in 1992 with sales of $1.1 billion.[133]

By the end of the decade, the video business was moving more towards the model set by the recording industry, with the majors handling sales for independent production companies. For example, in 1987, Warner Home Video bought Lorimar, and also made arrangements to distribute Cannon's films on video. Orion arranged to handle Nelson Entertainment films.[134]

Thus, the majors have mostly squeezed out the independent video suppliers. In the early years of home video, seven of the major Hollywood film distributors held over 90 percent of the market share for home videos (Twentieth, Paramount, Warner, MCA, MGM, Columbia, and Disney). By 1986, eleven top major and independent program suppliers received 91 percent of the aggregate dollar volume and 86 percent of unit volume.[135] And while the percentages have shifted over the years, the majors have generally held substantial portions of the business. (See figure 6.3 for market shares of suppliers in 1991.)

Some of the remaining independent companies moved to producing their own films, both for theatrical and video release. Vestron formed a theatrical division in 1986, and succeeded for a while, especially with their big hit, *Dirty Dancing*, which generated over $20 million in gross retail revenues for licensing products alone. But ultimately the company was unable to compete with the Hollywood big boys. As industry analyst Harold Vogel observed, "It is difficult to reap the full benefits of production except for major studios. It is hard to attract the talent to make the films. And even if you make films, it is hard to get the best movie theaters for the needed amount of time."[136] By 1987 Vestron had started laying off employees, and it eventually went under in 1991.[137] Other companies attempting production in the early nineties were Media Home Entertainment, Academy, and Vidmark.[138]

Yet other independent companies aligned with the major producing companies through either individual deals or mergers. For instance, in 1986 International Video Entertainment (IVE) arranged for the video distribution of Carolco's films by providing at least $6 million towards each film's production.[139]

Duplication Companies

Film to video transfers   Before duplication companies make the millions of copies of cassettes, a video master must be prepared of a film. Initially, films were transferred to tape by simply aiming a video camera at a movie screen. However, later techniques have been far more sophisticated film to video transfers. The quality has varied, as some video transfers produce noticeably inferior versions of original films. As *Video Review* magazine has pointed out, problems can include "poor color, scenes that are too dark or too bright, characters cut out of the frame when the widescreen movie image is cut down to fit the TV screen, tinny audio and mangled sound effects."[140]

A good transfer job, however, can cost as much as $20,000 per film, and uses either a special low-contrast print of the film or the interpositive and a flying spot scanner, such as the Rank Cintel (discussed in chapter 3). The process not only involves adjusting color and brightness, but fitting a widescreen film image with a 1.66:1 or 1.85:1 or 2.35:1 (CinemaScope) aspect ratio, into a basically square TV image with a 1.33:1 aspect ratio. When wide-angle shots are converted to TV images, a video transfer specialist either adds cuts or uses a process called pan-

and-scan, in other words, panning to another part of the screen. "When clumsily done, pan-and-scan moves are obvious to the discerning viewer; the sudden, lateral movement of the image looks artificial compared to a real camera pan."[141] A good transfer can be time-consuming and complicated. For instance, the mine chase scene in *Indiana Jones and the Temple of Doom* required more than 700 corrections.

Another option is to prepare a letterbox version of a film, which presents a smaller image (usually masked at the top and bottom of the screen) and less detail, but the complete image of the original film. Letterboxed versions, however, are less common than pan-and-scan cassettes.

During the video transfer process, the audio track receives close attention, too, as technicians may go back to the original audio mix for a film. The process also may include adding foreign language tracks for foreign release.

The result is a video and audio master, from which one-inch sub-masters are prepared which are used to produce cassette copies. The sub-masters also may include closed captions, and most often, an anti copying device which prevents tapes from being copied. The typical process used by most distributors at the end of the eighties was the Macrovision encoder, although at times the process was bypassed because of the additional time or expense required.[142]

The sub-masters, then, are sent to duplicating companies, where millions of copies are made on half-inch video cassettes.

Video duplicating companies While a few new companies have entered this sector, companies that have traditionally been involved in laboratory work in Hollywood have prevailed. But a wave of con-solidation took place toward the end of the decade. Technicolor was purchased in 1988 by London-based Carlton Communications, making the company the largest duplicator in the world. The British company, which is primarily involved in television production and post-produc-tion, also owned Modern Video, the largest high-speed duplicator in the USA, plus European facilities. Meanwhile, Rank Video Services bought Bell & Howell/Columbia/Paramount, and Video Technology Services (mostly in Europe). Thus, Carlton-owned Technicolor and Rank con-trolled 50–60 percent of the total duplicating capacity in the USA.[143]

Initially, several problems in the duplicating process held up produc-tion. The first was the process itself. Although master copies operated on a master unit controlling slave machines (sometimes, thousands) to mass-produce cassettes, copying was done in "real time," meaning a machine was necessary for each copy made. The second problem stemmed from the first: low duplicating capacity increased costs. In 1985, for instance, only 90 million units could be duplicated. By 1991, volume had increased to 300 to 310 million, and high-speed duplication processes plus features duplicated in the EP (extended play) mode made it possible to speed up production and lower costs. Nevertheless, by 1993 most duplication was in real time, using the SP (standard play) mode.[144]

Wholesalers

Wholesalers (also called distributors in home video) distribute videos for the manufacturer to the retailer. Wholesalers solicit a network of video dealers, then place orders with manufacturers, and deliver the tapes. The wholesalers sell to retailers at around 63 percent of suggested retail price.[145] In 1990, the wholesale price increased, with some releases priced at about $63 wholesale, before discounts.[146] Retailers are usually extended 30–60 days' credit by wholesalers, although retailers may typically need 60–90 days to recoup investment through rentals.

By 1988, margins for wholesalers were said to be 2.7–2.9 percent.[147] By 1990, 5–10 percent of video sales went to dealers.[148] In 1988, $2.1–2.2 billion worth of videocassettes were reportedly distributed through the traditional home video distribution network.[149]

Distribution activities are usually concentrated within specific geographic regions, although there are no exclusive geographic rights or domination over local areas. And generally, suppliers do not grant exclusive selling rights to a wholesaler for major films. One observer noted in 1983, "The result is that wholesaling is a free-for-all; firms compete intensely for orders from widely dispersed retailers."[150] However, in 1987, RCA/Columbia made industry news by restricting its distributors to geographic regions.

By the end of the 1980s, a small share of the business was direct distribution, but mostly to department stores and chains. Rack-jobbing companies place videos on a consignment basis in these outlets. The Handleman Company and Lieberman Enterprises have dominated the rack-jobbing business for a number of years.[151]

In addition to rack-jobbers, the threat of major manufacturers selling directly to larger retail stores also worries the wholesaler, as mentioned previously. This activity could lead to other changes in wholesaling, such as discounting product and wholesalers taking an even smaller profit margin.

During 1988, the distribution sector was shaken by several suppliers cutting back (without notice) on the number of wholesalers/distributors they used. (Examples: Fox had 104 distributors in 1980, and cut back to 14 in 1988. Other studios made similar moves.) The majors called it an attempt at more efficiency, although others hinted that it might be a prelude to direct distribution.[152] Certainly, the majors saved money by cutting distribution expenses. But most agreed that it was also a "muscle-flexing exercise aimed at asserting control over the way distributors do business."[153] While suppliers explained that it was a "natural evolution" of the business, the president of one company affected by the cuts expressed his opinion of suppliers accordingly: "They have all the attributes of a dog, except loyalty."[154] As explained in *Billboard*: "Industry insiders say the cutbacks are being engineered in an effort to pressure distributors into selling more of a given manufacturer's line. When distributors are axed, those remaining in the fold may be more inclined to go the extra yard."[155]

By the beginning of the nineties, many studios were directly distributing their cassettes to their large retail accounts, and very often using direct distribution in many foreign markets.[156] Not only have there been consequences for wholesalers, but retailers have experienced more inconvenience and higher prices.

Around the same time that the suppliers were dropping wholesalers, several large wholesaling companies also cut the number of independent producers they handled, concentrating on the major program suppliers' products.[157] For instance, the largest distributor, Commtron Corp., dropped over 30 suppliers and identified their remaining clients – primarily, the majors and a few others. While retailers worried about price increases and the quality of service, the action was only one in a number of moves indicating the growth of a "hits orientation" by wholesalers and retailers.[158]

In attempting to resist the dominance of the suppliers, retailers and wholesalers initiated partial boycotts, ordering only A-titles, and neglecting B-titles and C-titles (very often, independent productions). Their strategy is claimed to have succeeded, as some wholesalers were reinstated and territorial restrictions eliminated. However, the results also may have reinforced the emphasis on hits and undermined independent production. Already by 1988, those films grossing over $10 million at the box office (almost always distributed by the major studios) represented 70 percent of wholesale video revenues.[159]

In addition, when the market for B titles was specifically affected, the major suppliers began a form of block booking. As one distributor explained, "What they are really saying is: 'for the privilege of carrying our major titles, you've also got to carry all the other shit we put out.'"[160]

So the video battles continued. Although it might have happened without the suppliers' cuts, the wholesale sector of the industry became even further concentrated towards the end of the eighties. At one time there were over 100 video wholesalers in the USA, with around 20 major wholesalers accounting for half of the business. By 1983, there were 20–30, with the number "steadily declining."[161] At the 1989 National Association of Video Distributors meeting, 23 distributor members (and 35 program supplier members) were present.[162]

In the mid-1980s, Commtron represented 21 percent of the market, while Sound Video and Metro Video captured 5 percent each. By July 1988, Commtron was still the largest wholesaler. Ingram started by distributing to specialty outlets and bookstores. But by the beginning of the nineties, Ingram had bought Home Entertainment, and Major Video Concepts (the fourth largest wholesaler) and Video Trend (the fifth largest) had merged.

Thus, home video wholesaling represents yet another sector of the media business which began as a relatively differentiated activity, but became concentrated rather quickly.

The Business of Video Software: Retailing

The growth of video retailing The most visible indication of a home video "revolution" has been the appearance of video stores and video-cassettes for sale or rent in a wide variety of other business establishments. The number of videos rented or sold has steadily grown; the average weekly transactions in July 1987 stood at 64 million, and by July 1988 at over 74 million.[163]

The business of video retailing has gone through several stages. A period of direct sales at high prices was followed by one of mostly rentals. Then, with lower prices for direct sales (or sell-throughs), a mix of sales and rentals evolved. In the early nineties, however, the suppliers were pushing more and more towards sell-through, by continuing to offer low-priced cassettes for as little as $14.95, yet increasing the price to retailers for rental copies. In this way, it has been argued that the Hollywood majors will be able to gain more power over the video speciality stores, where rental revenues are beyond their reach.[164]

Industry reports for 1987 indicated a 4.3 percent increase in sales, accounting for 18.9 percent of total volume. In other words, rentals still accounted for 81.1 percent of the total business of video software. Sales represented 14.6 percent in 1986, and 18.9 percent in 1987.[165] However, the estimates differ according to the source: by 1988, the ratio was either 65 percent rentals to 35 percent sales (*Channels* magazine), 85 percent rentals to 15 percent sales (Video Software Dealers Association), or 92.4 percent rentals to 7.6 percent sales (*Video Store* and Paul Kagan Associates).[166] (See figure 6.1 again for *Video Store Magazine's* estimates.)

It seemed clear, though, that sell-though activity was increasing rapidly at the end of the eighties. In 1988, 60 percent of the 150 million cassettes sold to retailers were for sell-through. By 1990, 75 percent of the 270 million cassettes were for direct sales, and for the first time, sell-through exceeded rentals in revenues going to suppliers.[167]

In addition, retailers often sell their extra rental tapes after the initial heavy rental period, either to consumers or to tape brokers who sell them to other stores. Half of the tapes sold by retailers in 1988 were these used cassettes.[168]

The distinction between rentals and sales is important for both supplier and retailer. Suppliers' profits come from sales, either directly to customers or to retailers, who then rent to consumers. For a big hit, the supplier gains only from the initial sale of the cassette; the retailer, after expenses are covered, gains from each transaction. One account claims that typical retailer profit margins are 26–30 percent on major releases.[169]

Video stores   Early video stores were opened mostly in large cities and relied to a great extent on the sale of pornographic material. Dan Moret has compared video stores to the early nickelodeons, noting that both were "equally disreputable in both entertainment and clientele," with "a predilection for pornography and pugilism" similar to other new communication technologies.[170]

But the range of content available on cassettes expanded, as did the number of video stores. Since 1986, there have been over 25,000 video stores in the USA representing the "core of home video."[171] (See figure 6.4 for growth of video retail outlets since 1979.) In 1985, the average store made 1,000 transactions each week, for a total of $3,300, with rentals accounting for 98 percent of the activity. While sales transactions represented only 2 percent of all transactions, they generated 21 percent of total revenue. While rental prices may have started higher, by 1992 the average was around $2.62 (for a new release), although

Figure 6.4   Number of US video retail outlets, 1980–92

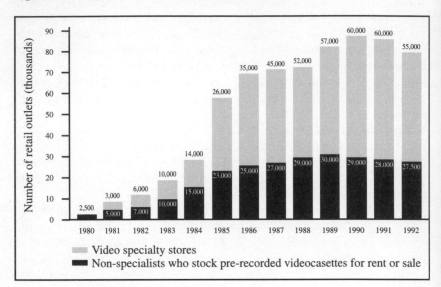

Source: Video Store Magazine, in *1993 International Television & Video Almanac*, New York: Quigley Publishing, 1993, p. 664.

prices vary widely depending on the time and place of the rental and what tape is rented.[172]

Although there is great variation between outlets, the average number of titles per store has varied over the years. In 1988, it generally ranged from 1,500 to 3,000. By 1992, the average rental inventory was nearly 6,000 units.[173] A "superstore," however, may carry as many as 15,000 titles.

One of the major issues for the business is the question of how many different videos a store carries, or *breadth of copy*. Another issue is the number of copies of a specific video, or *depth of copy*. Of course, suppliers argue that retailers do not carry enough copies and consequently lose customers. Retailers want to have enough copies of a hit available for customers, without getting stuck with too many copies of less popular films.[174] X-rated cassettes are still important sources of revenue for at least 75 percent of all video stores, yet they may not be as prominently displayed as in the past.[175]

While some video stores still charge membership fees, the practice was more prevalent in the early days of home video as a way for retailers to gain necessary working capital and customer loyalty.

At first opening a video store was relatively inexpensive, with an investment of about $20,000 required during the early 1980s. By the early 1990s, however, franchises were anywhere from $140,000 to $185,000. Blockbuster Video stores were considerably higher, with franchise deals at around $535,000 if stores were purchased in groups.[176] But there are payoffs for these investments: the average store in the top 100 video store chains received revenues of over $400,000 annually in 1989. Smaller stores, however, made considerably less, with the average gross annual revenue for all stores reported at $192,000 in 1992.[177]

In 1988, 60 percent of the stores in one survey were computerized.[178] Special computer software and hardware designed for video stores was particularly important in the attempt by the studios to introduce pay-per-transaction. Such a system, however, can be an expensive addition, with individual computers costing as much as $65,000.[179]

Another source of revenue for video stores is the rental of VCRs, which at one point generated around 10 percent of an average outlet's total revenues. Video games have been added to many stores' inventory, and game rentals alone accounted for 8% of the total revenue for video retailers in 1992. Video stores also have experienced some diversification, selling popcorn, candy, other food products, sports cards and publications, as well as offering video duplication, film-to-tape transfers, and photo developing. According to *Video Store*, 84 percent of video retailers offered at least one of these products or services by 1988, with these activities overall contributing around 7 percent of total revenues for an average store. Compact discs are another commonly found product sold in video stores and involve some of the previously mentioned video wholesalers.[180]

Video store chains   While the independent or "mom and pop" video store characterized the early video industry, many of these retailers experienced increased competition from video chains, mass merchandising outlets, and convenience stores in the late eighties and early nineties. During 1987, hundreds of shops were reported to have failed, only to be replaced by chain stores, thus keeping the total numbers of outlets relatively stable.[181]

By the mid-eighties, the video retailing sector started showing distinct signs of horizontal concentration. Regional chains and franchise operations multiplied, with the advantages of increased buying power, rotation of inventory, shared advertising costs, and direct dealings with suppliers. Surveys by industry trade publications indicated that while video store chains paid less for cassettes, they typically charged the highest rental fees.[182]

Table 6.3 Top ten US video retail chains, 1992

Company	No. of outlets		1992 revenue ($m)
	1992	1991	
1 Blockbuster	2,100	1,870	1,600.0
2 West Coast Video	516	510	157.9
3 Tower Video	77	69	70.0
4 The Video Connection	100	94	34.2
5 Video Central	35	34	34.1
6 Palmer Video	80	83	32.4
7 Mr Movies	91	86	26.7
8 Movie Gallery	54	54	24.5
9 Video Update	63	63	22.5
10 RKO Warner Video	19	30	19.0

Source: "The Top 100: An Annual Ranking of the Largest Video Retail Chains," *Video Store Magazine*, December 1992.

In 1987, chains and franchises represented 36 percent of all video speciality stores, with many chains continuing to grow.[183] During the following years, however, there was even further concentration, as the publisher of the trade journal *Video Software Dealer* explained:

> This business was built on the shoulders of "mom and pop." But look how they have changed. In 1982, the typical retailer owned one outlet. The 1988 VSDA study pegs the average "independent" with 6.8 stores. But just as the growth curve appeared to be peaking, the money-men discovered video retailing. Cash is pouring into the retail sectors from all corners. Investment bankers, cable TV operators, theatrical exhibitors, even studios, are investing in what is commonly called "the final frontier" of the (film) business.[184]

Video Store Magazine's annual Video Store 100 survey reported in December 1988 that the top ten chains in the USA represented 67 percent of the top 100 revenues; by 1992, the top ten received over 79 percent. Furthermore, the top three chains produced over 18 percent of the total national revenue in 1989.[185] (See table 6.3.)

As video franchising accelerated, the costs of opening and operating a store grew as well. In 1988, *The Franchise Annual* listed initial investments for some chains as high as $250,000–650,000. Franchise fees averaged $10,000–20,000, although the larger chains' fees were higher (Blockbuster's fee was $35,000). Royalty fees (paid to the franchising company, of course) ranged from 4 to 7 percent of revenues, not including mandatory advertising which averaged 1 to 2 percent. As the trade magazine, *Billboard*, concluded, "Video franchising with the big boys is no longer a poor man's game."[186]

Early chains included Atkinson's Video Station with 462 stores in 1982, National Video, which owned as many as 693 stores, and Adventureland with 565 stores by 1986, but bankrupt by 1988. The same year, the president of the Video Software Distributors Association (VSDA) called the dominant companies in video retailing "The Magnificent Seven," referring to Blockbuster, Erol's, Wherehouse, National, RKO, West Coast and Palmer. Since then, however, Erol's as well as numerous other chains have been purchased by Blockbuster and National has merged with West Coast.

Video McDonald's   But the leader of the video store pack at the beginning of the nineties was Blockbuster Video. Blockbuster Entertainment Corporation's first store was opened in 1985. Only one year and a half later the Fort Lauderdale-based company owned or had franchised 800 stores, and it has been growing steadily. By 1992, there were over 2,100 Blockbuster stores. (The next largest chain – West Coast Video – had only around 500 franchises.) There is no doubt that Blockbuster dominated the business by 1990. The company received $1.25 billion in revenues out of $2.3 billion received by the top 100 largest US video chains.[188] The company reported that their earnings had increased by 30 percent during 1991, when they controlled 12 percent of the rental market.[189]

By 1989, a Blockbuster franchise could cost as much as $78,000, with 7 percent royalties on revenues paid to Blockbuster, plus other expenses.[190] While individual franchises added to the numbers, Blockbuster bought out several competitors: Major Video's 127 stores in 1988 and Erol's 200 stores (for $30 million) in 1990. The company also attracted some big time investors as franchisers. Both TCI/United Cable and Cox Cable have invested in Blockbuster stores. (In addition, Cox bought 1.3 percent of Blockbuster's stock in September 1988.) Thus, in many markets across the USA, the same owners operate the local cable outlet, theaters and video outlets. The Blockbuster phenomenon also moved into global markets, with stores in Japan, the UK, Australia, Mexico, Ireland and Spain during the early 1990s. In 1992, the company reported 1,000 international outlets which generated $400,000 each.[191]

Plate 3 The Leader of the Pack Blockbuster Video is the overwhelming leader among video chains in the US, with $1.6 billion in revenues and over 2,100 franchises in 1992. Blockbuster also has diversified its activities, investing in cable, sports teams (the Florida Marlins), as well as sponsoring media events such as the Blockbuster Bowl. As indicated in the photo above, some individual video stores also have diversified beyond video-cassette rentals and sales, and often carry video games and other merchandise or services. *Photograph by Carlos R. Calderon*

At the end of the eighties, Blockbuster indulged in a huge promotional push with nationwide television advertising, sponsorship of the Block-buster Bowl (an end-of-the-year collegiate football game), exclusive rights to Major League Baseball videos and 1992 Summer Olympics on video. In 1991, Blockbuster's President, Wayne Huizenga, obtained a major league baseball franchise for Florida. The expansion team, named the Florida Marlins, played its first season in 1993.

The Blockbuster style has been similar to the successful McDonald's formula for quick food outlets: standardization and consistency. Yet, some of the company's policies have attracted harsh criticism. In 1989, Blockbuster's corporate management made headlines when they decided their stores would not carry the controversial film, *The Last Temptation of Christ*. Other chains offered the film to the public, as well as their opinion of Blockbuster. As Moret noted, "In an industry in which the motto has been, 'Watch what you want, when you want,' Blockbuster was roundly criticized for its refusal to carry the critically acclaimed film."[192] Blockbuster further damaged its reputation when announcing that their stores would not carry X-rated films. Then in January 1991, the company banned movies with NC-17 ratings, announcing that they would destroy those films in stock which carried the rating. The MPAA reacted, accusing the company of prior censorship.

Meanwhile, *Video Business* reported that Blockbuster had attempted to get exclusive deals for films from suppliers, another move that further illustrates the lessening of competition in the video industry.

Mass merchants Traditional video stores have increasingly had to compete with non-specialty outlets and mass merchants in the rental business, as well as in sell-through activity, which has been favored by distributors. The phenomenon caught on rapidly as drug stores, convenience stores, gas stations, grocery stores and supermarkets started renting or selling videos. One estimate claimed that there were 20,300 non-specialty stores selling videos by 1984.[193] By 1989, alternative outlets – that is, other than video stores – received 30 percent of rental revenues, but 70 percent of sell-through revenues.[194]

The real competition developed when rack-jobbers started placing videos on the shelves of discount and mass merchants, such as Target, Federated, Fedco, Sears, and Kmart, as well as supermarkets, drug stores, and sometimes even video stores. (Rack-jobbers are businesses that monitor product on stores' shelves, replacing titles when necessary.) In 1984, U-Haul added video to its 600 outlets, and in 1986, Southland Corp. added video rentals at 2,000 of its 7-Eleven stores, becoming one of the largest video retailers in the USA at the time.[195] By 1985, 25 percent of the mass-merchandise discount stores were carrying videos.[196] By the end of the decade, 9,000 out of the 11,800 mass merchants in the country were stocking videos, which attracted the largest share of revenue from sell-through videos ($480 million) in 1987.[197] Table 6.4 illustrates the importance of mass merchants such as Kmart and Wal-Mart in overall video revenue, for 1991 and 1992.

In fact, a new breed of rack-jobber evolved just to service stores such as 7-Elevens. Video rental centers were installed and operated by the convenience store jobbers, who either paid rent to the store or shared a percentage of the video rentals. The convenience store centers offered

Table 6.4 Top ten US retail chains ranked by total estimated pre-recorded video revenue

		1992 revenue ($m)	1991 revenue ($m)
1	Blockbuster Video	1,511.0	1,267.0
2	Kmart	211.1	180.0
3	Musicland Group	175.0	165.0
4	Wal-Mart	165.7	144.0
5	Wherehouse Entertainment	151.0	146.0
6	West Coast Video	140.5	132.5
7	Sam's	72.1	56.0
8	Price Club	65.1	50.0
9	Jumbo Video	63.2	51.2
10	Target	53.7	46.5

Source: *Video Week*, December 21, 1992.

intense competition to other video outlets for a while, not only because of their size, but because of their focus on hits, lower rental prices and low overheads. However, the market share for convenience stores declined towards the end of the decade to only 5 percent in 1989, perhaps attributable to the small number of titles carried by these outlets. By late 1989, 11,000 out of the 60,000 convenience stores in the USA carried videos.[198]

By 1988, wholesalers were complaining to suppliers about preferential treatment for rack-jobbers and mass merchants, who were said to be receiving better prices and more lead time. Eventually, however, some of the wholesalers started expanding into rack-jobbing, due to supplier pressures to get into sell-through, as well as to find new sources of profit.[199]

Rack-jobbers increasingly represent important players in the home video field. Video Channels is owned by the Rank Organization (also involved in video duplication) and is also involved in audio operations, due to its purchase of Olympia, an audio–video rack-jobbing company.

In the early 1990s, the largest rack-jobbing outfit was the Handleman Company, which also owned Video Treasures (a sublicensing company), Video Cassette Duplicating Corp., Video Loaders Inc., Video Cassette Sales Inc., Media Home Entertainment and a video store. Thus, Handleman represented a fully integrated video corporation.[200]

Meanwhile, supermarkets have expanded their video sections, as managers have been more than pleased with the profit margins from video rental activity and customers appreciate the convenience of incorporating video rentals with other shopping tasks. Promotional tie-ins between film and food companies (such as Disney and Nabisco) also were appreciated by store managers: "Linking such products increases their visibility to consumers, creating a stronger draw that builds super-market business."[201] (See Chapter 8 for more on tie-ins.)

Nearly 45 percent of the supermarkets in the country carried videos by the end of the decade. In 1988, these stores reported $650 million in rental revenues, and were expected to exceed $850 million the next year.[202]

Record stores The enormous success of Michael Jackson's *Thriller* tape around 1982 prompted nearly 2,500 record stores to sell music videos. By the end of the decade, around 77 percent of the music stores in the country carried videos. In 1985, video sales represented 62.2 percent, while video rentals were 33.8 percent of record stores' total video dollar volume.[203]

The competition from large record chains was especially strong, with a company like Wherehouse Entertainment, for instance, producing $118 million in video revenues for 1989. The advantage is having stores that represent complete home entertainment centers, selling audio and video products.

Other outlets A wide range of other businesses carry videocassettes, either for sale or rent. During the 1980s, relatively few book stores stocked videos (1,800 out of 15,000), with direct sales involved and virtually no rentals. By the 1990s, however, most of the larger book chains sold videocassettes. However, one video entrepreneur's predic-tion that half of the future home video business would be in bookstores had certainly not come true.[204]

In 1983, over 7,000 merchandising outlets, such as toy stores, sporting goods stores and spots, and exercise locations sold videos. By 1986, there were over 20,000, however mostly speciality videos were featured. Another outlet for video distribution was through direct mail retailers or video clubs, such as CBS Video Club. By 1987, these sources rep-resented $161 million in sales (third highest share in sell-through activity).

The truly automated video outlet, or video vending machine, also was introduced in the 1980s, allowing consumers to choose a tape from several hundred possibilities and pay by credit card. But, despite predic-tions of many hundreds of machines operating by the 1990s, only a few hundred were installed during the late eighties.[205]

The Business of Home Video:
Marketing and Sales

An important advantage for home video's ability to compete with other media is the great product diversity it offers. . . . Home video brings you not only *Star Wars* but *Casablanca* and *I Walked with a Zombie.*
David Waterman, "Prerecorded Home Video and the Distribution of Theatrical Feature Films" in Eli Noam, ed., *Video Media Competition*

Freedom of Choice – the control of one's own viewing habits – has been the major impact of home video on the leisure-time industry in America. Owners of videocassette recorders can view what they want when they want and are no longer subject to the programming schedules of the television networks and cable stations.
1987 International Television and Video Almanac

We have failed as an industry to diversify our product in the mind of the consumer. What we have, essentially, is what we started with – a movie-rental business.
"Orion Chief Predicts Tape 'Ice Age,'" *Billboard*

More movies Despite the claim that home video is revolutionizing America's viewing habits, the most common type of cassette rented or purchased is a movie. A Hollywood movie. They probably account for about 90 percent of tape rentals and 60 percent of tape purchases.[206]

By the end of the 1980s, an average store bought 27 new titles per month at an average price of $62.25 (less if the retailer owned more than one store). But it was estimated that around 77 percent of the movies ordered each month by video store owners were A-titles. As one owner explained, "First choice will be to buy 10 or 20 of the hot new A-titles like *Rambo*, *Ghostbusters*, or *Back to the Future*."[207]

Another study indicated that 56 percent of a video store's inventory will never have appeared at a local theater, and 40 percent may have never appeared on television; however, A-titles still accounted for 75 percent of videos rented by 1987.[208] Another estimate is that retailers make 80 percent of their revenues from hit films which comprise only 20 percent of their stock. While some attribute the growth of A-titles' popularity to viewer sophistication, many industry observers have noted the increasing interest by the entire home video industry in ordering and pushing big films. One indication is the increase in advertising for these titles – the video industry's expenditure on television advertising increased 70 percent in 1990 – from $25 million in 1989 to $42 million.[209]

Figure 6.5   Percentage of unit home video sales by genre

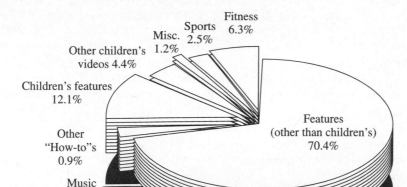

Source: Video Store Magazine, in *1992 International Television & Video Almanac,* New York: Quigley Publishing, 1992.

So, the retail end of the business has evolved as a "hit-obsessed market," with video stores, especially, stocking and promoting hit movies over other titles,[210] and the smaller, non-blockbuster film facing the problem of lack of exposure in many video outlets.[211]

The popularity of certain film genres has varied slightly over the years. (Figure 6.5 represents genres' popularity in 1992.) Interestingly, there has been a decline in the attraction of adult videos (13 percent in 1985) and how-to-videos (3 percent in 1985)[212] Stores also may carry foreign-language programming, especially Spanish-language tapes. And while a mix of genres by percentage is recommended by video consultants, decisions about which films and how many to order are most often made according to the success of a film in its theatrical release.[213]

Individual tape sales   The blockbuster mentality has been boosted by the increasing number of cassettes sold of individual titles. In 1983, any cassette that sold over 25,000 was considered a hit. A few years later, 200,000 copies sold represented a popular title. In June 1986, MCA shipped 425,000 copies of *Rambo II,* but demand was not as big as expected. Meanwhile, *Back to the Future* shipped 350,000 copies and

435,000 additional were ordered. By 1991, though, records were still being broken, as *Dances with Wolves* sold 649,000 units, while *Terminator 2* sold 714,000 units. But these numbers seem to be totally eclipsed by big blockbusters' sell-through records, such as *E.T.* and *Bambi*, each of which sold 10 million copies, and *Beauty and The Beast*, which had sold over 14 million copies by the beginning of 1993.[214]

Another indication of the blockbuster mentality was the estimate in 1991 that a typical blockbuster which had grossed over $100 million in theaters, would sell more than nine copies per video retailer. Films which typically received less than $5 million during a theatrical run would usually ship fewer than two copies.[215]

It is interesting to note that the awards for top-selling tapes, as well as the "official" tabulation of tape sales, are actually within the realm of the record industry. While lists of top-selling and top-rented cassettes are compiled by the record industry's trade publication, *Billboard*, the Recording Industry of America Association awards top-selling cassettes. Gold certification is awarded to theatrical tapes which sell 75,000 units or generate $3 million at retail prices. Platinum awards are for tapes that sell 150,000 units or generate $6 million retail. Non-theatrical tapes (not in theatrical release) receive gold for 30,000 units or $1.5 million retail, and platinum for 60,000 units or $2 million retail.[216]

Marketing strategies   Video entrepreneurs have been given advice that other businesses have long realized: "Marketing is creating a consumer need and then filling it through a particular video program."[217]

Marketing strategies for video involve all three sectors of the industry: manufacturing, wholesale, and retail. The program supplier markets to wholesalers, who in turn market to video retailers, who market to consumers. While promotional material is generated at every level, efforts sometimes overlap, i.e. the program supplier may send material to the retailer, even though the wholesaler makes the sale.

Marketing techniques include special promotions and sale incentives, trade and consumer press coverage, trade and consumer press advertising, point-of-purchase (POP) materials (in-store promotion, posters, banners, give-aways), video trailers, and trade conventions.

Merchandising and tie-ins with other products have intensified for films in general, as will be discussed in Chapter 8, but also for video release. As *Channels* magazine pointed out: "In 1988, the studios moved increasingly toward diversified marketing techniques, adapting much from the packaged-goods companies and in fact tying in with beverage, snack and prepared-food marketers to reach the studios' target audiences." Examples were Disney with Coca-Cola, P&G and McDonald's; Vestron and Nestlé; Nelson and Chun King, Tsingtao; MCA and Pepsi.[218]

The Threat of Piracy

For the Big Boys, the loss of control over video retailing was felt for a while, at least, to be one of the most harmful aspects of home video. However, some in the industry argued that the predicted harm from home video was greatest in the area of copyright protection. As Sidney Sheinberg, who led MCA's suit against Sony, commented:

> With the benefit of hindsight, I think it has been even more harmful than we thought. The harm is not only in the copying of material, which deprives us of subsequent potential revenues – all the arguments that we made in the litigation – but in the continuing degeneration of the concept of copyright. Whether it's people plucking the HBO signal off the air or not paying for taps on cable systems or whatever, it's caused and fed a deteriorating respect for a basic and constitutionally motivated right.[219]

As Sheinberg's statement implies, video piracy is only one example of what might be called *cultural piracy*, which includes audio piracy, cable or signal piracy, and pirate radio stations, as well as Captain Video (the lone pirate who invaded HBO's signals with his own message in the mid-1980s). After the Sony suit, the Hollywood majors were mostly concerned with those who copied videocassettes with profit motives. In the early eighties, professional pirates were able to make early copies of blockbuster films, including *Return of the Jedi* and *E.T.*, for which MCA filed and won a civil suit.[220]

At one point, the industry claimed that MPAA members "lost" between $300 and $400 million from video and cable theft, while non-MPAA members came up $1 billion short. By the early 1990s, the MPAA announced that the video piracy level nationally was between 5 and 10 percent, with an especially high incidence of pirating in specific states, such as California and New York.[221]

The industry has found some relief from pirating by creating various forms of anti-copying devices for videocassettes, as mentioned previously. However, technological progress means that there will inevitably be methods developed to invade, copy or break into even the newest prevention systems.

It is not surprising that the industry has again turned to the state for assistance in combating piracy. Such efforts have been led by the

MPAA's Film Security Office, which confiscated 14,000 tapes in 1984 and 25,000 cassettes in the first half of 1985. The MPAA, however, was still not pleased, noting that "it doesn't even make a dent in that illegal activity."[222] In 1989, there was a 51 percent increase in video raids, with nearly 660,000 illegal tapes seized in the USA. In addition, several states increased penalties for violators of copyright.[223] The industry also enlisted the help of the FBI and Interpol to serve as a kind of cultural police to prevent illegal copying. And, at least in the USA, rewards to individual citizens were offered for information leading to pirates' dens.

The industry has been seriously concerned about the lack of respect for copyrights in some Third World countries where a good deal of piracy takes place. Not to be denied their "fair share," the industry enlisted assistance from the US government to strengthen copyright laws in several countries. For instance, in the 1980s several Asian nations were threatened with trade restrictions, unless they tightened up their copyright enforcement.[224]

Home Video and Other Media

Unbundled advantages Home video has definitely had an impact on other entertainment forms, as it represents a lucrative market for film distribution with certain advantages over other markets. As David Waterman has observed:

> pre-recorded home video successfully competes as a delivery system by offering distributors more efficient, "unbundled" methods of pricing programs to consumers. This direct, unbundled pricing is far superior to that of advertiser-supported broadcasting and, in important respects, is superior to the "bundled" pricing of the subscription-supported pay-TV systems.[225]

In other words, home video provided Hollywood companies with another clear way to assess the popularity (and thus price) for a specific film, rather than the inexact estimates of audiences for over-the-air television and pay cable. Even if they do not directly control rentals, the suppliers know exactly how many tapes are being shipped and sold.[226]

Competing for the audience As home video became a reality, fear spread through other media sectors. Again, the end of movie theaters was predicted. And, indeed, the prospects looked gloomy at first: one study found that 48 percent of the early VCR owners went to movies in theaters less often than non-owners.[227] In 1985, it was claimed that the theater business was losing between 100 and 200 million admissions yearly because of home video and pay cable.[228] Some theaters even began selling cassettes in their lobbies, trying to cash in on the video boom, but also, perhaps, trying to prove that they did not fear the new competition.

Despite the gloom and doom forecast in the early eighties, the theater business grew during the late eighties, with new theaters, new screens and increasing box-office receipts (see Chapter 7.) Second-run theaters, adult movie sites and drive-ins were less fortunate and declined dramatically. And, of course, many have blamed home video. At least one observer attributed the changing demographics of drive-in audiences directly to home video and pay cable, claiming that the former "passion pits" were serving those segments of the population (specifically, working class and minority groups) who were unable to pay extra for these new technologies.[229]

But cable also felt the impact of home video's rapid growth, as VCRs were blamed for the slow-down in pay-cable subscriptions during the mid-eighties. By 1988, almost 80 percent of the homes that purchased HBO also had VCRs.[230]

But it probably was over-the-air television that suffered the most from the impact of the video boom. While there has generally been an increase in the total number of hours an average viewer watches television, increasingly viewers turned to the new alternatives to the once-dominant national networks. A 1990 survey found that VCR households spent around four hours a week watching videos and recording around two hours and 11 minutes of television programming each week, mostly while not watching the set. If this was not bad enough, most of the taped programming was viewed during network television's prime time.[231] Saturday night was especially affected, as the most popular night for video viewing.[232] Films that did make it to the networks typically performed miserably: one source estimated that the network screening of *Star Wars* would have drawn a 50 to 60 share if the film had not first appeared on pay-per-view, pay cable and in video stores. By the time the blockbuster reached television, it received a mere 35 share.[233]

Changing release patterns   It might be argued that home video's impact on these other media outlets also has been felt by the Hollywood majors in that they still supply those outlets (television and cable) with their films and television series. However, the majors have strategically adjusted their release patterns and marketing strategies to maximize revenues from all of these markets.

There were gradual changes in the typical release pattern during the 1980s, thanks to home video and cable. Prior to 1980, theatrical release was followed by theatrical reissue, then network and syndicated television releases. From 1980 to around 1983, pay channels followed theatrical release. But since 1983, home video has followed theatrical release by three to ten months, with pay cable airing within one year, followed (possibly) by network television within two years.[234]

As one industry observer summed up:

> We've come a long way from the days, not all that long ago, when the American studios released films in theaters here and abroad, milked them in second-run houses and drive-ins, then waited seven years for a handsome payoff for network airings on TV. The formula now is: American and foreign theatrical releases, followed from six to nine months later by a video release, followed a few months later by a pay-cable release, followed a year or so later – if anybody cares – by release on commercial TV.[235]

Thus, the tiered release – re-releases and second-runs – have become a thing of the past. The smaller movie houses which used to offer films at cheaper prices than first-run can no longer compete. So audiences who may want to wait to see a film at their local, less expensive theater generally do not have that choice, for those theaters most often are no longer there.

As a consequence, there are fewer theatrical films on network television. Although some films may be available at lower cost from the distributors, the networks and their advertisers may no longer be interested when a feature film is already available on cassette and has already been aired on pay cable. There have been implications for network programming, as we have seen more mini-series, made-for-TV movies, TV series, and syndication. As noted previously, we also have seen a dramatic decline of the networks themselves.

It might be noted that there were some early attempts to release films directly to cable or on video – in 1980, Twentieth Century boldly announced simultaneous video and theater release. And in 1983, *Pirates of Penzance* received a simultaneous pay-per-view and cinema release, while *Rocky IV*, *Cocoon*, *Jewel of the Nile*, and *White Nights* were among those films with similar simultaneous releases. Generally, though, the video release has followed theatrical distribution, as the box office provides a good indication of the future popularity of a film. (It also might be noted that the suppliers (the majors) have become theater owners; thus their interests may be better served by maintaining exclusive theatrical release. See further discussion in Chapter 7.)

In the late eighties, *Variety* reported that more new features were produced for video-only sales, sometimes bypassing theatrical release entirely. Some mainly-video companies have moved to producing films "to satisfy their movie-hungry video customers."

Video's Influence on Film Content and Aesthetics

> Home video is now a major force in shaping how movies are made and even what movies get made.
> Ed Hulse, "Hollywood's Video Invasion," *Video Review*, 1989

New/old genres Certain genres of film seemed to thrive in video. The word from someone who should know (Stephen King) is that, thanks to video, more horror movies are getting produced and financed than ever before.[236] *Nightmare* was one of the first films totally financed by a video company and it made tons of money. But video companies also made some bad decisions: video rights to *Santa Claus – The Movie* cost Media Home Entertainment over $4 million, and it turned out to be a huge box-office and video flop.

Although teenagers still seemed to be the dominant force in the movie market by the end of the eighties, many agreed that a variety of films were produced due to the expanded consumer base of video viewers. With the sense that adults were "returning en masse to movies," the studios seemed to be less hesitant to release adult-theme films, an activity that had been relegated to independent products and boutique distributors. By the end of the eighties, summer releases of such films also were not uncommon. Some examples were *The Kiss of the Spider Woman* (1985), *A Fish Called Wanda* (1988), and *The Last Temptation of Christ* (1988). As one observer pointed out, "[t]he distributors, driven by market forces that didn't exist 10 years ago, were supplying two essential demands. They were providing movies for adults who go to theaters year-round and they were putting into the pipeline titles that would be released on video the following winter and spring, when demand is greatest in that market."[237]

Nevertheless, some minor box-office films proved to do even better in video release. In other words, with more outlets for products, those films that may not "have legs" in the theater, may actually make it on cable or on cassette. Thus, there is at least the possibility that films with smaller audience appeal can survive. However, most sources agree that the biggest video hits seem to be the biggest theatrical hits, as movies still prove their value at the theatrical box office.[238]

Televisionization   Critics such as Vincent Canby have observed that home video has altered film aesthetics:

> Since the videocassette recorder has become, in effect, the second run of the theatrical film, there has been a televisionization in the look of movies. An interesting number of today's theatrical movies give the impression of being photographed almost entirely in the close-ups and medium shots that register best on the small screen.[239]

Televisionization means that directors shoot the main action in "an easily cropped area of the frame," thus minimizing the need to pan and scan. Anton Wilson, of *American Cinematographer*, has observed that:

> films shot with TV distribution in mind employ a full-frame camera aperture with both 1.85:1 and 1.33:1 markings in the camera viewfinder. By keeping all the pertinent action within the 1.85:1 markings, yet keeping the 1.33:1 area clean of microphone booms and the like, the final print can be used for . . . theatrical distribution, as well as TV distribution, without additional cropping.[240]

It might also be noted that pan-and-scan and letter-boxing, as discussed earlier in this chapter, are forms of televisionization of film, as well as less sophisticated techniques that simply take the best and largest images for video release. As Wilson argues, "all the techniques bastardize the original integrity and mood of the film and while it may make the film easier to view on TV, the percentage of missing image remains almost the same."[241]

Televisionization also involves differences in lighting. Film has a luminance or contrast ratio that is much wider than for video (128:1 for film compared to around 25:1 to 32:1 for video). Thus, scenes shot for film often lose subtle lighting nuances when screened via video. Anton Wilson uses the example of *The Godfather* to explain the differences:

> Coppola created the magnificent "underworld" texture by extensively exploiting the shadow detail capability of film. Most of the action in many

of the interior scenes existed in the lowest regions of the exposure curve. In my opinion this subtle feel of the texture was lost when the film appeared on television as the medium could not cope with the range of exposure, especially the shadow details.[242]

Film connoisseurs and critics may bemoan the bastardization of the film image on video, but the trend continues. As one film scholar has noted: "Cinema might well be the artistic, aesthetic 'important thing,' but increasingly, the market-driven exhibition possibilities of broadcast, cable and videocassette have a greater and greater say in production decisions."[243]

While some directors and camera technicians are bothered by the consequences of televisionization, still others consider it a necessity. As the director of *Nightmare on Elm Street 4* explains, "Today's young audiences have grown up with TV and they watch a lot of videos. So it's important to shoot a movie that will look good on TV."[244]

The Death of the Video Industry?

The tremendous growth of the home video industry is an interesting case in itself. Yet, it is possible that the entrepreneurs who fought the majors to preserve control of their businesses may be wiped out by more than just the blockbusters of the video world. Rather than becoming a concentrated industry with a few large video store chains, as some have predicted, the home video trade may suffer dramatically by the paving of new "electronic superhighways" into consumers' homes, offering features such as video dial tone or video-on-demand. Whatever forms these new systems take in the future, it is very likely that motion pictures will play a key role. In other words, consumers will be able to enjoy movies in the convenience of their homes, viewed at their leisure but delivered via electronic systems, rather than via videocassettes picked up and returned to a local video outlet. Thus, the home video business that has emerged as a successful enterprise since 1975 may find it difficult to survive into the next century.

A Video Revolution?

Home video has become a way of life in millions of homes around the world. The convenience and ease of viewing entertainment at any time of day or night has been accepted and celebrated by millions of VCR owners. How can one quibble with this technological breakthrough?

After considering the development of home video in this chapter, we can conclude that, similar to media technologies in the past, some very familiar patterns have emerged with this "revolution."

There is no question that the consumer has gained more independence from the schedules of those who control cultural and informational output. But, again, there is still nearly total dependence on that output. In other words, home video recorders for the most part are used to record and playback information and entertainment *created for* audiences. Though the technology is available, audience members have not been encouraged to develop truly two-way communication via new video equipment. Again, communication and culture have been conceived as one-way processes.

An interesting development of the video revolution has been the use of home video recording equipment, but camcorders and other video systems have been used by the public mostly as a replacement for still cameras and 8 mm film equipment to document family activities. Nevertheless, there is still some hope that video can become a new medium of communication and art. For instance, video artist Nam June Paik envisions "a channel devoted solely to video art showcasing the best of the millions of videotapes made by consumers every year."[245] So far, however, the type of activity we have seen in the USA is represented by ABC's *America's Funniest Home Videos*, which became the number one prime-time television program in the USA in March 1990. The show relies on audience members to send in funny videos, but chooses mostly those that capture people (or animals) in awkward or embarrassing moments. Another notable (and sometimes disturbing) use of camcorders has been for recording crimes or unlawful activities, thus turning ordinary citizens into video vigilantes. It remains to be seen whether or not the 500-channel universe will provide the opportunity and impetus for other uses of video technology.

While the convenience of home video is hailed by those pointing out the inconveniences of going to a theater, it still seems remarkable that the public has adapted to a rental system that actually does take them out of their home, not once, but twice, to pick up and return rented cassettes. Certainly, the cost of renting a film and sharing it with the rest of the family or a few friends is appealing. But, again, we are isolated from larger groups of people and increasingly experience culture in our homes. Culture increasingly is narrowed to a private rather than a public experience.

And there are those who also bemoan the quality of the viewing experience with video. As Steven Spielberg once stated, "Movies should be seen in dark, hallowed halls."[246] There is no doubt that encountering a film on a 20-inch box via electronic technology is a qualitatively different experience than viewing a film on a large screen via celluloid technology and more sophisticated audio systems. The conversion to video involves a loss of picture size and quality, thus the original intention of the creators may be virtually lost when viewed on even the best video systems. And then there's the difference in the viewing environment: a theater should provide a more ideal setting to view a film, uninterrupted by household noises and telephones (unless you happen to sit next to someone who brings their cellular telephone to the theater). The special nature of "going out" to a movie also may contribute to the experience of theater viewing (although there are those, of course, who might argue that in many urban environments, it is increasingly dangerous and risky to venture outside the security of one's home for any reason).

But there have been signs that the VCR has not been such a hit with the entire population for other reasons. As the sales of video equipment started declining in 1989, there were widespread reports of a decline in the amount of time spent using a VCR after its initial purchase. Some even admitted that the technology had "limited utility." An EIA representative explained: "There are a lot of people out there who simply don't want to buy a VCR, either because it's too difficult for them to operate, or because they don't watch much TV, or some other reason."[247]

Another reason may be that those without the resources to purchase a video recorder – those who may have chosen in the past to view a film when it is presented on over-the-air commercial television – may not have that option, as the film may never even appear on network or syndicated television, with cable and video options more lucrative to distributors. Perhaps it is a small problem, but might there be an "entertainment" or "cultural" poor, in addition to an information poor?

In essence, home video has been yet another communication technology developed primarily as a commodity. Those corporations involved with entertainment, especially, have echoed the sentiments of Madison Square Gardens, when they explained the creation of their home video label as "a *natural* extension of our core business."[248] Indeed, the truly *revolutionary* characteristics of home video – control over the creation and retransmission of information and cultural creation – has been overshadowed by the acceptance of the technology as a *natural* development of the commodified form of information and entertainment and consequently, control of home video's development has remained in the hands of those corporations which previously dominated these activities.

Again, we have seen the potential for more competition and diversity developing around home video technology. Yet, again, as with most other areas of cultural production, concentration and consolidation have been apparent, and perhaps inevitable, in light of the corporate and industrial character of home video's development. And it follows for many that the consolidation of the home video industry has meant less diversity, at least among those voices heard. As one writer for *Video Business* simply stated, "In a universe of fewer players, there will be fewer programming choices."[249]

While there are still advantages for alternative and truly independent production through less expensive and more accessible video formats, there is still the age-old problem of distribution. Even if an independent producer successfully gets a film to the video stage, how is it possible to reach audiences when video stores accept a Hollywood "blockbuster" mentality, an attitude which is (not too surprisingly) picked up by consumers. The result? Audiences equate home video to yet another, sometimes more convenient, outlet for Hollywood products.

But what is the big problem? Are we not still offered hundreds, possibly thousands, more films to choose from, to view in the convenience of our home? Yes, of course, but those products available in our local video stores are the same products which have been available in the past, only in a different form. On the one hand we are getting simply more of the same, but on the other hand, we are also getting less of the same. As noted earlier, the number of new Hollywood films has decreased rather than increased, despite high box office and video revenues.

Yes, there still are exercise and documentary videos on some of the shelves of video stores and retail outlets. Yes, it is possible to find videos for a wider audience (children's programming, for instance). But, for the most part, the home video industry is fueled by, dominated by, driven by Hollywood products. And, increasingly, *BIG* Hollywood products.

And who benefits? Audiences are offered more entertainment – for a price – and a great deal of money is made through the sale of video equipment and the video release of films, both new and old. One might ask why that seems to be such a problem. After all, that is capitalism. And it is also the commodification of culture. The point is that there is not so much really new here, despite those who want us to believe that there has been a revolution.

7

The Silver Screen: Theatrical Exhibition in the Information Age

Long ago Hollywood came to appreciate distribution outlets other than movie theaters, moving beyond the silver screen to other profitable markets. As we have seen, home video revenues now far surpass theatrical box office receipts, while cable and other markets provide even further income. Nevertheless, theaters still play an important role for the film industry and in the life of a major motion picture.

The chapter will discuss the exhibition sector of the traditional film industry, outlining the competitive climate for theaters faced with popular new distribution outlets, the majors' move back into exhibition, and the influence of technological developments in theatrical exhibition.

Motion Picture Theaters in the 1990s

The report of my death was an exaggeration.

Mark Twain

Common sense would lead one to conclude that movies on cable and videocassettes would take business away from theaters. But this depends on when and where Hollywood distributors actually decide to release their products.

The major distributors did indeed release their films to cable, pay cable and home video, and as these newer distribution outlets emerged, the demise of theaters was again predicted as it had been with the introduction of television.

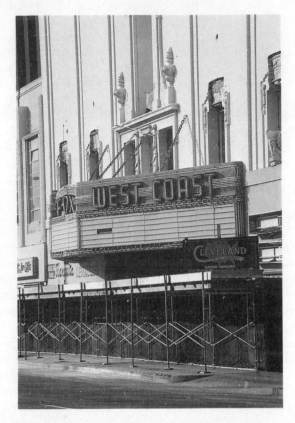

Plate 4 The End of an Era The West Coast Theater in Long Beach, California, undergoes a dramatic transformation. While some older theaters like the West Coast have been demolished, others have been converted to multiplexes, with many screens under the same roof. *Photograph by Mark Walters and Gary Cohn*

In the early 1980s, along with complaints about getting their "fair share," some Hollywood executives were extremely excited about these new outlets, making public statements that should have sent shivers down the spine of any theater owner. Alan Hirschfield, as head of Twentieth Century Fox, was especially enthusiastic about establishing distribution systems in the home, such as pay-per-view. For instance, when he considered the potential distribution methods for videodiscs, he noted, "I don't care if the milkman brings the disc. You can't sell milk without cows, and I've got the cows." It didn't encourage theater owners, either, when Marvin Davis, the owner of Fox at the time, announced that he would not even take his family to a local movie theater.[1]

Meanwhile, Frank Rosenfelt, another Hollywood executive, did not seem to mind distributing his films to the home market either: "I don't own a screwdriver, I don't even know how my television set works. All I know is they need programming and I have the programming. All I care about is that it's my product and I get paid for it."[2]

As it turned out, though, videodiscs and pay-per-view were not the eventual culprits – it was the VCR and pay cable that claimed to draw audiences away from theaters. By 1982, as home video increased in popularity, the head of the National Organization for Theater Owners (NATO) confessed that "near-panic" prevailed among theater owners.[3]

Living (competing) with home video   However, by 1986 the head of NATO was vociferously deriding the popular press for announcing the death of theaters.[4] After a few years of living with competition from home outlets, some of the industry reports were less gloomy. Based on a two-year study of 50,000 customers, General Cinema, the largest theater chain in the USA, announced in 1987 that VCRs were beneficial to the film business, renewed people's interest in feature films, and could elevate the taste of the mass public. The study also found that 73 percent of GCC patrons owned a VCR. As GCC's chairman, Richard Smith concluded: "Audiences will become more discriminating and more sophisticated in their moviegoing and movie viewing patterns. . . . As a result, Hollywood will be encouraged to make larger investments for films that will appeal to mature audiences, not just a youth-culture audience."[5] It might be added that General Cinema had reported a "disappointing" year in 1986, but blamed unpopular films rather than VCRs.

Further, the GCC study found that VCR owners gradually decreased the number of movies rented and eventually came back to the theaters – a phenomenon called the extinction curve.[6] Other exhibitors claimed that the home video boom also helped more than hurt theaters, emphasizing that a new market had been added – those people who had lost interest in movies in general. On the other hand, many argued that there is a key movie-going group that will always support theatrical film exhibition.

A few exhibitors believed the new outlets were helping the industry by helping producers. Larry Moyer, a Northwest theater owner, noted: "What people who are not in the industry are finally beginning to realize is that every one of those 'innovations' [radio, TV, VCRs, pay TV] has added to the income of the movie producers. And when they're healthy, we're healthy." In other words, more movies meant more movie theater construction and expansion. At the same time, however, Moyer had added a video store chain (First Stop Video) to his theater business, which accounted for 28 percent of the company's income around 1986–7.[7] Other exhibitors were even so bold as to rent and/or sell videos in their theater lobbies, treating video as an opportunity rather than a threat.[8]

Honey, I shrunk the theater With the growth of VCRs and the perceived loss of control by the majors, Hollywood representatives like Valenti made a plea for a better theater experience. And, indeed, some theaters did expand and improve during the eighties and into the nineties. As the *Los Angeles Times* observed: "To compete with each other and lure people away from their videocassette recorders and cable programs, theater owners are offering bigger, cleaner, more technologically advanced, comfortable and architecturally interesting facilities than have been built during the past couple of decades."[9]

Yet, more often than not, the expansion was still in the form of multiplexes – theater centers with several screens in smaller auditoriums with fewer seats, and, most would argue, much less luxury. During the eighties, the total number of screens increased (from 17,675 in 1980 to over 23,000 in 1990), but not the total number of theaters.[10]

Some have argued that the small screens were characteristic of the type of films shown. "Movies like *Total Recall* and *Die Hard 2* are, to a large extent, the product of the architecture in which they're presented. For one thing, they fit a relatively small screen, since they don't depend on majestic images, grand scale or detail."[11] The increase in the number of screens also was cited as one of the contributing factors to the rising cost of launching a film, i.e. the number of prints necessary and more advertising expenses.

But by the end of the eighties, theaters were not the only shrinking feature of the exhibition sector. Three of the largest chains experienced dramatic losses. United Artists Entertainment Co., the largest circuit with 2,766 screens, planned to shut down 17 percent of its screens. General Cinema's operating income plunged 44 percent from 1989. (See table 7.1 for numbers of screens for the largest circuits in 1991). Although the box office was higher (see table 7.2), there had actually been a decline in the number of tickets sold and much of the added box office was due to increased ticket prices, from an average of $1.65 in 1970 to $4.11 in 1988.

In addition, because of the increase in the number of screens the

Table 7.1 Largest theater chains, USA and Canada, 1993

Chain	Parent company	Number of screens
United Artists[a]	United Artists Theatre Circuit Inc.	2,378
Cineplex Odeon[b]	Cineplex Odeon Corp.	1,619
American Multi-Cinema	AMC Entertainment	1,585
Carmike	Carmike Cinema	1,570
General Cinema	General Cinema Corp.	1,396
Cinemark	Cinemark USA	996
Loews	Sony Corp.	868
National Amusements[c]	National Amusements	725
Act III Theatres	Act III Theatres, Inc.	533
Famous Players[d]	Paramount Communications	474
Hoyts Cinema Corp.	Hoyts Corp.	460
Cinamerica	Paramount Communications & Time Warner	382

[a] Includes some screens in Hong Kong.
[b] About 50% owned by Matsushita Electric Industrial Co., Ltd. Includes about 575 screens in Canada.
[c] May include a relatively small number of theaters in the United Kingdom.
[d] In Canada.
Sources: *Hollywood Reporter; Variety; Forbes Magazine*; company reports; Standard & Poor estimates, presented in *Standard & Poor's Industry Surveys*, 11 March 1993, p. L17.

demand for films had grown, but the supply had not. Theaters increasingly had to deal with stiff demands from distributors, including a tougher bidding process, a larger share of the box office gross, and (sometimes) per capita minimums on film rentals.[12] In addition, a few distributors refused to book their films in theaters that ran advertising. (There will be more discussion of advertising in theaters in chapter 8.)

Another change in the exhibition sector was the demise of second-run or sub-run and repertoire theaters.[13] Although some of the blame has been placed on the TV generation or the changing tastes of younger audience members, the availability of videocassettes of films previously featured at revival houses was more likely the problem. As an *American Film* writer noted, "The 'window' – the amount of time between a film's theatrical release and home exhibition – is closing, and in the new era of exhibition, the last theaters to get the product will be the first casualties."[14]

Table 7.2   US theatrical film industry profile

	Box office		Admissions		Average ticket price		No. of screens
Year	Billions $	% change	Billions	% change	Dollars	% change	
E1992	4.923	2.5	0.977	(0.5)	5.04	3.0	25,000
1991	4.803	(4.4)	0.982	(7.1)	4.89	2.9	24,570
1990	5.022	(0.2)	1.057	(6.7)	4.75	6.9	23,689
1989	5.033	12.9	1.133	4.4	4.45	8.1	23,132
1988	4.458	4.8	1.085	(0.3)	4.11	5.2	23,234
1987	4.253	12.6	1.089	7.0	3.91	5.2	23,555
1986	3.778	0.8	1.017	(3.7)	3.71	4.6	22,765
1985	3.749	(7.0)	1.056	(11.9)	3.55	5.6	21,147
1984	4.031	7.0	1.199	0.2	3.36	6.8	20,200
1983	3.766	9.1	1.197	1.8	3.15	7.1	18,884

E: Estimated.
Source: Motion Picture Association of America and Standard & Poor estimates, presented in *Standard & Poor's Industry Surveys*, 11 March 1993, p. L17.

The privileging of theaters   Though relations sometimes have been strained, distributors and exhibitors ultimately work together to get the most out of the theater market. And, despite the harsh words and dire predictions, distributors still tend to release their films first to theaters, as theatrical exhibition still brings in the largest share of revenues and serves as a major determinant of a film's value in other outlets, such as home video, cable, and foreign markets. This may partially explain why advertising expenses during the theatrical release of major films increased drastically during the last decade. As one advertising publication observed in the early nineties: "Box office figures open windows a year down the road. If you spend a lot of money, you get better box office. And the higher the box office, the better the movie looks to the cable channels and the video dealers."[15] This reasoning may be partially faulty, however, as some deals for ancillary markets are made long before theatrical exhibition.

At any rate, there is still a heavy emphasis on the theatrical release of a major motion picture. Frank Price, in otherwise exuberant remarks about pay-per-view, commented: "Theaters are the goose, even if pay-per-view is the golden egg."[16] Exhibitors have pointed out that theaters are the only place where distributors can be assured of receiving payment for each viewer who sees a film. While distributors may recall instances of exhibitors misrepresenting box office numbers and illegally splitting the product, there is still some validity to the argument that theaters offer the most profitable and strategic initial distribution outlet for major films.[17]

The Majors and Theater Ownership

In August 1982, *Variety* reporter A. D. Murphy valiantly defended theaters' role in presenting films to the public. He concluded, however, that structural changes were inevitable, hinting at an electronic future for theaters:

> Exhibition's future will require broadly-based nationwide organizations to maintain and upgrade the quality of theater operation. (Dish antennae on the roof to receive a signal from a distrib's transponder won't be cheap; nor will the high-density electronic screen, etc.) If, however, the new leaders of exhibition don't grab the ball, some distribution companies in the coming post-Consent Decree era will do so. If not in the form of direct ownership, then partial ownership or (official) affiliation.[18]

Oh, how prophetic. Indeed, the majors did more than just grab the ball; they nearly took over the whole game. During the eighties, the exhibition end of the industry became increasingly more concentrated, with a handful of large chains controlling a majority of the theaters in the USA and Canada.[19] But in 1986, this consolidation process was compounded. During that year, $1.62 billion and 4,357 screens changed hands, and the major Hollywood distribution companies were actively involved in these transactions[20] (see table 7.3).

While the distributors gave numerous explanations for their purchases of theaters, it was generally agreed that they wanted more control over their own product – the type of control that they did not have with home video and pay cable. With theater ownership, the majors could "nurture" their films, building an audience for an otherwise overlooked product. Murphy explained: "It's not mollycoddling; it's marketing."[21] Others agreed that it was vertical integration, pure and simple – "a feeding frenzy that has got everybody in this town scared to death."[22]

Despite the Paramount decrees (see chapter 2, note 25), which supposedly severed exhibition from production and distribution, several of the major distribution companies were technically allowed to own theaters if competitive bidding for new film releases prevailed. Several

Table 7.3 Distributors' theater acquisitions, 1986–7

Major	Theaters	No. of Screens
MCA	Cineplex Odeon[a] (50%)	1,550
	Plitt	692
	Septum	48
	Essaness	41
	Sterling Recreation Organization[b]	100
	Neighborhood	76
Columbia	Walter Reade Organization	11
TriStar[c]	United Artists Communication	1,200
	Loews	300
	Music Makers	65
Cannon	Commonwealth	425
Gulf + Western	Trans-Lux	24
	Mann	360
	Festival Enterprises	101
Theaters previously owned:		
G+W	Famous Players	469
G+W/MCA	Cinema Intl Corp.	76

[a] A separate subsidiary of Cineplex Odeon also owns the RKO Century Warner chain, including 97 Cinema Five theaters.
[b] The Sterling Recreation Organization also licenses pictures for 30 other screens.
[c] 35 percent owned by Columbia.
Source: *Variety*, 7 January 1987; Gerald F. Phillips, "The Recent Acquisition of Theatre Circuits by Major Distributors," *The Entertainment and Sports Lawyer*, Winter 1987, p. 20.

companies were not restricted from owning theaters by the Paramount decrees in the late 1940s: Paramount was not limited by its early agreement, while Universal, United Artists and Columbia were not involved with exhibition at the time. Only Warner, MGM and Fox were restricted, yet could receive special dispensation from the Department of Justice to engage in exhibition activities.[23]

The 1980s was an ideal political climate to make such moves, as antitrust enforcement was relatively lax, especially when it concerned vertical integration. The Department of Justice reviewed the consent decrees after Reagan came to power in 1981, yet slowly the majors went ahead and made their purchases. In July 1986, the Department of Justice announced that it would not oppose any acquisitions, but was "monitoring" distributors' activities.[24]

Of course, the majors' actions did not go unnoticed by the industry. But while NATO issued its opposition to distributors' moves into theater ownership, exhibitors were not really united. *Variety* expressed a somewhat stronger reaction, noting the implications for a competitive marketplace:

> As small, independent distributors have found, it is traditionally difficult to obtain wide theater bookings, obtain the best theaters or find playtime in crowded seasons (let alone be able to hold screens for more than one or two weeks) if one doesn't have a steady product line to deliver.
>
> With integrated suppliers/exhibitors in the marketplace it will become even more difficult for the smallfry who own no theaters and have no upcoming stream of additional product to enter the marketplace.[25]

To prove the point, *Variety* did a survey and found that 53 percent of the independently produced films had failed to appear in the domestic market.[26]

But with no real opposition forthcoming from the government, the majors moved on. At one point, Warner even advanced the idea of franchising theaters as *exclusive* outlets for their films. And other communications companies jumped into the game, as well. Tele-Communication Inc. (TCI) bought United Artists Communications Inc. (renamed United Artists Entertainment Co.) in 1986, as well as several other chains. Thus, as we have seen in previous chapters, TCI became an entertainment powerhouse with large holdings in theaters, and cable and video sales, even though there were those who worried out loud about the effects of such consolidation on deals made between studios and distribution outlets.[27]

In response to the majors moving into the theater sector, some exhibitors ventured into distribution, deliberately or through acquisition. Cineplex formed Cineplex Odeon Films to distribute features in the USA and added Canadian distribution operations, while National Amusements linked with Viacom.[28]

Obviously, the moves by the majors, as well as general consolidation in the exhibition sector, represented a threat to a competitive film industry. While the top ten exhibitors still owned fewer than 30 percent of the screens, their share of the "showcase screens" increased to at least 50 percent.[29] And, again, the strongest corporations in the industry were involved with the production, distribution and exhibition sectors, with distributors able to arrange preferential deals for their own theaters. As one industry commentator noted:

> Representatives of the new Hollywood may insist that monopoly is the last thought in their minds, but many independent producers and exhibitors remain skeptical. They see further theater acquisitions on the horizon, fewer independently produced and distributed pictures, a re-establishment of the majors' power over all aspects of the industry.[30]

New Technologies and Theaters

> The whole medium of motion pictures – which is strips of plastic, with sprockets and cams and mechanical movements – is totally archaic, relative to the technical base that we have available today.
> Pat Dowell and Ray Heinrich, "Bigger than Life," *American Film*, 1984

Computers and automation Despite the threat of new distribution outlets competing directly with theaters, technological developments in exhibition seem to have been slower than in other sectors of the film industry.

The business of exhibition has been influenced by computers in a similar way to other businesses, and includes computerized business records and management, as well as automated teller systems. Computerized systems for movie tickets by phone also have been introduced. Teleticketing technology in the USA currently is dominated by two companies, Pacer/CATS and MovieFone, who agreed to refrain from competition and pool their resources in 1992. MovieFone and Pacer already provided their services to the top exhibitors in the USA, but together planned to expand a teleticketing system which would link a phone reservation system to box offices. Pacer/CATS is the largest box office automation equipment company in the USA, but part of the UK-based Wembley PLC, the diversified company that includes Wembley Stadium in London. MovieFone is the largest telephone movie guide and reservation service in the USA and a member of a privately held group of companies involved in merchant banking and financial services called the Falconwood Group. The banking connection is an interesting one, as a standard teleticketing system is important to pave the way for financial services to enter the $6 billion-a-year teleticketing business. Perhaps this explains why such systems have been subsidized for exhibitors, who pay less than the usual $17,000 to $50,000 installation fees.[31]

As noted previously, exhibitors also tried to make their theaters more comfortable and enjoyable, and sometimes computers were used to help plan and design these improvements. An example was the AMC Theaters complex in Century City, built in 1986: "computerized so there is optimum sound from each seat" with "computer-designed, state-of-the-art floors – so there are no bad seats."[32]

Another technological change has been the proliferation of automated projection systems. Such systems make possible the multi-screen phenomenon, but may affect the quality of the viewing experience. With no live projectionist supervising a screening, there is at least the chance that there will be no adjustments made to a poor picture, etc. Obviously, automated projection systems have led to fewer projectionist jobs. In 1990, Michael Nielsen estimated that non-union projectionists, or personnel other than projectionists, operated equipment in over 60 percent of all theaters.[33]

Bigger sound In the past, most of the new technologies influencing exhibition, such as new sound and projection systems, have been initiated by producers, as theaters must be assured that films will be produced in the new formats or with new processes before investing in expensive technological upgrades. This seems to be the pattern with the new audio systems introduced in theaters during the last few decades. Dolby sound systems are gradually making their way into theaters, with a few more featuring films released with digital tracks (*Dick Tracy* was one of the first, as mentioned in chapter 3).[34] Meanwhile, by 1990 around 500 cinemas worldwide offered George Lucas' THX system, introduced in theaters by a trailer which concludes, "The Audience is Listening." (A Home THX Audio System was also available for $5,000 around the same time.)[35]

Bigger and better images Theater owners sometimes have added more sophisticated, curved screens. But further improvements in film projection are still awaited. Over the last few decades, advanced projection systems have been introduced, but most have been only showcase affairs and not widely adopted by theaters or accepted by the production sector. A wide array of possibilities has been introduced, including systems offering larger screen formats (Imax, Omnimax, etc.), better film quality (Showscan), plus added features such as holography, interactive systems, and the integration of video into film.

First, there are projection processes which present larger images than the standard 35 mm. The use of 70 mm is not that unusual and has been used for big blockbuster films. But newer systems, based on the 70 mm format, offer even more detail and more realistic images.

The Imax system, premiered at Expo '70 in Osaka, was one of the first large screen formats. While printed on regular 70 mm stock, the image runs horizontally through the camera and projector without the use of sprocket holes, at an accelerated rate (5.5 feet per second). The film format is ten times the size of an ordinary 35 mm frame and three times the size of 70 mm, and images are projected on huge screens (the Smithsonian Air and Space Museum exhibit featured a screen measuring 50 by 75 feet). A similar process is Omnimax, which is projected on a dome surrounding the audience.[36]

While these systems have been used successfully at museums and special exhibitions, there has been little sustained interest for feature film production. The main problem has been the cost of both shooting with these systems and converting or building new theaters.[37]

Showscan is another system utilizing 70 mm film, but shown at a faster-than-normal speed (60 frames per second rather than 24). The process was developed in the late 1970s by Douglas Trumbull while he was president of Future General Corp., a research subsidiary of Paramount. Trumbull had been involved with special effects for films such as *2001* and *Star Trek*, and eventually left Paramount to develop Showscan on his own (although the studio still apparently received royalties on the process).[38] Trumbull's system presents flickerless, life-like images on a larger-than-normal screen. Despite the minimal modification to projection equipment, the problem has been convincing producers and exhibitors that the change is worth the transition. The dilemma was explained by Trumbull in 1984:

> No studio will commit fifteen or twenty million dollars to produce a film unless there are hundreds of theaters to show it in. No theater owner is going to put a hundred thousand dollars worth of new equipment in his theater unless all the movies coming out of Hollywood are produced in the process – they only reluctantly put in a $700 Dolby card.[39]

Another system is Envirovision, featuring a 360-degree spheric projection process with theater seats that can be repositioned. There also have been numerous attempts to revive 3-D, one of which received backing from Eastman Kodak and United Artists Theatre Circuit.[40]

Perhaps the ultimate movie experience will involve one of the sophisticated 3-D processes, presenting some form of cyberspace or virtual reality. Since the late eighties, science fiction fans have enjoyed the exploits of cyberspace adventures in novels such as William Gibson's *Neuromancer* and *Mona Lisa Overdrive*. Simulated experiences have been common in the training of astronauts and pilots, with systems such as NASA's VIVID, making it possible to explore and interact within a 360-degree, synthesized environment. Other experiments dealing with virtual reality appeared at the end of the eighties, including some entertainment venues. The "Star Tours" ride at Disneyland featured a virtual reality element, as did the "Tour of the Universe" in Toronto.[41] Meanwhile, an Imax process, called 3-D Solido system, featured special goggles giving audience members close-to-real-life experiences. The Japanese Broadcasting Company (NHK) introduced a form of 3-D television, using the same principle.[42] Showscan also introduced a Dynamic Motion Simulator, using high-definition film and a moving platform to simulate the experience of skiing downhill or racing a car.[43] Meanwhile, another company, VPL Research Inc., has created a DataSuit, utilized at the moment by actors to help with more realistic computer-generated effects, but designed to allow users to create their own worlds. One of DataSuit's creators envisions virtual reality networks using telecommunication links, enabling users "to communicate long-distance, not to escape into their own canned, pre-set metatelevision realities."[44]

However, some predict that it will be far in the future when we see actual cyberspace or virtual reality films. As one experimenter observes, "We have created all this technology, but we haven't made the leap as entertainers to utilize it."[45]

The electronic theater   In the early 1980s EMI opened four video theaters in England, reporting some success at keeping costs down. The industry as a whole, however, did not rush to convert to the new process, which had been developed by the same company which had perfected airline video projectors.[46]

But for nearly a decade now, HDTV (high-definition television) has been looming as a viable possibility to take motion picture theaters into an electronic age. As Valenti noted in 1987, "We look forward to a single worldwide standard for TV program distribution. HDTV coupled with high quality projection systems now in development and large-capacity communication satellites may bring about the development of 'electronic theaters' with significant benefits to distributors and exhibitors."[47]

An electronic theater would offer some benefits to the industry, including increased quality of image and sound, and the costs saved in prints and distribution, as well as in production. However, one of the questions at the beginning of the nineties was whether HDTV would be seen first in theaters, or in private homes, thus becoming another threat to theaters.[48] Decisions at the FCC seemed to push towards HDTV in the home, as individual TV stations were to be encouraged to transmit using the new format, and the industry was showing signs of cooperation by adopting a standard digital HDTV system in May 1993.[49] Another possibility was that cable companies would serve as distribution outlets for HDTV signals to receivers installed by cable companies.[50] Then again, some wondered whether HDTV would actually take hold anywhere, as the cost involved seemed prohibitive to all these parties.[51] The electronic theater holds out the advantage of large screen size for larger-than-life images, thus theaters may be able (again) to offer something other outlets cannot.

Different HDTV systems have been proposed for electronic theaters, including fiber optics as the mode of delivery for HDTV, thus involving cable and satellite technology. One vision involves electronic cineplexes, featuring taped or closed-circuit programming including first-run movies, as well as remote cultural events.

But the prevailing opinion is that if HDTV does reach theaters, it will be "driven by movies." Along those lines, James McKinney of the White House Military Office stated that "the HDTV medium will be controlled by videotape manufacturers and Hollywood programmers."[52]

If an electronic theater emerges, there will be real problems for many film employees in laboratories, film exchanges and projection booths. As Nielsen concludes:

> For the film technicians, however, the fact remains that there presently exist no plans to retrain projectionists, lab technicians, and film exchange employees to take advantage of these new production jobs, nor is there the appropriate economic geography to even make such a plan feasible.
> The goal in development of electronic cinema is toward efficiency in organization and production. The film unions, like unions bargaining for workers in many other US industries, seem to be unable or unwilling to resist the demands for increased automation and elimination of jobs.[53]

Conclusions

While the major Hollywood distributors are adjusting to and benefitting from the changing technological climate, the same rosy picture may not be painted for most exhibitors. Unless major changes in the way that films are distributed to theaters take place, many argue that exhibition will suffer further decline in box office and profits.

Despite the dependence on theatrical release before other outlets, one should not go too far in predicting how loyal the Hollywood majors will remain to the theaters, even with their ownership interests in theater chains. These days, at least, the theaters need the distributors' films far more than the distributors need theaters to reach an audience.

If theaters are to survive, they must walk a fine line between the distributors' rising demands and pricing tickets beyond the reach of most of their customers. In other words, if distributor demands force exhibitors to continue raising ticket prices (and concession prices, as well), theaters may indeed lose even more of their customers to the cheaper home technologies.

Exhibitors may eventually have to employ their own schemes, incorporating new technologies where they can in order to survive in the new world of home video, for the small "cracker-box" theaters ultimately may not be enough to lure viewers away from their comfortable home environments. We may see movie theaters in the future with even better and larger screen images, further enhanced audio systems, or new multi-media experiences or interactive presentations.

While these innovations may prove to be only novelties, they may attract audiences back to the theaters for video images beamed to theaters and screened on high definition TV systems or virtual reality experiences. One way or another, though, exhibitors will most likely depend once again on distributors to provide the product. And for distributors with product, there are, even now, a wide range of other options beyond the silver screen.

8

Hollywood Meets Madison Ave.: The Commercialization of US Films

Hollywood motion pictures have long been recognized as commodities. Yet, these days motion pictures also are the vehicles for even further commercial activity in the form of advertising and merchandising.

It is as difficult to ignore the brand-name products scattered throughout a typical Hollywood blockbuster, as it is to avoid the ever-present tie-in campaigns featured at supermarkets and quick-food outlets. Meanwhile, there is a proliferation of toys, games and other merchandise based on Hollywood films. While there are numerous studies of movie advertising, few have considered the implications of the growing trend of advertising within films and merchandising activities which surround them.[1]

This chapter examines the growth of advertising and marketing in and around Hollywood films and argues that these marketing strategies have become more deliberate and carefully coordinated than in the past. These developments, furthermore, enhance the commodification of culture and promote a consumer society. The chapter will consider product advertising, tie-in campaigns, and licensing and merchandising activities. The creative, economic and cultural implications of these developments will then be discussed.

Product Advertising

The notion that US films stimulate demand for US products has long been acknowledged.[2] By the 1920s fashions seen in films were being promoted by stars and retail establishments and the cigarette industry was lobbying performers to smoke on screen.[3] Placement of name brand products within major motion pictures is not a new phenomenon; just one example is Joan Crawford drinking Jack Daniels whiskey in the 1945 production, *Mildred Pierce*.[4]

However, in these earlier times product placement was a much more casual, even haphazard endeavor. Property masters would call the local Jack Daniels distributor and ask for some product to be used in the film, or simply go to the store and buy the product themselves. The Jack Daniels distributor would more than likely send a couple of cases so that the property master would not only have enough product for the film but plenty left over to spread among the cast and crew, thus engendering a measure of goodwill toward the company.

Today the system of product placement is much more deliberate and sophisticated. Indeed, the vast majority of Fortune 500 companies are involved in product placement activities,[5] and the process has become an industry in and of itself. There now exist somewhere between 15 and 30 companies whose sole purpose is to secure placement for their clients' products.[6] Jack Daniels itself employs a product placement firm.

This section will explore the recent trend of product advertising in the Hollywood film industry and argues that as Hollywood continues to search for additional sources of revenue, the commodification of the film industry will continue to accelerate. This process has manifested itself not only in terms of product placements within films, but in such practices as advertising on videos and within motion picture theaters. Each of these areas will be analyzed separately, but it should be remembered that they are tied by a common thread. When considered as a whole, evidence indicates that the Hollywood film industry is rapidly becoming a major advertising medium.

Product Placement

Arranging the appearance or mention of specific brand names in motion pictures has become a multimillion dollar business. Firms charge clients fees ranging from $5,000 to $250,000 for guaranteed placement in a contracted number of films with escalation clauses for particularly extensive or prominent appearances.[7] Some companies (e.g. Coca-Cola, Pepsi, Anheuser-Busch) have formed their own in-house divisions dedicated specifically to product placement and/or Hollywood advertising activities.

Product placement firms and corporate in-house divisions typically review 400–500 movie screenplays per year looking for opportunities. One such company, Creative Film Promotions, utilizes a computer program to search scripts for product placement ideas. On average the firm claims the computer will discover at least 50 potential placements in a given screenplay; for example, adding a dresser with a client's brand of clock radio and cosmetics whenever a script reads "INTERIOR: BEDROOM."[8]

Such efforts have resulted in significant product placements in Hollywood films. The Pepsi-Cola Entertainment Marketing Group (Pepsi's in-house placement division) reported placing the Pepsi trademark in approximately 70 feature films in 1989, while another private firm, Entertainment Marketing Group, placed products in 150 films the same year.[9] Another firm, Associated Film Promotions, claims to have placed clients in more than 175 features.[10] It has been estimated that current movies contain, on average, 30–40 minutes of screen time given over to product plugs.[11] This translates to approximately one-third of a typical movie containing product advertisements.

Why the current growth in product placement activity? From Hollywood's point of view, product placement means added revenues. On the other hand, product placement equals effective advertising for corporate sponsors. According to Twentieth Century Fox Licensing and Merchandising Corporation (Fox's subsidiary responsible for product placement), the studio will charge anywhere from $20,000 to $100,000 or more for a product appearance in a major motion picture.[12] If one assumes 20–50 potential promotional opportunities per film, it follows that a producer could easily realize well in excess of one million dollars from product placements in a given production. The amount charged for placement is directly correlated with the level of prominence the product achieves in the film. If the product merely appears in the background, the fee is significantly lower than if the product is actually handled by the movie's star.[13] Verbal mention of a product, as in the film *Wall Street*, where Martin Sheen's character yelled to the waitress, "Get this kid a Molson Light," also pushes the fee higher.[14]

One result of the acceleration of this type of activity is that placements have become standard operating procedure; simply part of the negotiation that can reduce the cost of production.[15] Negotiations do not always revolve around a straight cash fee, however. Often placement deals involve product, equipment and its maintenance, or advertising commitments. Paramount's *Days of Thunder*, in which star Tom Cruise drives a neon Chevy Lumina stock car named for Coca-Cola Company's Mellow Yellow soft drink, serves as an appropriate example. The placement agreement provided that General Motors would not only provide the necessary car(s), but also mechanics to make sure they operated properly. In addition, both Chevy and Coca-Cola committed themselves to extensive promotional campaigns tied to the movie. Such media expenditures can literally add tens of millions of dollars to a movie's promotional budget.[16] Joe Allegro, co-owner of the Entertainment Marketing Group, estimates that of the placements his firm secures approximately one half are for cash and the remaining 50 percent are for media or equipment.[17]

Meanwhile, corporate marketing departments are equally enthusiastic about product placements. In an era of generally rising media costs, motion pictures with their new afterlife of videocassettes and pay television are increasingly attractive from a cost standpoint. If a movie grosses $50 million, the advertiser has reached an audience of 13.7 million in theater viewers.[18] The industry generally assumes that if a movie grosses $50 million, it will likely sell 200,000 videocassettes. If the movie grosses over $50 million, it could easily sell 300,000 videos. It is further assumed that a top feature film will be rented five or more times per week, thus adding an additional (over theater) 25–30 million impressions per placement. And when pay cable and network TV are added into the equation, the cost to advertisers is literally pennies per thousand.[19] In addition, advertisers feel as though they are reaching an otherwise hard-to-reach audience: the 12-to-24-year-old market.[20]

But most convincing is evidence that movie placement works. The most cited example is Hershey Company's Reese's Pieces, when sales levitated 85 percent after *E.T.: The Extra Terrestrial.* Another case is little-known Mumford High School in Detroit, which sold $1 million worth of T-shirts after Eddie Murphy appeared in one in *Beverly Hills Cop.*[21] Patrick Denin, marketing coordinator for Zane Management, which handled local product placements for the movie *Rocky V*, asserts that product placements "are more credible than endorsements because they portray someone using a product in everyday life."[22] A critical factor here is product *usage* as compared to the mere appearance of a product in the film. Research by one product placement firm found that nearly 60 percent of respondents recalled (3–5 day delayed recall) Sylvester Stallone eating Wheaties in the movie *Rocky III.* However, only 1 percent remembered a quick shot of a William Grant and Sons Glenfiddich scotch bottle.[23]

It seems reasonable to assume that such findings will provide impetus for advertisers to further intrude into the creative process. Sandra Locke, the director of the film *Impulse*, relates such a conflict. During one scene, a TV set was supposed to be blaring a commercial, which was contracted to be on screen. Locke says her view of the scene did not

accommodate the commercial on screen, so she asked if audio placement would be sufficient, i.e. allowing the audience to hear but not see
the commercial. She was told that if the TV with the commercial did
not appear on screen, "we don't get the money."[24] In reality, product
placers increasingly view themselves as agents for products and,
therefore, view their function as getting "parts" for their clients. If
obvious opportunities for placement are not available, then placers are
wont to rewrite scripts to fit in product plugs. "I'm part screenwriter,"
says placer Larry Dorn, "I'm a creative artist."[25] Associated Film
Promotions claims it had a salad-making scene added to the film *North
Dallas Forty*, simply and specifically to promote Bertolli salad oil.[26]
Another example is the use of Mumm's Champagne in *Moonstruck*;
originally another brand of champagne was to be used.
    Lois Sheinfield has suggested the following:

> The movie industry may not realize the legal problems attendant upon
> this "valuable resource" [corporate America] and the commercialization
> of film. Take for example a movie version of Macbeth. What if Lady M.
> tries to get the damned spot out with a can of Ajax? If Ajax is Kovoloff's
> client and has to be presented in a positive manner, then naturally the
> Lady will get the spot out. Well, that's a problem. No matter that Shake-
> speare didn't want her to get the spot out. He's dead and can't complain.
> The problem is Truth in Advertising. Can Ajax get out a blood spot on
> the brain? Aye, there's the rub![27]

    Such anecdotes point out the very real danger of product placements
dictating production content. Peggy Charren, president of Action for
Children's TV, says, "It has gotten to the point where it (product placement) influences the story, where they'll say, 'Let's do this instead of
that, so we can make 20 deals.' It affects the content of editorial speech.
That's one reason you're likely to see films set only in the present,
instead of historical subjects. You can't make Marie Antoinette eat
Domino's Pizza."[28]
    Movie producers generally argue that they choose subjects of interest
and then listen to product placement appeals. Further, they argue that
product placements do not unduly influence artistic interpretation and
point out that placements often end up on the cutting room floor. Finally, it is suggested that such placements allow an element of reality by
providing real products in realistic settings. A product placement firm
executive explained that, "They used to go to great lengths not to have
a known product name in the movies. But now, a generic name would
detract from a scene. Unless you wanted it to look camp, like *Repo Man*,
with all those cans that said 'Food.'"[29]

Recent developments and knowledge of the intricacies of the system challenge these disclaimers. First, while it may be true that topics are contemplated without regard to product placements, it also seems increasingly likely that in an age of rising production costs consideration of potential revenues will be analyzed before the undertaking of any project. While it can be stated that a topic matter, in the abstract, may be beyond the purview of advertisers, can the same be said of the presentation in terms of individual scenes?

Second, the efficacy of the "cutting room floor" argument has recently become considerably more tenuous. Black and Decker has filed a $150,000 lawsuit naming Twentieth Century Fox and Krown-Young and Rubicam as defendants. The basis of the suit is breach of promise, in that a Black and Decker drill did not appear in the movie *Die Hard 2*.[30] If other manufacturers pursue this course of action, and given the quantity of expenditures that often support product placement, it seems inevitable that they will, then producers may be much less inclined to leave placements on the cutting room floor.

An additional permutation is the fact that product placement firms represent more than one branded product, leading to family deals where for a given amount of money the entire family, or some subdivision thereof, is placed in a film. Reality, in this case, has nothing to do with the vision of director or producer but rather with what products happen to be represented by a given placement firm.

In addition to recommending products and creating scenes to depict those products, script screeners also function to warn their clients of possible negative consequences for their products. Thus warned that a product is going to be used in a manner that may reflect adversely on the firm, corporations have a chance to lobby a producer to make changes or threaten a lawsuit before the film reaches the theaters.

The level of intrusion by advertisers into motion pictures has come under scrutiny by both citizen and legislative bodies. The concern of many is that product placement is a form of advertising that is largely unregulated. Congress is looking at placements by the cigarette industry with the intent of banning such "paid advertisements" in feature films.[31] Meanwhile, the Center for the Study of Commercialization, sponsored by the Center for Science in the Public Interest, a consumer advocacy group, has gone even farther and advocated the use of subtitles to identify every paid appearance or mention of a product or brand in a movie.[32] The group recently filed a petition with the Federal Trade Commission to declare product placements "an unfair business practice and require on-screen disclosure of products advertised in films."[33]

Certainly this practice has not been restricted solely to motion pictures.

A recent survey by *Advertising Age* found 818 "free plugs" over a 24 hour period on the three networks.[34] There is even a case of a product placement within a novel.[35] But for motion pictures, the phenomenon is becoming more and more entrenched. As president of marketing for Walt Disney Pictures, Bob Levin, recently observed, "I believe it's a long-term relationship that's now going to exist [between] the movie industry and product marketers."[36]

Advertisements in Theaters

Movie production is not the only area within the film industry that has seized upon the revenue opportunities presented by advertisers. Exhibitors are exploring ways to increase revenues, as advertisers and marketing agents are providing theater owners with opportunities to derive monies not directly related to the box office.

The most obvious vehicle is the practice of paid screen advertisements before the showing of a film. While this practice is common outside the USA, paid product endorsements are becoming more and more lucrative to American theater owners, as well. One company, Screenvision Cinema Network, has been packaging advertising for theaters since the late 1970s, although the advertisements were seldom the hard-sell commercials more common at the end of the 1980s. By 1989 the company produced commercials for a 5,700 screen system and sold approximately $25 million annually in advertising time.[37] Screenvision charges advertisers $20,000 per thousand viewers for a one-time 60 second shot, or $600,000 to $700,000 for a 28 day run that carries the guarantee of 31 million viewers.[38]

Advertisers are willing to commit such sums for two basic reasons: (1) they believe that commercials specifically designed to run in theaters are effective; and (2) moviegoers are, in general, relatively light viewers of television and therefore are exposed to fewer ads than the majority of the American populace. Moviegoers thus represent a prime (untapped) target for advertisers, especially a younger audience that (supposedly) does not watch as much television.[39]

The perception that theater audiences are, by and large, a captive, under-exposed (in terms of advertising) target market is indicated in the following examples:

1   The "Popcorn Report," a series of short subjects produced by West Glen Communications. These advertiser-sponsored newsreels are approximately ten minutes in length and cover a variety of subjects,

such as the 100th anniversary of peanut butter, sponsored by CPC International, the parent company of Skippy peanut butter. This might be an example of the infomercial trend, more commonly used in television advertising.

2   *Movies USA*, an entertainment magazine distributed primarily in theaters and supported by advertising. The magazine is currently 32 pages in length, of which 10–12 pages are advertising. Publisher Todd Macrae hoped to double distribution to 2 million copies and increase advertising support to expand the length to 64 pages by 1992. The magazine carries a cover price of $1.50, but is distributed free in theaters.

3   National Cinema Network's On-Screen Entertainment, a slide program including advertisements currently distributed to approximately 3,000 theaters. The slide show is shown during intermissions and currently runs at about 13 to 15 minutes. A four-week run costs advertisers $250,000. Long-term goals call for advertising slides to comprise a maximum of 20 percent of the program.

4   Turner Broadcasting System's Cable News Network's planned advertising-sponsored newsreel that would run prior to feature films. The company recently completed a two-minute test version that was distributed in twelve Manhattan theaters.[40]

5   Various merchandising programs within theaters. *Model* magazine has started distributing samples of products advertised in its publication in theaters nationwide. Screenvision Cinema Network has initiated a program offering moviegoers the opportunity to test-drive new cars parked directly outside the theater. Meanwhile, theater owners themselves are beginning to sell merchandise, such as clothing and other products, inside the theater. Terry Laughren, president of Screenvision, predicts that by the end of the decade, movie theaters will offer a wide range of products for sale to consumers who will have seen these products in the movie or commercials that precede it.

Screen advertising has engendered a modicum of controversy, most specifically in the advertising bans carried out by Disney and Warner Brothers, in which they mandated that no advertising messages be shown prior to their films. The companies' stated reasons for instituting the ban was their research (principally Disney's) indicating that theatergoers do not like, or want, advertisements played in the theater. The two companies claim that their ban is an attempt to conform to the wishes of the market and to differentiate the theater experience from in-home viewing. But again, these claims can be challenged.

First, Disney's findings are highly questionable. Basically, the company asked moviegoers if they "want commercials shown in movie theaters?" It is unlikely that even a minority of theater patrons would respond to this question in the affirmative. Why would anyone necessarily *want* commercials shown in theaters? It seems likely that the results of Disney's poll were exactly the results that Disney wanted to generate. This point is illustrated by the results of a poll conducted by the Gallup Organization for *Advertising Age*, claiming that opposition is milder than indicated by the Disney poll and that such resistance declines rapidly if the alternative to advertisements is higher ticket prices.[41]

In addition, both Disney and Warner Brothers specifically exempt trailers from their ban. Thus it is assumed that it is acceptable to advertise one's own products, and viewers object only to advertisements for others' products. Also exempted are slides projected during the intermission and messages for approved charitable purposes. In addition, the ban does not apply to short subjects, newsreels, or such vehicles as *Movies USA*. The idea that the ban will insulate moviegoers from advertisements is, obviously, ludicrous.

The final hypocrisy is that neither company has broached the subject of product placements within their movies. Both companies continue to accept and solicit product placements. For example, around the same time as the ban, Disney sent a letter to product makers offering placements in its film *Mr Destiny*, ranging in price from $20,000 to 60,000.[42]

The final say on in-theater advertising may be the province of the government, as the FTC is currently investigating the studios' ban as possible restraint of trade.[43] Regardless of any FTC action, in-theater advertisements in one form or another are likely to continue to increase in US theaters for the foreseeable future.

Meanwhile, theater owners are developing new schemes to bring in advertising revenue. One involves distributing samples of products in theaters, and was tested in selected UA theaters during 1991.[44]

Advertisements on Video

Commercials on home video find their genesis in the same bipartite mechanism that motivates product placements and ads in theaters: extra money for companies that release video movies and an attractive market for advertisers. Of course, advertising is not new to videocassettes – trailers for movies and other videos have been part and parcel of video movies since their inception. As video became more and more an alternative to commercial TV, it naturally followed that advertisers would be attracted to the medium.

Video advertising began with the video release of *Top Gun*, which included a Diet Pepsi advertisement. As mentioned previously, Paramount priced the cassette at $26.95, and sold almost 3 million units. Although other commercial sponsorships were initially turned down, by mid-1988 industry sources were concluding that "commercials in videocassettes are here to stay."[45] Money is paid by the advertiser to the supplier, with a variety of pricing arrangements. Sometimes pricing is similar to broadcast television (cost-per-thousand), although set fees can be charged: $2 per tape sold, or a single payment of $30,000.

Historically, from the advertisers' point of view, commercials on video were not so much an attempt to increase exposure as to maintain the level of exposure for those viewers who were deserting TV for video. More recently this trend has changed, as advertisers have started creating advertisements specifically for videos that relate thematically to the film, targeting specific audiences, and increasing cash fees for advertisements and promotional commitments. While exact figures have not been published, it is estimated that the Diet Pepsi advertisement on the *Top Gun* video was worth $8 million in promotional value to Paramount, and Vestron reportedly received between $50,000 and $100,000 from Nestlé for its advertisement on the *Dirty Dancing* video.[46]

Such sums are committed to video because, as an advertising medium, it is no longer perceived as merely supplementary to TV. In fact, advertisers are increasingly viewing video as a separate market comprised of a disparate audience that in many ways is more attractive than traditional TV audiences. One study determined that viewers recall commercials on cassettes ten times better than on commercial TV.[47] Such research cannot but provide impetus to the growth of video advertisements.

Further motivation is likely to be provided by Nielsen's home video ratings which have recently come on line. Data from Nielsen will allow advertisers to compile demographic information and more accurately assess viewing and response tendencies.[48] Preliminary tests conducted by Nielsen indicate that the vast majority of video viewers watch the advertisements, particularly those that are tied to the film either thematically or by using stars from the film.[49] Such data serves to validate video as a primary part of the advertising media mix.

Tie-ins

Joint promotions can help defray the cost of marketing a movie ... and they help us reach broader demographics. With joint consumer product

promotions, we can touch an audience that we don't normally reach with traditional movie advertising.
Jan Kean, national director of promotions for Orion Pictures Corporation

The boundary between what constitutes a tie-in and merchandising is at best indistinct. In this text, tie-ins will be considered as promotional campaigns tied to specific films, but associated with products not in the movie per se, nor based on characters or objects in the movie. Thus, the availability of a "special edition Rambo knife" selling for $2,250 falls under the category of merchandising, whereas the inclusion of a 60 second Pizza Hut commercial and coupon book good for $20 in food and Pepsi products at Pizza Hut restaurants on the *Teenage Mutant Ninja Turtles* videocassette constitutes a tie-in.[50] While it is true that the Turtles are renowned for their voracious appetite for pizza, Domino's Pizza, through a product placement deal, is the one that appears in the movie. The tie-in between pizza and the Ninja Turtles is a logical one, but instances of such things are not always as clear-cut. For instance, in order to promote the introduction of Paul Newman's salad dressing to its outlets, Burger King offered the videocassette of his film *Absence of Malice* to customers at a reduced price when they purchased salads.[51]

With so many promotional activities associated with a film, sometimes it becomes unclear who is promoting who or what is promoting what. To gain a clearer understanding of what is involved, a more in-depth look at specific instances is warranted. It is recognized that these are high profile, big budget examples. But rather than being aberrations from the norm, these examples are actually in the vanguard of tie-in practices and thus serve more as models than brief one-offs to be discounted.

"*Willow*"   George Lucas' film *Willow*, about a race of little people, sparked off a rash of tie-in activity. It is estimated that over $50 million in marketing tie-ins was riding on this one feature. Quaker Oats Co. alone committed $26 million in promotional programs. Other companies involved included General Foods, Hunt-Wesson, Kraft, Wendy's International, Tonka Toys, Parker Brothers, and Random House.

While the advertising budget of the distributor, MGM/UA Communications, was in excess of $6 million, Lucas Film Ltd promised a further $20 million in advertising and promotional support for its licensees. But these figures pale in comparison with the accumulative amounts coming from these licensees. Not only are the amounts of money being thrown around impressive, but the number of products tied to the film are equally overwhelming. Although the biggest media budgets were tied to Quaker's children's cereals (such as Cap'n Crunch and Oh's), the promotion also was extended to adult brands, including Aunt Jemima pancake mix, Rice-A-Roni side dishes and Quaker 100% Natural Cereal. The Quaker promotion kicked off on June 12, 1988, with a free standing insert (FSI) including coupons for free milk and a *Willow* spoon-and-dish premium. A second FSI offered $6 in coupons, plus other *Willow* premiums for consumers purchasing a variety of Quaker brands. In addition, these tie-ins were the focus of a five-week flight of TV spots for Cap'n Crunch.

Kraft Inc.'s multibrand cheese promotion – its biggest of the year – kicked off with a national FSI on May 22nd offering *Willow* products. Kraft's involvement included virtually all of its cheese products group: Cheez Whiz, Cracker Barrel, Kraft Singles, 100 percent Natural Cheeses, Philadelphia Brand cream cheese and Velveeta. The latter contained free *Willow* tickets in packages during May and June.

Meanwhile, Wendy's spent an estimated $5 million on a children's meal promotion tied to the film, and featured *Willow* magic cups with heat-sensitive decals depicting scenes from the film. This was backed by network TV and print advertising support. Beatrice Hunt-Wesson ran a back-to-school promotion for Peter Pan peanut butter tied to the film, while Dow Chemical Co.'s Ziploc brand had in-pack character trading cards in its sandwich bags. In addition, children were able to get free school folders at Dow's in-store displays. General Foods Corporation's Jell-o brand sponsored a give-away of 2 million *Willow* activity books in support of the Children's Miracle Network fund-raising telethon. Finally, there were toy tie-ins through Tonka Corporation, a board game from Parker Brothers and book versions for both adults and children from Ballantine Books.[52]

Although *Willow* did not materialize into the anticipated box office smash, Quaker exceeded its promotion objectives by 50 percent.[53] Thus for Quaker, at least, the tie-ins clearly worked, despite the movie's limited success at the box office.

It is apparent, then, that most of the tie-ins came from companies which had no literal connection with the movie – after all, no one in the film actually eats any Velveeta cheese (on screen, that is). The benefit to these companies comes from their association with a potentially successful movie which gives their essentially dull products (in terms of image) the chance to be thought of as part and parcel of a world of mystery and wonder. The purchaser can be involved in the fantasy world of *Willow* through the cards, figures, cereal bowls, etc., offered by these manufacturers.

For the movie, these kinds of tie-ins mean additional (free) TV and print advertising, point-of-sale advertising in every major supermarket in the country (which would be difficult to arrange without such tie-ins), and the chance to be associated with "good" promotional campaigns which tie themselves in turn to charitable causes (as in the case of Jell-o) or freebies for the kids associated with back-to-school (as in the case of Hunt-Wesson and Dow Chemical).

"Oliver & Company" and "Land Before Time"   When we look at the release and marketing strategy for two other films that hit the screens in late 1988, the complexity and interdependency of marketing tie-ins becomes clearer. *Oliver & Company* (Disney) had exclusive promotional tie-ins with Sears, Roebuck and Co. and McDonald's Corporation. *Land Before Time* (Universal/Amblin) went with J. C. Penney, Pizza Hut, and Dow Chemical Company. The unusual situation of two major animated features from major distributors scheduled for Christmas release meant that advertising and promotional tie-ins were even more crucial than normal. Because of the need to successfully break into the lucrative Christmas market, neither studio took any chances.

Marketing consultant for Universal and Amblin Entertainment, Martin Levy, acknowledged that they were doing somewhat more in their overall marketing effort because of competition from the Disney movie. Besides the tie-ins, Universal sent about 40,000 dinosaur "education kits" to schools across the country. In each kit were activities such as running twine out thirty feet to better understand how big the prehistoric beasts really were (note: another example of "good" marketing through schools, similar to the *Willow* examples). As one might expect, Universal was not solely concerned with the children's education, and thus each kit also included photos from the movie and a one-sheet display poster.

The campaigns by both sides were informed by the tremendous success that Universal had had with *An American Tail* (1987). Although the film was pitted against a re-release of Disney's *Cinderella*, it grossed $48 million at the box office, breaking records for the initial release of an animated feature. And, as of November 1988, *An American Tail* had sold over one million videocassettes. This success has been credited to one of the industry's most extensive merchandising and promotional deals (at that time) with Sears and McDonald's. Noting this phenomenon, Disney wasted no time in snapping up exclusive merchandising deals with Sears and McDonald's, starting with *Oliver & Company*. The deal was no doubt helped by the successful campaign run by Disney in the summer of 1988, with limited merchandising deals set up with McDonald's and Coca-Cola for Spielberg's *Who Framed Roger Rabbit?*. McDonald's and Coca-Cola spent $12 million and $10 million respectively on campaigns associated with the movie.[54]

The marketing strategy employed by Universal for *Land Before Time*, however, serves as a model for this type of enterprise, although obviously there are variations depending on the company involved. As Levy explains, "the first thing you do is establish the film." The $12 million campaign – featuring the slogan, "Here's the new one from the creators of *An American Tail*" – was a straightforward appeal and contained no mention of merchandise. The bulk of the advertisements were on network, spot and cable TV, targeting young women with children. After the movie broke, the advertising baton was passed to partners J. C. Penney and Pizza Hut. Penney's, which had $50 million worth of everything from plush animals and kids' clothing to sheets and wrapping paper tied up in the promotion, supported the licensing deal with a $6 million corporate advertising budget. This included two weeks of national TV and five holiday pre-prints, including an eight-page newspaper insert with a *Land Before Time* pop-up. The advertisements included movie clips for in-store advertising, for which Penney's created jungle-like shops to house dinosaur merchandise themed to the movie. In this jungle environment Penney's ran a videotape of select scenes from the film and listed local theaters showing it. Pizza Hut, for their part, spent an estimated $10 million, including four weeks of TV, direct mail and print. The only restrictions placed were that no advertisements were to break until November 16, two days before the movie's release. Thus, there was a tightly organized advertising campaign from early November through Christmas. In January, Dow Chemical stepped in with Ziploc bag advertisements touting its exclusive *Land Before Time* plastic glass promotion. Universal sustained its own campaign during this period, but as Levy notes, "the biggest bulk of TV was from them [the tie-in partners] not us and that is why we developed the spots with them so carefully."[55]

The exact nature and extent of cooperation between the tie-in partners and the studios certainly varies, according to the film and the participants. When Universal planned to release *An American Tail*, they were forced to change the release date (which in many cases, is of crucial importance) by Sears and McDonald's, who felt that the licensing risk was too great if they were given only a few weeks to sell their wares during the all-important Christmas season. Thus, instead of breaking the film when children's Christmas vacations started in mid-December, the release date was brought forward to mid-November. Although in the past, movie companies had been reluctant to share plots and character developments before release (Disney, in particular, still holds off from this), Amblin, although known for its secrecy in the past, gave the *Land Before Time* script to Penney's and Pizza Hut about a year before release on a confidential basis.

More examples could be cited, but the nature and extent of tie-ins for big budget films, particularly those aimed at children, is essentially the same. As Belinda Hulin-Salkin notes,

> Consumer promotions have gone Hollywood. In the continuing quest to cut through the media clutter – and rise above eroding network television ratings – marketers increasingly have set their sight on what may be the last captive media audience in America: moviegoers. And as film industry executives place more and more emphasis on bottom-line results, these partners are now welcomed onto movie sets with air kisses and open arms. The days when film makers could afford to snub tie-in proposals from manufacturers are clearly over.[56]

But lest one think that all we have here is a flurry of merchandisers beating down the doors of Hollywood in order to tie their products to the latest hot movie, this is indeed a two-way flow. Pamela Ellis-Simons notes that "movie studios, fully realizing how much an extra $20 million or so in advertising can help their film, are now courting marketers with the lure of exclusive deals. Overfield (Penney's) reports that several studios have already come to Penney's about future tie-ins."[57]

Some films released during the summer of 1990 were reported to have received $30–40 million in tie-in revenue, with the "Dick Tracy Crimestopper Game" promotion by McDonald's purported to be the largest movie tie-in ever at $40 million. However, 1991's big summer movies boasted only "modest" support averaging around $10–15 million per film.[58]

Clearly the situation is beneficial to all parties involved. No budget-conscious studio could pass up the chance for the extra advertising clout that tie-ins can furnish. However, it is unclear to what extent the desire for this extra exposure influences the studios' conduct or the content of the films. Marketers will not be willing to invest or promote films that they do not feel can guarantee a return. Stung by past failures, such as *Howard the Duck*, marketers will wish more and closer involvement with the studios, as indicated with *Land Before Time*. Thus, it would seem that only the safest of commodities will be the recipients of the tie-in goldmine, and consequently variety and innovation may be pushed aside. Moreover, as we noted with the involvement of Disney with Sears and McDonald's, some of the most lucrative outlets have already been tied to exclusive contracts, further restricting the ability of other studios to exploit the potential of these symbiotic relationships should they so desire.

Since 1988 the studios have intensified their marketing strategies of videos, as well, incorporating techniques similar to packaged-goods companies. Tie-ins with beverages and packaged foods mean valuable display placements in supermarkets, convenience stores and restaurants. An example is Disney's 1989 holiday campaign, which included cross-promotion of its videos with Coca-Cola, Procter and Gamble and McDonald's. Other studios made similar arrangements with other companies, allowing their products to be seen much more widely than in video rental stores.[59]

In a new merchandising wrinkle, Paramount Pictures announced a tie-in arrangement with Kmart, which would promote all of its summer films during 1991. The promotion – entitled "Passport to Summer Entertainment" – involved scratch and win cards redeemable for prizes at the stores. While not unusual in itself, it marked the first time a complete list of summer films would be tied to a single promotional partner.[60]

Meanwhile, *Advertising Age* reported that home video marketers spent $85 million during the second half of 1991 to market movies to children. Distributors aligned with promotional partners to share the costs. For example, Fox Video's *Home Alone* was backed with a $25 million promotional campaign shared by Pepsi-Cola and American Airlines, while New Line Home Video, Burger King and Nabisco devoted $20 million to promoting the video release of *Teenage Mutant Ninja Turtles II*.[61]

Merchandising and Licensing

> Merchandising! We put the picture's name on everything. Merchandising, merchandising; that's where the real money from the movie is made.
> (Just Plain) Yogurt, played by Mel Brooks, in *Space Balls*

> Warner Communications – Licensing the World.
> Seen on a shopping bag carried by a woman in San Francisco airport

The distinction between tie-ins and merchandise is often blurred, as some merchandise is produced for tie-ins. This study will consider merchandise as commodities based on movie themes, characters or images which are designed, produced and marketed for direct sale, and not connected to other products or services (as with tie-ins).

Licensing has been described as a "legal mechanism by which one party legally obligates itself to pay the holder of a copyright or trademark a specific royalty in order to use a name, likeness or image."[62] Thus, licensing is the legal act – the process of selling or buying property rights to produce commodities using specific copyrighted properties. On the other hand, merchandising can be thought of as the mechanical act of making or selling a product based on a copyrightable product.

There is an extremely wide variety of movie-based merchandise, including items based on a specific movie, character or theme, or on-going movie characters and themes. While there has been a strong emphasis on children's toys, games and other items (lunch boxes, school supplies, etc.), other movie-based merchandise includes home furnishings (clocks, towels, bedding, mugs, telephones), clothing, jewelry, stationary items, print material (novelizations, trading cards, posters, etc.), food (especially cereals and candy), and decorations (such as Christmas ornaments).

Other more unusual, less mass-produced items sometimes accompany (or follow) movie releases, including "art objects" such as prints, sculptures, ceramic figures, and animation sets (an example is the set of five Bugs Bunny animation cels available from the Warner collection at $3,250). Other examples would be a replica of Rambo's knife ($2,250), Bugs Bunny greeting calls (1-900-VIP-BUGS), and *Gone with the Wind* wine.[63]

Other merchandise is based on the celebrity status of Hollywood stars. While successful actors and actresses in the 1940s started independent film companies, celebrities of the 1980s pitched their own brand of salad dressing (Paul Newman), line of clothing (Brooke Shields), or perfume and cologne (Elizabeth Taylor). Though not based on characters or themes from specific films, these items draw on the status of the film star to sell products, and thus should be considered Hollywood-related merchandise.

In addition to specific film- or character-based merchandise, some of the larger entertainment companies now offer generic movie or studio merchandise. Examples include Warner Brothers hats, jackets, and mugs, miniature movie clapper boards, and mock Academy Awards. These items are sold through the studios' catalogues or "entertainment stores," such as Suncoast Motion Picture Company. The Hollywood Chamber of Commerce has joined in, marketing trading cards based on stars featured on Hollywood Boulevard's "Walk of Fame." Thus, Hollywood increasingly has been selling itself in merchandisable forms.

While movie-based merchandising can be viewed as part of the proliferation of commercialization in Hollywood, this type of activity is
part of a larger merchandising and licensing trend. Licensed products
represented $66.5 billion in retail sales in 1990.[64] TV programs and
characters – especially those aimed at children – are an obvious and
prevalent form of merchandising, while sports teams and players, rock
stars, and musical groups have long histories of licensing and merchandising activities.[65] For instance, the growing phenomenon of sports cards
dates back to the 1880s, when tobacco companies included baseball
heroes in packets of tobacco.[66] These days products are based on well-
known images, brands and even companies, e.g. Coca-Cola clothes,
Harley-Davidson sunglasses. Even non-commercial organizations in the
USA are now offering merchandise, such as the products available from
public broadcast stations. *Signals* is a catalog published by the WGBH
Education Foundation, which offers videos of PBS series, plus T-shirts,
mugs, books, jewelry and other educational, comic, or "tasteful" items,
sometimes, but not always, connected to PBS programming.

Movie-based merchandise is especially motivated by the proliferation
of such activities, as well as the massive, coordinated merchandising
campaigns – often started months before a film's release – associated
with a few blockbuster films. This merchandising bonanza represents
sizable profits. Sales of merchandise licensed from movies and stage
shows in 1985 brought in $3.5 billion, although only $2.2 billion was
received in 1987.[67]

Some recent examples include *Batman*, which grossed $250 million
and earned $50 million in licensing fees, *Rambo III*, which involved 50
licensing agreements for more than 75 products,[68] and *The Jetsons*, which
also attracted 50 licensees. Meanwhile, the *Star Trek* television series and
films have generated a $500 million merchandising bonanza for the 35
companies which produce various products.[69] Merchandising successes
have not only featured cuddly, heroic characters: Freddy Krueger of
Nightmare on Elm Street has generated more than $3 million in licensing
fees for Freddy posters, T-shirts, and other items.[70]

Universal's *Jurassic Park* may represent the ultimate model (at this
point in time) for blockbuster merchandising/tie-in/product placement
activities. The dino-tale made over $50 million at the box office during
the first weekend of release in June 1993, and reached $750 million in
gross worldwide revenues before the year ended.

But that was only half the story. As one reporter announced, the
feature film "has unleashed a wave of dinosaur-mania across the US."[71]
More accurately, Universal Pictures and producer/director Steven
Spielberg unleashed a wave of Jurassic Park products, playing into the

already-existing interest in dinosaurs and prehistoric creatures. The film was accompanied by over 1,000 products identified as official Jurassic Park merchandise, distributed by 100 official Jurassic Park manufacturers around the world. The products included the usual: T-shirts, toothbrushes, and school supplies. Also available were $15 boxer shorts with images of velociraptors, a $1 Jurassic Park jawbreaker ("take eons to eat") and a line of 30 toys (featuring "Dino Damage") from Kenner. The tie-ins included McDonald's and Toys-R-Us, which distributed free Jurassic Park boxes including sample products and coupons.

Interestingly, the film itself was a tie-in, with the Jurassic Park logo in the film repeated on official Jurassic Park merchandise, plus a scene in the film featuring the park's gift store displaying Jurassic Park merchandise – the same merchandise available outside the movie. Thus, Universal and Spielberg neatly combined Jurassic Park merchandising, product placement and tie-in activities into one process.

The recent proliferation of movie merchandising may be related to the current upswing in general merchandising, as well as an increase in animated features and the re-release and remakes of films with readily identifiable, on-going characters and themes. But while these recent developments may reflect a new stage in Hollywood's commodification of entertainment, merchandising is not really a new game in Tinseltown.

Until the 1960s and 1970s, relatively little merchandising activity took place in Hollywood, except for Disney. For the Disney company, merchandising started almost simultaneously with the tremendous success of Mickey Mouse's *Steamboat Willie*. Although various histories claim that Walt Disney was not necessarily interested in licensing his characters, merchandising activities still provided needed revenue to continue producing expensive animated films.[72] In 1929 the company was offered $300 to put Mickey Mouse on writing tablets, and by January 1930, Mickey appeared in a comic strip distributed by King Features (Hearst-owned). During the 1930s, the George Borgfeldt Co. was authorized to handle the licensing of Mickey and Minnie products, which included handkerchiefs, drums, rubber balls and other toys. But in 1932, Herman "Kay" Kayman took over and began to flood the market with Disney products. "Mickey's likeness soon appeared on everything from soap to ice-cream cones to Cartier diamond bracelets ($1,250)."[73]

During the depths of the depression, the Disney merchandising bonanza supposedly saved the Lionel Co. with the sale of 253,000 Mickey Mouse handcars and the Ingersoll Waterbury Co. with the sale of 2.5 million Mickey Mouse watches. By 1934, annual profits on films and merchandise brought in over $600,000 for the Disney company. Mickey is still claimed to be the most popular licensed character in the world today, appearing on more than 7,500 items, not including publications.[74] (More on Disney later in this section.)

But the Disney company has been the exception, rather than the rule. While the motion picture industry may have been relatively slow to pick up on merchandising activities, television was less hesitant. Since the 1950s, there have been numerous examples of licensing and merchandising successes from children's shows to westerns to action adventure programs. But the current phase of film-based licensing can be traced back to the merchandising successes of *Star Wars* and *E.T.* in the 1970s.

According to one industry source, "[e]ntertainment licensing is a very small and closely knit community."[75] The *owners* of licensable properties are most often the major entertainment corporations which distribute a wide range of entertainment commodities and hold copyrights and trademarks for movie-based characters and themes. Special licensing divisions often are organized to handle these properties (and those owned by others, as well), e.g. Warner's Licensing Corporation of America (LCA) and Disney's Consumer Products division. But even smaller successful film producers sometimes are involved in licensing, as represented by Lucasfilm Licensing.

Licensees include a wide array of individuals, companies, and firms which buy the rights to produce merchandise based on a copyrighted character or image. Larger companies usually do their own research before licensing a character or product, although information is available (for a price) from *research companies* such as Marketing Evaluations/TVQ, which measures consumer attitudes toward celebrities, brand names, and cartoon characters.[76] *Retailers* are those companies which offer the products for sale to the public. Five *trade magazines* covering the licensing industry have started since 1979, thus indicating the rapid growth of the merchandising business.

Licensees usually pay royalties based on a fixed percentage (typically 5–15 percent) on the wholesale or retail selling price of the licensee's products.[77] Other promotional deals involve a fee, ranging from $25,000 for an average film to $100,000 for a major film or sequel. In addition "the marketer pays royalties or a percent of premium sales (the average is 6% or 7% of the manufacturer's selling price)."[78] Another source explains that most licensers add an 8–15 percent fee on top of the normal price of a licensed product.[79] While there are sometimes complications over the sharing of ancillary rights, creative control (i.e. how a character is used), or quality standards for products,[80] the arrangements often are advantageous for all parties concerned.

The benefits for studios are the increased profits – "easy dollars . . . all bottom line and very clean."[81] Such revenues also contribute to production costs, which continue to rise dramatically for Hollywood productions. In addition, merchandising typically helps to promote a film, especially when linked to other activities, thus creating synergy within a corporation. It is even claimed that for some films, merchandising is necessary for success at the box office. A recent example was the weak release of *Teenage Mutant Ninja Turtles* in Japan, which was blamed on the lack of merchandising back-up.[82]

For merchandisers, the obvious advantage is to be linked to a successful movie. "A film has the potential to be a big event that will produce a product to break out of the pack," explains James Pisors, director of licensing and entertainment for Tonka Toy Co.[83]

However, it seems that Hollywood wants the toymakers more than the toymakers want Hollywood, as indicated by the toy industry's $16 billion retail revenue in 1989 (three times the revenues received at the box office for Hollywood films).[84] Products based on a movie can be considered risky for merchandisers, as they often have short lifespans connected to the box office release of the film.[85] Some toy companies are not even interested in this type of merchandise, noting that "[a]s soon as the movie is pulled from release, the corresponding property usually becomes ancient history on toy shelves and unless it's timed for Christmas it isn't worth the financial exposure."[86]

Licensees may have to take further risks initially by sinking money into a film that is not completed (or sometimes not even started). There also is criticism that movie companies put "too much emphasis on box office at expense of merchandise."[87] Thus, some conclude that "the risk of a licensing failure falls mostly to the manufacturer of the product, not to the company selling its name."[88]

At worst, a studio may need to change a release date, especially to coincide with the lucrative Christmas season.[89] But for the most part, licensing represents an attractive proposition to movie makers who can offer merchandisable properties.

But what is merchandisable? And why do some products succeed while others fail? As one industry insider notes, "[t]he licensed property per se is relatively insignificant . . . for the most part it doesn't matter whether it's a film or TV character or a toy or a hot new band. It can be anything from a rock to a raisin."[90] Another industry executive offered advice for television, which also seems applicable to film: "A program must have a sense of adventure and create an environment which the child or adult can relate to on many plateaus. In other words, the situation must develop into *toyetic applications* – characters which have a personality that can be easily transferred to dolls and playset environments" (emphasis added).[91]

However, there seem to be as many examples of merchandising failures as there are of successes. Some are connected to unsuccessful (in terms of box office) films, like *Howard the Duck*. When the film flopped in 1986, LJN Toys was reported to have written down $1 million.[92] Other films have been successful at the box office, but not in terms of merchandising (i.e. *Jaws, Back to the Future, Who Framed Roger Rabbit?, Rambo, First Blood: Part II*).

The editor of *Toy and Hobby World*, Larry Carlat, has suggested four basic reasons for these "bombs."[93] The first element is timing. Carlat notes that there is a "merchandising window of opportunity" during which the movie is doing well at the box office. There also are seasonal variations, with summer and Christmas as the hottest marketing periods of the year for both movies and merchandise. Another tricky timing problem is coordinating merchandise availability with the film's opening. While *Batman's* pre-exposure campaign seemingly worked well, the strategy used for *Dick Tracy* (merchandise mostly timed with the film's release) may have contributed to the disappointing performance of Tracy merchandise, at least according to many merchandisers. (The Disney company seemed to be quite pleased, however, as discussed in the case study to follow.)

Another factor suggested by Carlat is competition, as he argues that there are only a few "hot licenses" at any one time. However, one successful film may start a "feeding frenzy," during which symbiotic relationships are formed. He notes that "[i]n entertainment licensing, everyone feeds off each other, at least until the consumer can't stomach it anymore." In addition, Carlat points out that movie licensing is streaky or cyclical, as indicated, for instance, by contrasting the total sales from 1985 ($3.5 billion) and 1987 ($2.2 billion).

Some companies are trying to overcome this problem by focusing on characters or images that endure. An example is *The Simpsons*. Although originally a television-based merchandising phenomenon, the Fox strategy of "playing licensing for the long haul" also translates to movie-based properties. Al Ovadia, vice-president of licensing and merchandising for Twentieth Century Fox, explains that "[w]e're really looking five years down the line . . . We're not just putting their pictures on a T-shirt. We're trying to sell the whole attitude."[94]

The final factor mentioned by Carlat is the kiss of death to merchandisers – no market demand. Although there are many merchandising success stories, there also is the real difficulty of translating film fantasy to popular products. One way of overcoming part of this problem is creating merchandise not dependent on people seeing a film,[95] or not directly linking the merchandise to a specific film. The main problem, however, is the creation of merchandise that consumers are interested in buying, whether or not they have actually seen the films on which the products are based.

Copied or pirated merchandise is another issue which might be added to Carlat's list, but mostly pertains to successful merchandising efforts which attract imitators and copyright infringers.[96] Obviously, the companies involved in licensing are strong supporters of stringent copyright and trademark protection.

Video Games

The importance of video games as ancillary products for Hollywood films has grown dramatically in the last few years and deserves more careful attention. The current video game boom has been built over the last eight years by two Japanese companies: Nintendo and Sega, relying primarily on a faithful market of pre-teen boys.[97] But strategies aimed at other market segments (sports-oriented games, etc.) and the use of new techniques to enhance the reality of game scenarios have attempted to expand the video game market beyond just young boys. Thus, Hollywood, as well as other companies, is paying much more attention to the $5.3 billion video game business in the USA, where a single hit can reap $500 million in sales. Meanwhile, revenues from worldwide game sales for 1992 exceeded $10 billion.

But the potential for interactivity on new information systems has directed even more attention to the video game phenomenon. Time Warner and TCI already offer a Sega channel on their cable systems. And these companies, along with AT&T and Matsushita, have invested in new video game companies which promise to offer the latest interactive games that may help sell new home information systems. In other words, video games have become an appealing and important product that these corporations hope will attract specific market segments to the fiber-optic 500-channel systems of the future. "Suddenly a new medium – and a new market opportunity – has opened up in the place where Hollywood, Silicon Valley and the information highway intersect."[98]

But the video game/Hollywood connection is not a new one. In the past, cartoon and film characters were licensed to video game makers for 5–10 percent of net sales, thus video game sales contributed to merchandising revenues for some films. Warner Communications was intimately involved in the early video game business through its ownership of Atari. But the relationship proved sour when the business collapsed in 1984, not helped by Atari's disastrous production of an *E.T.* game for $23 million. Since then, video games have been seen by Hollywood as part of overall merchandising efforts, and it has continued to license its characters to companies such as Nintendo and Sega for video game development.

Today, with an expanded video game market and the potential for even further expansion, Hollywood has rediscovered video games as an obvious element in their synergistic strategies. As noted in chapter 4 in the discussion of Sony and Columbia Pictures, video games are no longer afterthoughts, but are developed and produced simultaneously with a feature film. The majors now have video game components or subsidiaries, which check out the potential of new films for game versions, may even alter film scripts to make more exciting games, and shoot footage for video games at the same time the film is shot. Computer and video technology make it possible to produce a game more quickly, and also to present increasingly realistic landscapes and to use real actors in game scenarios.[99]

Hollywood has made a few video game characters into feature film and television programs, including Super Mario and Sonic the Hedgehog. But more often, appropriate movies become video games, just as they become T-shirts, CDs and trading cards. Christmas offerings for 1993 included new games based on *Cliffhanger*, *Last Action Hero*, *Bram Stoker's Dracula*, and, of course, *Jurassic Park*. Already available were game titles such as *RoboCop*, *Terminator 2*, *RoboCop versus Terminator*, *Star Wars*, *Beauty and the Beast*, *The Little Mermaid* and *Aladdin*. Which brings us again to Disney.

Case Study: Disney

The Walt Disney Co. represents the premier movie merchandising company. Not only has the company been at the merchandising business longer than most other film companies, as previously discussed, but also Disney has a reputation for licensing and producing only quality products.

Disney also represents the ultimate example of synergism in action. As discussed in chapter 4, in addition to producing and distributing Disney, Touchstone and Hollywood films and Disney television programming, the company owns a pay-cable channel, home video division, independent TV station, and numerous theme parks, hotels, and resort complexes. Not only does Disney actively create licensable properties, but the company is able to reinforce their merchandising efforts throughout their extensive business empire.

Even though some merchandisers were disappointed with the results of Disney's (actually, Touchstone's) *Dick Tracy*, the film still represents an excellent example of this synergistic cycle. According to Disney sources, *Tracy* was reported to be the top grossing film licensing program of all time for the Disney company, garnering twice the revenues of their previous champ, *Roger Rabbit*.[100] The premiere of the film was staged at the MGM/Disney park, followed by daily *Dick Tracy* shows and store windows featuring Tracy merchandise. All this activity was in addition to the merchandise offered by 84 licensees, numerous tie-in deals, and "boutiques" featuring Tracy products at top retail chains.

Even the competition was in awe. "*Dick Tracy* was certainly a very, very effective job of bringing together, synergistically, Disney's cross divisions," admitted David Weitzner, president of worldwide marketing for MCA's recreation services.[101] One of Disney's executives echoed Weitzner: "When you combine the right film with the right products, there's a terrific synergy that takes place."[102]

Generally, Disney's licensing activities are handled by their Consumer Products division. Their job is to "license the name of Walt Disney, its characters, its visual and literary properties and its songs and music to various consumer manufacturers, retailers and publishers throughout the world." The division also becomes "actively involved in the creation, design and approval of licensed merchandise. . . . The company also continually seeks to create new characters to be used in licensed products."[103] Thus, the Disney company produces some merchandise itself, but also sells licenses to others to produce Disney merchandise.

One estimate claims that 3,000 companies manufacture 14,000 Disney-licensed products, which were sold at retail for more than $1 billion in 1987.[104] According to the company, the value of Disney retail products in the USA topped $2.5 billion in 1990.[105] Revenues for the Consumer Products division reached $573,800,000 in 1990, 40 percent higher than in 1989, which was 67 percent higher than 1988. Operating income for 1990 was $223,200,000.[106] It has also been reported that the Disney company reaps $100 million annually in foreign sales of merchandised products.[107]

The Consumer Products division supervises an extremely wide array of outlets in which Disney characters may be featured. Publishing activities include comic books, children's books, and other printed material. The addition of new comic book titles typically follows the release of new Disney films (example: *Roger Rabbit* was added in 1990). *Disney Adventures Magazine* appeared in stores in October 1990, and includes a mix of stories and Disney comics. The publishing arm also handles Disney Books by Mail, and arranges long-term deals with other publishers. Disney Audio Entertainment produces book and audio cassette read-alongs, which proved especially lucrative for *The Little Mermaid* – more than one million copies were sold in only six months after its release.[108]

Records, audio products and music publishing offer further opportunities to feature Disney properties, and are especially lucrative for animated features, given the important role of music in these films. Disney sells music-related products through domestic retail sales and direct marketing (catalogs, coupon packages and television).

In 1988, Disney spent $61 million on Childcraft, a New Jersey company that owned two of the biggest mail order lists in the country.[109] And by 1990, the company was mailing over 45 million Disney, Childcraft (direct mail subsidiary) and Just for Kids! catalogs. Products offered included infant merchandise, featuring Disney character brands (the Disney Babies Brand with Baby Mickey, Baby Donald and friends). The company represents 10 percent of the $2.2 billion infant products market.[110]

In addition, Disney Educational Productions created 47 films, videos, and film strips for schools, libraries, and other institutions in 1990. The company also produces educational toys, play equipment, and classroom furniture for children, as well as posters and teaching aids. Disney licenses its properties to software producers through the Disney Software Licensing division.

The Consumer Products division is in charge of new retailing activities, which also contribute to the synergistic emphasis of the Disney empire. The newly added Disney Store chain promised 100 outlets by the end of 1991, providing centralized sources for Disney merchandise, both in the USA and in foreign locations. The stores are consistent with Disney philosophy: "The core strategy behind The Walt Disney Co.'s retail endeavor, The Disney Store, is to be both entertainer and merchant."[111] The outlets include Disney characters in costume, videos, animation, and other attractions, carefully coordinated with the racks of merchandise in each store. By 1991, sales volume had doubled each year since the opening of the first store in 1987.

These Consumer Services activities link with other Disney businesses to provide the ultimate synergism for merchandising maximization. Disney cartoons and features are distributed via film, television, cable, and home video. The theme parks offer ready-made opportunities to feature new Disney characters and themes, as well as to sell merchandise. Recent additions to the parks have included shows and revues based on the Muppets, Roger Rabbit, The Little Mermaid, Aladdin and the previously mentioned Dick Tracy.

The company has been highly successful in merchandising activities in international markets. The most recent examples include an outlet on the French Minitel home information network which provides information about Disney publications, TV programs, home video and films. It has become the most popular channel for children aged 6 to 12.[112]

Disney magazines and comics were recently introduced in eastern Germany, Czechoslovakia, Poland and the former USSR, where 200,000 copies of the first Russian-language Mickey Mouse comic books sold out within hours after being released in 1990. And in Japan, a quarterly magazine and merchandise catalog (*Disney Fan*) is distributed at Tokyo Disneyland.

Disney also is known as one of the toughest enforcers of copyright, as attested by the large number of suits filed against infringers of their products and characters.[113]

Merchandising Madness

It has been pointed out that some movies have become one long merchandising pitch, just as children's cartoons on television have. But what about other less obvious influences on the creative process and film content?

Synergistic links may mean the influence of marketing decisions on the creative process. The advice cited previously about creating toyetic characters or situations was supplemented as follows: "The licensing arm of your business must be in constant touch with the producers to give advice and to encourage the inclusion of licensable elements in the weekly shows. This action will aid in creating a most beneficial licensing factor for the show."[114] One might imagine the same advice being given to filmmakers. Indeed, at a symposium for writers and producers held at UCLA in the late 1970s, a merchandising executive from one of the companies handling *Star Wars* products blatantly advised screenwriters to *write in* characters which have merchandisable characteristics.

Carlat also has suggested that merchandise is formula-driven, relying on established genres and characters.[115] Thus, creativity may be minimal when film scripts and characters must fit into these formulas in order to land valuable merchandising contracts. And Kathleen Kennedy, of Amblin Entertainment, has called attention to the timing of licensing activity connected with a film, noting that there has been "a real acceleration in the need to analyze what your market is earlier in the film production process, especially given the long lead time required by licensing and merchandising to launch production and film tie-ins."[116]

Other concerns revolve around the proliferation of merchandise and products. Some ask what is wrong with audiences consuming merchandise featuring their favorite character or movie theme? If consumers are willing to pay, so what? Some speculate that people have dull lives and want to identify with heroes (or villains), movie stars, or romantic or exciting situations. Others claim that nostalgia and patriotism are expressed through such merchandise.[117]

Meanwhile, the only fear of merchandisers and filmmakers – other than products not selling – seems to be overmarketing or saturation. A Disney executive has explained that "the company is very aware of the dangers of commercialism."[118] Yet, the expansion continues with little or no concern about the effects on the society and culture as a whole.

So What?

While product placements, tie-ins and merchandising are not characteristic of all Hollywood films, it is clear that these commercial activities have accelerated dramatically over the last decade. Blockbuster films and those oriented to children are the most common examples of these trends, although films appealing to a more narrowly targeted audience are not exempt (e.g. Nike shoes in Spike Lee films).

It also seems obvious that there is far more coordination of these activities, thus the potential for more profits but from fewer ideas. In other words, there is much more deliberate commercialization surrounding the production and distribution of Hollywood films than in the past. The potential consequences of these developments can be discussed in terms of creative, economic, and cultural implications.

While it is impossible to say with any absolute certainty how the growing trends of product placement within films and of merchandising possibilities affect creative decision-making, a number of conclusions can be inferred. In several instances cited in these case studies, manufacturers and those involved with joint promotions were privy to script details well before release date. Although there is little evidence that they were able to change the script in any way, it is not inconceivable that in the future (given the highly lucrative and often risky nature of merchandising and tie-ins), manufacturers and joint promoters will demand more and more knowledge of the film before release and may indeed even try to influence the productions in order to maximize the benefits accruing to them by such deals.

In the case of independent producers, the ability to offset production costs by use of tie-ins and product placement is an even thornier issue. While it is true that most product placement and tie-in activity is associated with the big budget, mass appeal films, independent productions which cater to minority or select audiences also are very attractive to manufacturers and advertisers. The ability to place products in such films enables the manufacturer to target a sizable audience in more direct and quantifiably measurable ways than afforded by more conventional advertising avenues. Clearly the prospect of knowing that you are targeting a large audience which is generally not catered to by mainstream media is a great incentive to manufacturers to push for product placement.

While in the short term this may be beneficial to independent filmmakers because of the greater availability of funds, in the long term it may have adverse effects, as the cultural identity and specificity of minorities become co-opted by the all-embracing power of the marketplace, which after all, serves to buttress and perpetuate the dominant society. Hence the minority becomes just another part of the larger culture and a consumer of its products and aspirations.

It might be argued that identifiable brand products add an aura of verisimilitude to a film. This may well be true, but it is important to note that the products placed are only those of the largest and most powerful producers and thus are not a true indication of the variety or use of products in the marketplace. In this sense, they actually become unrealistic. For example, not everyone in the Afro-American community drinks Miller's beer, but if one takes the example of *Do the Right Thing*, it would seem as though they did.

One result of this general acceptance of movies as a viable advertising medium (product placements, in theaters, and on video) is that advertisers are likely to get involved in the whole process at a much earlier stage. In product placement by means of script searches, in advertising and product promotion in theaters, and in advertisements appearing on cassettes, advertisers will attempt to promote specific themes and deliver consistent messages. Throw in promotional tie-ins and merchandising efforts, and it may not be too far-fetched to predict the day when advertisers approve scripts and stars and modify all elements of the motion picture process to suit particular advertising goals. As one writer concludes, "where the economic stakes are high, the pressures to subordinate professional integrity to the sales agenda of the highest bidder are irresistible."[119]

In this sense children's video may offer a view of the future. Certainly it is hard to imagine most children's videos (as with TV cartoons) as anything other than one long commercial. One series of tapes, "Dyno-Riders," are not only essentially a commercial, they intersperse the "plot" with advertising breaks exactly like the format of commercial TV – an "ads within an ad" technique that takes audience manipulation to new levels.

Further, although it is true that the marketplace controls the types of films made, an increasing reliance on the revenues from the sources discussed in this chapter may actually limit the types of film considered for production, as possible spin-offs, tie-ins, and product deals come to play a more important factor in pre-production planning.

The most obvious economic consequence is the further commodification of motion pictures. Similar to other forms of mass media, film now represents not only a commodity in itself, but also serves as an advertising medium for other commodities and increasingly generates additional commodities. These developments provide additional sources of capital (and possibly profits) for film companies, advertising agencies and product manufacturers.

It seems clear from this discussion, then, that American entertainment generally stimulates the US economy as a multiplier for other products and businesses, including advertising, toys and games, consumer electronics, fast food, etc. This effect has been noted by the Chief of the US Census Bureau of Economic Programs, who claimed that "the role of entertainment as a multiplier is probably as great as, or greater than, any other industry's." While there are difficulties accurately measuring the impact of this effect on the economy, some economists estimate that over $500 billion in sales are generated from entertainment-related activities in the USA alone.[120]

It has been suggested that placements may aid independent film production and thus create diversity by pouring money into needy projects. Certainly the potential for such an eventuality exists. However, product placement, despite its potential returns, is still by and large a gamble. An advertiser that buys a significant amount of time on network TV is likely to receive a credit if ratings on sponsored programs fail to live up to expectations. But a manufacturer that pours money into a Hollywood dud is essentially out of luck. Therefore, placement firms by and large recommend placement based on proven track records – who is producing, starring, directing and distributing.[121] Such conservativeness does little more than perpetuate the status quo.

It might be argued that at least more capital and profits would lead to more films produced. However, there is little hope for such a development when the typical companies able to successfully participate in these activities are the larger dominant corporations interested primarily in big, blockbuster films. These firms are better able to attract advertisers and merchandisers, thus (again) limiting competition for these new sources of capital and profits.

Finally, there are cultural implications related to these creative and economic consequences. Perhaps the most obvious is the contribution made by these developments to an enhanced consumer culture. Reminiscent of Thorstein Veblen's concept of "conspicuous consumption,"[122] Hollywood films increasingly provide the vehicle and inspiration for the display of brand-name products and culturally identifiable merchandise. In sometimes disturbing ways, both individual and cultural identities become bound up in this type of consumption. Indeed, the way in which these "real world" commodities are introduced in the fantasy world of film is another disturbing element that deserves more attention.

The amount of advertising in our society is disturbing enough, but even more ominous when directed at children. As Ronald Collins recently argued,

> The advertisers' catechism teaches vulnerable children to worship materialism. The product push in turn begins a chain reaction of peer pressure, which then is eased only by purchasing the product. Everything from the cartoons kids watch to the comics they read, from school studies to sports activities, from movies to malls, is colored by the consumptive bias of commercialism.[123]

It also might be argued that the repetition of themes, images, and characters, across media, as well as into other areas of daily life, severely limits the expression of ideas and values, or what Eileen Meehan has called the "cultural fund."[124] Indeed, the principle of synergy in the business sense might be extended to popular culture; in other words, a form of *cultural synergy* results from this overlapping of cultural images and ideas. (This idea will be further discussed in chapter 10.)

While this chapter has only tentatively addressed these issues, it seems clear that the various activities described work together to enhance the commodification of culture and the intensification of consumer society.

We will return to these themes in the final chapter, but first there is a great deal to Hollywood that is beyond the borders of the USA. Thus, the next chapter will discuss the global expansion of the US film industry.

9

Around the World in Nanoseconds: International Markets for Filmed Entertainment

From Hollywood – the entertainment capital of the world...
Introduction to *The Comedy Hour* on the Arts and
Entertainment Channel

The USA, while no longer the unchallenged industrial giant it once was, still excels in producing missiles, and selling entertainment commodities. It has been estimated that in 1986 the US industry received around 30 percent of total revenues from film, pay cable, TV and video from foreign markets. By the early 1990s, that amount had increased to 43 percent. The industry received an estimated $11.5 billion from all these markets in 1991.[1] (See table 9.1 for worldwide film revenues for US companies in 1986 and 1991). While international markets are not foreign to Hollywood, the dramatic growth in revenues from these sources is an important element in understanding the film industry in the 1990s.

US dominance in entertainment and media worldwide has been scrutinized, analyzed, dissected and bisected by critics, media researchers and scholars. But a reassessment of its growing strength is especially germane given recent political events and technological developments. Thus, a closer examination of Tinseltown's economic muscle and its global strategies in today's rapidly expanding markets is even more essential. This chapter will focus primarily on Hollywood companies' activities in Europe; however, similar strategies and expansion have been employed in other parts of the world.[2]

Table 9.1 Worldwide film revenues for US companies

	Revenues ($m)		% of total		Annual growth rate
	1986	1991	1986	1991	
Worldwide					
Box office rentals	2,701	4,629	40.2	34.5	11.4
Home video	2,411	5,714	35.9	42.6	18.8
Television	1,609	3,075	23.9	22.9	13.8
Total	6,721	13,418	100.0	100.0	14.8
Domestic	4,366	7,132	65.0	53.2	10.3
Foreign	2,355	6,286	35.0	46.8	21.7

Sources: Veronis, Suhler & Associates; Paul Kagan Associates; Wilkofsky Gruen Associates; presented in *Standard & Poor's Industry Surveys*, 11 March 1993, p. L23.

What's New? Europe's Expanding Markets

In addition to fluctuations in the value of the dollar and the general economic climate, there are several major factors which did not exist a decade ago, which have given Hollywood more power in foreign markets: first, the privatization of media; second, the unification of the European market; third, the revolutionary changes in Eastern Europe; and, fourth, the development and proliferation of new technologies, mainly satellite and cable television and VCRs.

Some forms of deregulation or privatization of media operations have been developing since the "Reagan–Thatcher revolution" of the 1980s, which unfortunately also affected the Continent. These changes have had the greatest impact, not so much on the celluloid industry, but over the air waves, in broadcasting, which is the most dominant form of popular culture. Several countries restructured their public service broadcasting institutions to either allow more privatization or lift restrictions on the purchase of foreign programming. The result has been that new commercial channels sprouted up all over the European landscape, which greatly expanded the broadcast programming and advertising markets.[3]

The European Community's decision to create a tariff-free single European market with 336 million consumers by 1992 was viewed by the US industry as a major development influencing the marketing of media and entertainment products. Global corporations looked forward to the creation of "the biggest and richest market in the world," evidently because of the uniformity of trade regulations within the region, as well as the benefits for their foreign subsidiaries and properties.[4] In addition, political upheavals and changes in the Soviet Union and Eastern European countries opened new markets, described as "virgin territory" for entertainment and media products.

Also, technological developments continue to enhance the European market, as newer distribution systems, such as cable, satellite, and home video, translate into further sales of entertainment products.

For these reasons, the European media and entertainment market has expanded and will continue to do so over the next few years. Looking at some demographics and figures clearly shows why Europe is such a profitable market. Europe currently contains the largest single concentration of television sets in the world (nearly 248 million).[5] In addition, the number of broadcast channels increased from 83 to 105 during the year 1991–2. Broadcast output, or the aggregate of all TV programming on the air, expanded from 325,000 hours in 1988 to 483,000 in 1989,[6] while one study concluded that European television channels will require 16,000 hours of prime-time fiction over the next five years, but are capable of producing only 2,500 hours.[7] While there were 60 satellite-delivered channels in Europe at the end of the 1980s, 74 services were projected by the end of 1990, reaching approximately 24.6 million television households.[8]

Then there is the development and proliferation of VCRs, which varies from country to country. By mid-1989 there were nearly 50 million VCRS in Europe, which resulted in sales of more than 132 million prerecorded videocassettes in that same calendar year, with sales expected to reach 223 million units by 1992.[9]

And in the cinema business, theater expansion and the "multiplexing of Europe," i.e. the construction of multi-screen theater facilities, has led to a boost in ticket sales prompting predictions of a future box office bonanza.

Thus, in a nutshell, the development and proliferation of new technologies, together with privatization and deregulation actions, have combined to further enhance an already lucrative market for Hollywood. And the formation of a unified European market and events in Eastern Europe have wetted the American entertainment industry's appetite for even further revenues.

Are the (European) Media still American?

How prevalent is Hollywood in Europe? Obviously, more accurate and thorough information is needed. However, some estimates may provide a partial insight into the situation.

Domination of American films at European box offices varies according to year and country. However, the Institut de L'audiovisuel et des
Télécommunications en Europe (IDATE) has estimated that American
films represented 77.4 percent of European revenues in 1990, while in
1985 they held 64 percent of the market.[10] The increase in American
penetration over the last decade is evident in individual markets: in
1991, US films represented no less than 58 percent in any EC country,
and 68 percent of the market in Italy, 58.7 percent in France, 91.5
percent in Ireland and 93 percent in the UK.[11] It is also estimated that
60 percent of the European film distribution industry is in the hands of
US companies – in other words, American companies not only distribute American films, but also many European films, as well as other
media products.[12]

European television also has come under the influence of the Hollywood spell, especially in the area of dramatic programming or fiction.
While again there is great variation between countries, a 1985 Unesco
report contended that 30 percent of European television programming
was imported. Of that total, roughly half (44 percent) was imported
from the USA, with 10 percent of total transmission time imported
from the USA.[13] While the Unesco study is probably the most often
quoted in international television flow discussions, Preben Sepstrup and
Anthony Pragnell present similar overall patterns, although Sepstrup
argues strongly (and persuasively) that there are considerable variations
between individual countries.[14]

Despite the need for better statistics and more accurate documentation,
it is not difficult to conclude that US entertainment conglomerates have
been successful in marketing their products in Europe, and in many
cases, dominate – at least economically – individual markets.

Covering the Risk or Passing the Gravy?

How important are international markets, and European markets, in
particular, to the US entertainment industry? It is generally acknowledged that entertainment is the second largest net export industry for
the US, after aerospace.[15] In 1986, total revenues from audiovisual products (film, pay cable, TV and video) totalled an estimated $2.5 billion.
As noted previously, that amount had grown to $11.5 billion by 1991.[16]

For motion pictures, in particular, the overseas box office revenues
increased from $2.43 billion in 1988 to $3.13 billion in 1989.[17] According

Table 9.2 International box office samples (gross revenues in $m)

	USA	Overseas
Rain Man (MGM/UA)	170	233
Fatal Attraction (Paramount)	157	189
Who Framed Roger Rabbit? (Buena Vista)	154	180
Black Rain (Paramount)	48	52
Cocktail (Disney)	77	89
Frantic (Warner Bros)	17	34

Source: From film studios, as reported in Geraldine Fabrikant, "When World Raves, Studios Jump," *New York Times*, 7 March 1990.

to the MPAA, foreign revenues for motion pictures constituted about 38 percent of the total industry revenues, up from 30 percent in 1980.[18] However, the major distributors received far more of their revenues from foreign markets, as international film rentals alone represented 40 percent of their total cinema revenues during 1990.[19]

Lately, the importance of the international film market has been attributed to the higher expenses of American filmmaking. An average film budget in the late 1980s was $23 million, with an additional $10 million invested in prints and advertising (P&A). This means that overseas markets were increasingly important, or in one film executive's words, "a safety net" for many film companies.[20] A vice-president of international marketing at one of the majors explained, "The costs of doing business are so high these days that we need to be involved in every possible profit center."[21] The international revenues from some films, however, seem to indicate that the majors are doing more than just covering costs (see table 9.2).

International distribution of television programming also is becoming an important consideration in production strategies. The aim, although it sometimes does not work, is for international distribution revenues to help make up production deficits before programs go into domestic syndication.[22] Estimates of the majors' revenues from the worldwide sale of television programs grew 63 percent between 1986 and 1988, and totalled $3.27 billion in 1991. Meanwhile, the independent companies' organization, the American Film Market Association (AFMA), reported its members' sales at $227 million.[23]

Another important profit source is the release of motion pictures, and sometimes television programming, on video. The American majors received around $1.8 billion in 1990 from international video sales and rentals, while the AFMA members added another $228.5.[24] Hollywood established an early lead in the international distribution of video-cassettes, holding about 60 percent of the world's pre-recorded video-cassette market in 1985.[25] However, it is still difficult to obtain complete and accurate data for international video markets.

While the global markets represent major revenue sources for Holly-wood, especially high revenues come from the distribution of American media products in the European Community. The major US film corporations received $1.8 billion in revenues from the distribution of US films, TV shows and videos in the EC countries during 1988.[26] Meanwhile, the AFMA reported that over 60 percent, or $561 million, of its members' total sales of theatrical film, television, cable, and home video products, were in European countries during 1988.[27]

Individual European countries regularly rank high in the majors' global film markets. Nine out of the top 15 major export markets for the US industry were located in Europe in 1989. In addition, the European market for television programming was worth nearly $1 billion in 1990.[28] Newly formed private channels are likely to provide even further sales.

Meanwhile, new distribution outlets are providing additional revenues for US companies in Europe. Most of the US majors (Fox, Warner, CIC) distribute videocassettes through their own home video distribution outlets in European countries, and some expect the European home video market eventually to be larger than the US market. There is already a higher average number of tapes purchased per VCR home in some European countries.[29]

New satellite services also represent lucrative new markets for US products.[30] Both Sky TV and British Satellite Broadcasting (BSB) have "output deals" with US majors for films and television programming. By 1990, BSB was said to have spent around £550 million on programming,[31] while Sky Channel has acquired 3,000 films, paying from $150,000 to $1.5 million per title in 175 separate deals.[32] CIT Research predicted that Sky and BSB would spend (combined) £400 million a year on programming and marketing, with US companies receiving a lion's share of these expenditures.[33]

Generally, revenues from the European media market are expected to double during the next decade. One study projects revenues from broadcast, film and video businesses to reach $58 billion by then, with special growth in the pay-TV business and in Eastern European markets.[34] As Gary Lucchesi, president of production at Paramount, explains, "The European market is expanding in leaps and bounds. When you combine the people in Eastern Europe with the Common Market countries, you have close to a billion people who will be longing for good entertainment." Another film executive exclaims, "For Hollywood in the 90s, it's once more Eastward Ho!"[35]

But how are Hollywood-based companies waging their crusade in European markets? The strength of the American industry and its global strategies will be discussed as follows: (1) Hollywood's historical legacy and current advantages; (2) breaking down protectionism, including lobbying strategies and state involvement; (3) marketing and distribution techniques; (4) direct investments; (5) production activities; (6) content strategies; and (7) supporting services.

Once upon a Time, there was a European Film Industry . . .

"There has been a long history of US activity in film and television markets in European countries and elsewhere.[36] The example of the post-war marketing of US films in Europe is illustrative and relevant, in that most of the global distributors of American entertainment products began as motion picture companies.

The export of American films and the domination of some global markets can be traced to the periods following World Wars I and II. Both wars left the European film industries in shambles, creating a void which US film companies quickly filled; the position they achieved then has never been surrendered. The cataclysmic events of World War II were especially effective in cementing Hollywood's grip on the European celluloid market.

As post-war Europe recovered, though, so did its film industries and so did opposition to Hollywood's domination. Many European countries imposed restrictions on their film markets, including issuing quotas on the number of foreign films screened, blocking funds earned by foreign companies, and supporting indigenous filmmakers through various subsidy schemes.

While Tinseltown seemingly had run into trouble, the Hollywood majors were extremely successful in overcoming such opposition through lobbying by the international arm of the MPAA, the Motion Picture Export Association (the MPEA) and government officials (primarily the State Department), as well as employing a variety of strategies such as boycotts, co-production activities, and creative financing mechanisms. As Jack Valenti has stated: "Really, the mission of the MPAA can be simply stated: to make sure the American film, television and home video program can move freely and unhobbled around in the world in marketplaces that are competitive."[37]

One industry observer has claimed that "the splinterized nature of the European film market – divided among many languages, copyright law, union regulations and distribution systems – has helped Hollywood to dominate the continent."[38] However, the US dominance also must be understood in the context of this historical legacy in which Hollywood established an early and strong presence in these global markets.

Cartel Power and the Home Field Advantage

Many of the historical strengths of the US entertainment industry still persist. Through worldwide film distribution cartels – United International (MCA, MGM/UA, Paramount), Warner (Warner, Disney) and Columbia – the Hollywood-based companies not only market their own products but other countries' products as well.

As a French producer explains, "the majors have been laying the foundation for future domination by infiltrating countries with cartel power. As a result, audiences get accustomed to US production values and *voilà*, the Yanks control the world." Another French filmmaker remarked that "Americans have educated people throughout the world for 75 years to appreciate their films. For many of these years, they did it at a loss. Now it's paying off."[39]

In contrast, it is estimated that 80 percent of European films never leave their own country.[40] Television program exporting is similarly parochial, according to a study by the British Screen Advisory Council, which found that only 10 percent of European television product is sold outside the country of origin.[41]

Of course, the US companies also rely on their home market for distribution of all entertainment forms. And since the US represents one of the largest markets in the world for entertainment products, there is a tremendous home market (or home field) advantage for the US-based companies.[42] Although this market also is expanding because of new technological developments (cable, video, etc.), foreign products are still not favored and indeed are often blocked from entry.[43] European and Canadian companies trying to compete with the vast American market have described this dilemma as the "Los Angelization of the unconscious."[44]

As we have seen, the US industry also has experienced considerable consolidation, thus enhancing the ability of these large corporations to act forcefully and effectively in global markets.[45] Indeed, some combinations (such as Time Warner) have been supported by the industry and the state because of the perceived need to "fight foreign competitors on their own terms."[46] Ironically, other takeovers have involved direct foreign investment, as discussed in chapter 4.

All in all, the Hollywood majors – and whoever owns them – are especially well prepared for their foreign crusade. As a media observer noted a few years ago, "Put it all together and the inescapable conclusion is that the unregulated, happily diversified majors are, despite the high cost of features and TV programs – and despite the critical deficit problem – poised for long-term clout and prosperity."[47]

Fortress Europe: Survival or Protectionism?

Although the European market offers a potential bonanza for entertainment corporations, the doors to this lucrative market are not wide open, as various governments and intergovernmental institutions continue to block or restrict foreign investment and imports. In one of the most potentially important actions, the European Community adopted its "Television Without Frontiers" directive in October 1989, imposing program quotas limiting the broadcast of non-European programs and restrictions on advertising by the end of 1990.[48] Meanwhile, the EC's actions have been echoed in attempts to include limits on imported entertainment as part of General Agreement on Tariffs and Trade (GATT) negotiations in Geneva.

Other national restrictions already existed. Sometimes referred to as non-tariff trade barriers, they have included import quotas, limits on foreign broadcast programming, taxes on theaters, videocassettes, and film/TV production companies, dubbing licenses, and regulations on shipping prints, equipment, etc.[49] Other annoyances for the companies have included paperwork for transporting prints and equipment, requirements for translating and filing distribution contracts, and restrictions on using foreign workers for dubbing imported programs. Some countries without such policies were considering them in the early 1990s.[50] The stated aim of most of these provisions has been to prevent domination by American companies. Jack Lang, Minister of Culture and one of the strongest advocates of such policies in France, explains, "our destiny is not to become the vassals of an immense empire of profit."[51]

Protective measures also have been devised to encourage and support European production. A wide variety of national production subsidies exist, as well as a few new proposals from the European Community at large. The European Film Distribution Office, for example, is an EC project involving $305 million to be invested over five years in production and distribution partnerships.[52] European Media '92 aims to strengthen the competitiveness of the European film industry, by training, technological development, investment opportunities, and exports.[53]

Fighting the "Cancer": The US Industry Fights Back

One explanation of the US response to such developments comes from a European media professional: "There's a feeling that a party is being given that the Americans have not been invited to."[54]

But the Americans are not so flippant; their responses have been straightforward and strong. Olivier Philippon, president, CBS Fox France, sums up the American point of view: "Any kind of regulation that attempts to rule a market is, by nature, bad. The consumer should be the ultimate judge. Film producers should take risks and release films that will please the public, rather than rely on subsidies."[55]

MPEA officials have even attributed the slide in cinema attendance to restrictive practices, calling the anti-free trade measures a form of "cancer," which is "murderous."[56] MPAA head, Jack Valenti, called the EC directive, in particular, a "maimed, disabled theory which honors restriction above public choice," while a *New York Times* editorial referred to the "absurd efforts to regulate public taste."[57]

The directive received especially strong resistance from the US industry, which objected to the quotas on imported TV programming, as well as to measures pertaining to copyright issues (which affect video piracy and satellite distribution to unlicensed territories). If the directive is taken seriously, claims MPEA president, Myron Karlin, "The only way that the cinema, home video and TV businesses would be protected was by 'country-to-country' sequential distribution."[58]

However, the actual legislation is said to be vague and difficult to enforce, especially Article Four which specifies that member states should ensure "when practicable" a majority of European works. There are also difficult questions pertaining to what is a European work.[59]

Nevertheless, the MPEA waged an intense campaign against the directive . . . and lost, although the battle was said to have given Valenti "a crusade and a cause."[60] Meanwhile, the MPEA has upgraded its

European offices, adding more people with US State Department experience, and one executive in Paris to focus especially on EC matters.[61]

With a Little Bit of Help from our Friends

But the industry does not just rely on its own resources. Lobbying is
carried on at the highest level of the US government and has included
special attention from US Presidents, including Reagan, Bush, and now
Clinton. As Valenti explains, "The President of the United States, the
Secretary of State, the Secretary of Commerce and the United States
Trade Representative have all been supportive. They have made it clear
to the chancelleries of Europe that the imposition of this quota is an
intolerable thing for the US."[62] More recently, President Clinton and
his staff have been enlisted to fight against GATT's inclusion of restrictions on imported film and television programs, as well as trying to
stiffen the agreement's provisions on piracy of video tapes, audio cassettes and satellite signals.

Indeed, the EC's directive triggered a strong response from the US
Congress as well, where in October 1989 the House of Representatives
denounced the proposed quotas and urged Bush and Trade Representative Carla Hill, "To take all feasible and appropriate action under
its authority . . . to protect and maintain US access to the EC broadcasting market."[63]

Previously, Congress had included provisions in the Omnibus Trade
Bill of 1988 to give the industry some support when denied access to
foreign markets. As one MPEA official commented, "Congress did this
because they saw the value of films and TV programs as a great US
trade asset. And, because of the nature of our product, a number of
countries choose to label movies as 'cultural,' and we have different
kinds of problems than most US exporters."[64]

Of less importance, perhaps, was Congressional lobbying by the film
industry to revoke the law which requires a propaganda label to be
placed on certain imported films that received government funding (for
example: the Canadian film, *If You Love This Planet*). Yet the law
essentially contradicts the US film industry's efforts against import quotas
and other restrictive practices in other countries.[65] As another MPEA
representative explained, "There are quotas around the world, and we
have to live with them until they become so onerous and discriminatory
that we simply have to confer with that country's government, as well
as enlist our own, to remedy unacceptable situations."[66]

The industry also has worked closely with the US government on other issues such as copyright and piracy, identified as major trade barriers by the US entertainment industry.[67] Pressure has been placed on various countries (especially in Southeast Asia) to adopt stronger copyright enforcement in light of the piracy problems in those countries. Indeed, the industry–government partnership has been quite successful in countries such as Malaysia, Indonesia, and Singapore, where trade sanctions were used as pressure for copyright adherence[68] (as mentioned in chapter 6). Other forms of pressure were experienced in Korea, where US pressure forced the Korean film industry to open up to American distribution companies.[69] In light of these instances, it is not surprising to see the industry–government alliance at work in Europe, which currently represents an even more lucrative market than Southeast Asia.

Thus, there is still heavy dependence on the state to clear the path for global marketing, especially in response to protective measures adopted by other governments and agencies, as well as when markets experience stress from new technological developments (as in the case of pirating).

Taking Care of Business

This is a market you can't afford to ignore.
Jeffrey Kruger, "Europe 1992 Brims with Possibilities," *Billboard*, 1989

The crusade against quotas and piracy is not the only strategy of the US entertainment companies. While Valenti and the politicians await more specific guidelines from the EC on production and distribution agreements, cable retransmission, and copyright, the industry is pursuing the opportunities presented by expanding European markets. As NBC's international vice-president J. B. Holston remarked after the EC passed the "Television Without Frontiers" policy, "Let the directive go forward. The substance is much less than the rhetoric. Instead, let's get down to the business of production and working together, rather than fighting trade wars."[70]

Despite these various forms of resistance, US companies continue to successfully market their products in European countries. While the actual process of international distribution and marketing of entertainment products needs more careful research (as Philip Schlesinger pointed out several years ago), it is still possible to note a few of the more obvious developments in this area.[71]

Some claim that the Americans are able to flood the market with a surplus of low-priced programming (films and television series) that benefit from the home field advantage mentioned previously. In other words, American products – often already amortized – are sold at prices much lower than the cost of producing national products.[72] But it is still difficult to assess these claims without direct access to actual production costs and prices – information that is often difficult to obtain.

Another development which needs more research attention is the role of film and television exchanges or markets, sometimes attached to film festivals, but often planned simply for buying and selling products and making industry contacts (or "smoozing" as it is known in the trade).[73] While these events have definitely increased over the last decade, the most popular markets seem to be, for film, Cannes, MIFED (in Milan) and the American Film Market (Los Angeles), and, for television, MIP-TV and MIPCOM.[74] Another important television exchange is the National Association for Television Producers and Executives (NATPE), where in January 1993, over 700 buyers and sellers paid as much as $100,000 for sales booths. While the price may seem high, the gathering was spartan compared to previous years where booths were even more elaborate and gimmicky, with free champagne, giveaways, etc. – up to $1 million expense for some companies.[75] A good proportion of the deals for films and television programs are made at these events, and thus, the ability to participate in them may affect a production or distribution company's ability to sell its products in international markets.

In addition to these efforts to sell products to theaters, television channels, and other media outlets, film marketing has intensified, with more money spent on advertising and promotion, and the increased use of sneak previews and test-marketing trailers.[76] Not only is there pressure on theaters to run films as long as possible, but theatrical features are opening earlier in foreign markets. Earlier release is seen as a way to prevent piracy, but also to cut costs.[77] An example was Universal's *Back to the Future II*, which opened in markets around the world at about the same time, rather than being delayed the typical six months after its US debut. A Universal executive explained, "We took in $85 million overseas six months earlier than we would have otherwise. That meant we saved millions in interest costs right away."[78]

Yet, as cinema people know quite well, there are no guarantees when it comes to the success of a motion picture. Despite sophisticated marketing techniques, films sometimes do not do as well as expected.

Despite, or perhaps because of, the intense marketing campaign before it opened, *Batman*, for instance, did not do as well as anticipated in some foreign markets. The industry has come to appreciate the importance of different strategies for different products in different markets. "You can't just blanket Europe. It's a market-by-market approach," says the head of Warner Brothers International's theatrical division. The strategy followed by Warner, at least, is "maximum distribution and careful territory by territory marketing."[79]

An example is the marketing of *Innerspace* in 1988 by Warner Brothers International: "We had five different campaigns working internationally, depending on what they wanted. In Japan, for instance, we emphasized the special effects, while it was different in Italy where we focused on the comedy."[80] *Innerspace* grossed $75 million in foreign territories that year.

The head of UIP, Michael Williams-Jones, has observed that a film's US success (or lack of it) is "not a good predictor of its fate in foreign release. A film's success abroad can hinge on a fresh marketing approach, including stumping by stars and directors." He cites the example of *Willow*, which did not do well in the USA in terms of box office, at least, but was an international smash. For the film's Japanese run, an original campaign was designed by UIP and Japanese collaborators. In addition, director George Lucas and cast members "stumped" the promotion trail in Japan. Williams-Jones explains: "Stars' visits to individual countries generate incredible publicity at extremely low cost. That allows us to cut back on straight advertising. All our research proves that editorial coverage, whether in newspapers, magazines or on TV or radio, is more believable to the general public."[81]

Other examples of careful marketing are the low-key campaigns by the Hollywood majors in France, in light of the strong French position on the question of quotas. Indeed, many US companies are deliberately not investing in production companies, but trying simply to encourage the rebuilding of the theatrical box office.[82]

The choice of trading partners also has become an important factor. The advice from one promoter is: "Make deals with European companies that have extensive marketing and distribution contacts in the Common Market countries."[83]

Other strategies include the use of management consultants, especially in orchestrating publicity campaigns and to round up customers for new media markets. An example is a US company active in Europe called Video Flash, which opened a campaign to combat the slow market for video rentals in the UK in the early 1990s. The company literature explained the problem: "The culprit seems to be the 'lapsed renter,' a uniquely English expression for the home video patron who now rents less frequently, if at all." Despite heavy competition from satellite and cable TV, Video Flash had the answer: "We have designed field work that will identify who this lapsed renter is. We want quantitative information: where do they live! If we can find them, our clients can sell them."[84]

Different strategies have emerged to deal with Eastern Europe and the former Soviet Union. The "political remake" – as the industry describes it – means that these countries are "virgin territory" for Western entertainment products.[85] The MPEA, represented by Jack Valenti, negotiated a deal to distribute American films in the Soviet Union in 1988.[86] The Hollywood majors also have expanded their offices and activities in Eastern European countries, where film distribution contracts are now being arranged as percentage deals, rather than on the previous flat fee basis. Thus, the distributors will now receive a share of the box office as in other countries.[87]

Expanded television sales are also expected. One analyst estimates that the Eastern European market could bring in $6.6 billion in the next decade, noting that "from chaos and black marketeers we shall see clear regulatory standards, stabilized currencies and a serious TV market emerging throughout the Eastern bloc."[88]

If You Can't Lick 'em, Join 'em

Direct US investment in European TV and film companies has increased, although companies may be more cautious than in the mid-80s, when American companies were making heavy investments in cable and satellite projects.[89] "Europe poses a complicated opportunity for American companies today," says one TV executive who has learned from past experiences of investing in satellite projects.[90]

Although they may be cautious, as well as facing competition from other transnational companies, US-based conglomerates are still investing in Europe. Several of the major film distribution companies and television networks are investing in production companies. For instance, ABC Video Enterprises has equity stakes in German, French and Spanish production companies, while NBC and Westinghouse are involved in several French production enterprises.[91]

US companies are involved in cable, as well, especially in the UK. ABC is involved with Screen Sport and various US film majors have invested in Premiere, Mirrorvision, and Bravo. Viacom, of course, owns

MTV Europe, while United Artists Entertainment (UAE) has interests in the European Discovery channel.[92] In 1990, North American cable TV operators (led by UAE) proposed setting up three national TV program services for UK cable, to be delivered via low-power satellite.

European theater construction (especially multiplex set-ups) is on the rise, with active participation by some of the US majors. Britain has been the forerunner of such activity, with American Multi Cinema, National Amusements, MCA and others adding 350 new screens in the UK during the last few years. More new theaters are planned for other European countries. Specifically, United Cinemas (MCA and Paramount) plans outlets for Germany and Spain, while Time Warner is looking to build new theaters in Germany and the countries of the former Soviet Union.[93]

The general consolidation of European cinemas also favors US distributors. According to one report, "They have fewer exhibitors to deal with and can more easily control release patterns."[94] And, of course, the more theaters, the more pictures are needed. As the head of Warner Brothers International's theatrical division reports, "Business has improved tremendously. Before, you'd be in line to get your films into the two theaters in town. Now you can get them out much earlier and feed off a lot of the publicity coming out of the United States."[95] An MCA spokesman claims that "the multiplexing of Europe will enable us to release twice as many movies."[96]

Another type of activity by several Hollywood majors is the construction of theme parks in Europe, as discussed in chapter 4. This is another strategy to enhance the popularity of the majors' other products, as well as (hopefully) providing even more profits. EuroDisneyland, located near Paris, opened in 1992, while MCA's proposed studio/theme park was to be built for around $4 billion, probably also outside Paris.[97]

Cause the Yanks are Comin', the Yanks are Comin'

In addition to direct investment, production activities have increased on both sides of the Atlantic. US studios are opening new offices and producing more films in Europe, while European companies are at least attempting to make deals in the USA. Both Twentieth Century Fox and Paramount have added London-based European production and acquisition units. Fox also opened Comedy House, a London-based production company, "angling to spawn clicks of the stature of *A Fish Called*

Wanda."[98] Production activities are especially lively in Eastern Europe and the former Soviet Union, where new and newly privatized companies are offering a wide range of production services.[99]

But the big news in the late 1980s was co-production. Actually, co-operative production ventures have been prevalent in the past, and US film production in Europe has a long history, albeit with numerous ups and downs. However, in the latest round of cooperative projects, companies were not just picking up films for distribution or simply financing projects, but becoming active in "creative partnerships." As a Disney executive explained: "We are actively exploring shooting films in Europe as real co-productions with French and Italian companies, no phony co-productions that were simply disguises for distribution arrangements."[100]

Distributors and sales agencies were "increasingly originating or participating at the very early stages in the development, preparation and assembly of the film package."[101] Often complete funding was provided, through a combination of pre-sales and a domestic US distribution agreement. Financing was available from distribution companies, pay-TV (such as HBO) and cable companies (such as Turner and the USA Network). As one industry observer noted, "An independent producer with a quality film package can often find financing from these companies, provided that the film package has overseas possibilities and a theatrical 'feel' at a reasonable budget."[102]

The American television networks also became more active in European production. In response to potential quotas, they were seeking "broad, global partnerships" involving "the major players in the industry around the world." One executive's advice for European activities was, "First, produce with Europeans for Europeans. Second, find investments and partnerships."[103] A few of the networks working in Europe were looking towards programs produced especially for American cable, rather than relying only on network and syndicated release.[104] But Europeans also tried to make sales to US television producers and cable programming companies. And private companies in Eastern European countries became especially active in making deals with the West.[105] Co-production activities may have been easier to arrange, according to one industry representative who claims that the demise of some companies "has served to centralize decision making in a smaller number of production financing sources and US theatrical distributors."[106]

While different arrangements on financing and distribution emerged, the question of "genuine creative partnerships" again became a concern for many Europeans. Some wondered "whether the tastes and sensibilities of European talent will be respected."[107]

Ya Gotta Have a Gimmick

The products of US-based entertainment companies also are influenced by globalization. A few of the international strategies that influence creative decision-making will illustrate the point.

The international angle is described well by an Associated Press reporter: "Before going ahead with a project, studios are increasingly trying to consider how movie scripts, and the actors they envision for the main roles, will play not only in Peoria but in Pisa, Perth and, now, Prague."[108] As the president of Warner Brothers explains: "American movies that do not travel are getting more difficult to make."[109]

Of course, tailoring films for international markets is certainly not a new Hollywood strategy. Joseph Phillips observed several years ago that "the American industry's search for formulas with international appeal has led to an increasing reliance on standardized "spectaculars."[110] Hollywood seems to have changed little over the years. Today, as in the past, internationally famous actors are one of the most important elements of an international film package, although their salaries are often mind-boggling. In industry terms, big names get big bucks but attract boffo coin (i.e. lots of money). As another industry observer noted,

> Stars like Sean Connery, Arnold Schwarzenegger and Eddie Murphy are able to command huge salaries in part because of the certainly that their presence in a movie will give it greater appeal around the world. . . . The films of certain stars, like Mr Schwarzenegger and Sylvestor Stallone, translate well abroad because they rarely depend on the subtleties of dialogue.[111]

Internationally famous directors and culturally sensitive scripts (or script variations) also are important elements of international film projects. An example is the Japanese version of *Fatal Attraction* produced by Paramount, which ended with a suicide. As a Paramount representative explained, "We thought it might work because there is a ritual in Japan in which a person who is dishonored commits ritualistic suicide. But the Japanese wanted the same ending that the rest of the world got."[112]

Genre is an important consideration, as well. Although foreign markets have different characteristics, the studios have found that comedies (with visual humor) and adventure films seem to be popular everywhere. Action films are especially profitable in global markets, prompting some American companies to follow the international formula: "make it simple and keep it moving."[113]

In the late 1980s, Hollywood started producing more animated features and television series (as discussed in chapter 3), which were extremely popular in international markets. It has been estimated that more than 50 percent of the investment in animated projects can be gleaned from foreign sales. It also might be noted that most of the work for animated projects was done in Asian countries, where labor is cheaper than in the USA.[114]

The other unmistakable trend in the film industry is the proliferation of remakes or sequels of successful films. For instance, the list of sequels released during the summer of 1990 seemed endless, but included *Robocop II*, *Back to the Future III*, *Die Hard 2*, and *Gremlins 2*. Several others were scheduled for fall release the same year.[115] Even remakes of foreign films have became popular, as Hollywood attempts to cash in on "sure bets," especially in foreign markets.[116]

Television production also is becoming increasingly more international, especially youth-oriented programming, which is extremely lucrative in foreign markets. Viacom's MTV Europe, for example, has a potential audience of 90 million homes in 26 countries. The Nickelodeon channel also sells well in international markets, and has found that selling program formats in other countries is another profitable endeavor.

Of course, the Disney enterprise continues to hit international markets in every possible way, dispersing "Disney magic" through a wide variety of entertainment products, merchandising activities, and theme parks, as discussed in chapters 4 and 8. Disney Clubs, for instance, are now tailored to individual countries. As *Channels* magazine has observed,

> They not only spread the Disney culture and build brand recognition, they spur demand for Disney merchandise and theme parks.
>
> In essence, by taking winning American product and tailoring it country by country, Disney and Viacom are helping shape the taste of Europe's first generation of commercial-TV watchers. As new European productions begin to flood the screen over the next decade, viewers who grew up watching Disney, Nickelodeon-inspired game shows and MTV will have already established their viewing habits. For Viacom and Disney, the sales boom was only the beginning.[117]

The Supporting Cast Goes Global

Supporting services for the entertainment industry's activities are growing increasingly more international, as well. In the past, the industry has been able to depend on international banking and financial support for corporate and production activities.[118] But as one US banker explained, "With the acceleration of satellite, cable and private television and multiplex cinemas, companies will need more bank or institutional financing."[119]

New financing schemes include off-shore placement of copyrights and pre-sales of theatrical, video, and television rights. An example is the $60 million budget for *Total Recall*, which was partly recouped from overseas rights before the movie went into production.[120]

With more international activities, accounting firms with international experience and expertise became even more important for the usual services, as well as handling tax advantages and tax shelter deals, which were still possible in some countries. As one accountant explained, "Many film companies are calling on the financial and consultancy services of large international accountancy firms."[121]

Internationally oriented legal firms also have been needed, and several Hollywood law firms opened European offices. As a group of Los Angeles lawyers observed:

> With the movement of film forging the global marketplace, attorneys will be faced with a myriad of problems within their expanding role. They will be asked to address issues of international law governing distribution and piracy, conduct diplomatic negotiations over the sensitive issue of perceived cultural erosion via international television, and comprehend international financial transactions, including currency repatriation restrictions.[122]

Although there may be less paperwork in EC countries, "On-the-spot expertise will come in handy for US clients in dealing with these new European arrangements, tax shelters and government subsidies, and well as currency transfers."[123]

Other support activities include new European offices for US talent agencies. And apparently, there are some real differences between European and American talent representatives. US agents are said to be generally more aggressive, putting together packages, etc., while working for less and with fewer restrictions than European agents.[124]

Cultural Domination Revisited

In light of these economic, technological and political developments, a reconsideration of the cultural imperialism thesis seems timely and relevant, and it is a task which already seems well underway. A number of scholars have challenged the cultural imperialist position, which argued that the international flow of media products is primarily one-way, Western-originated, and planned to ideologically or culturally dominate third world or non-industrialized countries.[125] Critics have pointed to the lack of a theoretical base and/or empirical grounding for some of the "classic" studies of media transnationalization. Others call for a stronger, more independent role for the audience.[126]

Preben Sepstrup, along with his critique of the "classic" cultural imperialist studies, suggests a more complex conceptual framework, first carefully examining the effect of international flows on transnationalization, and then analyzing the effects of transnationalization on culture, the economy, and consumption.[127]

The foregoing analysis of Hollywood's global strategies, therefore, addresses the first level of Sepstrup's model: the analysis of international flows and transnationalization. But this is a necessary *first* step in understanding the cultural impact or substantial effects of transnationalization. The question it has tackled is that of *economic* dominance of cultural products, but it has not considered the question of *cultural* dominance. The discussion is not intended to underestimate or neglect the audience for cultural products or the reception process – it is only to establish more carefully and accurately the structural framework in which these cultural encounters occur. This is consistent with a point made by Graham Murdock, when he noted that the economic determines in the first (rather than the last) instance, "and that it is a necessary starting point for analysis but not a destination. Economic dynamics are crucial to critical inquiry because they establish some of the key contexts within which consumption takes place, but they do not negate the need for a full and separate analysis of symbolic determinations."[128]

Yet Another Crusade . . . the Universal Market?

This study has not looked at texts, products or audiences, per se. However, as international markets become increasingly more important, the question of cultural domination not only disappears but becomes even more urgent. And the extent of transnationalization still is the necessary foundation for assessing cultural domination.

Certainly from this study it is possible to argue that Hollywood has become more global than ever before. And with its economic strength tied to on-going political support, we can look forward to even further attempts to dominate world markets. However, it is also important; to acknowledge that there are no guarantees that US-based entertainment corporations or products will succeed over others. Competition is heavy from transnationals based in Europe (backed up by political efforts to protect European industries), as well as from other international players.

Again, we might ask what is so surprising about all of this? And again, the answer is not a lot. Hollywood is a capitalist enterprise, competing with other capitalists. It is the nature of capitalist enterprises to expand and seek wider markets. Indeed, the world market may not even be the last crusade, but a prelude to the quest for the universal market (complete with Disneyland-Mars and multiplexes on the moon?).

For the moment, however, global markets continue to evolve, and Hollywood (and capitalism) continue to adapt, although not by employing "free" market strategies, but with help from the state to clear any obstacles, and often by working non-competitively with other US-based corporations in foreign markets.

The struggles around the GATT negotiations provide the latest example of Hollywood's hypocritical call for free and open markets, while at the same time relying heavily on the state to protect its interests. In addition, the US industry is still relying on basically economic arguments, neglecting the relevance of film and other entertainment products as forms of cultural expression and worthy of protection.

On the other hand, it is certainly possible to defend the protective measures of the EC and individual nations on economic reasons alone, as cultural production contributes to a country or region's economy as well as providing a certain number of jobs.

Also, while more attention and research may be necessary to establish a clearer picture of the influences of imported popular culture, it is not difficult to defend a country's right to preserve space for its own cultural expression. For this reason at least, film and other cultural products must be viewed differently to other commodities. However, it seems unlikely that Hollywood will easily be convinced of this point, and thus the quest for global markets continues.

10

Hooray for Hollywood: Moving into the 21st Century

It should be remembered that every step in modern media history – telephone, phonograph, motion picture, radio, television, satellite – stirred similar euphoric predictions. All were expected to usher in an age of enlightenment. All were seen as fulfilling the promise of democracy. Possible benefits were always easier to envisage than misuses and corruptions, and still are.
Erik Barnouw, *The Sponsor: Notes on a Modern Potentate*

Despite the new "rational" structure, the expensive talent, irrational consumers, and government regulations can still greatly influence this immature and socially irresponsible industry.
John Micklethwait, "The Entertainment Industry: Raising the Stakes,"
The Economist, 1983

When Hollywood contemplates the future of entertainment technology, the optimists see a world of profit and delight. But skeptics see an expensive future that is difficult to make a reality.
Anthony Ramirez, "High-tech TV: So Near, Yet So far Away,"
New York Times, 1992

Yes, There Have Been Changes

One cannot deny that there were some pretty dramatic changes in the distribution and exhibition of Hollywood films and other entertainment products during the 1980s. While the introduction of new technologies was responsible for some of these changes, the political-economic context in which these innovations were introduced is crucial. Indeed, deregulation and globalization tendencies have set the stage for Hollywood in this era as much as technological development, and it seems clear from this study that these various factors can scarcely by separated.

New technologies – new outlets   Audiences of the 1990s experience
mass-mediated culture differently to earlier generations. VCRs have
made viewing time more flexible and convenient, and cable has provided a range of new programming possibilities with special interest
channels catering to smaller audiences. In addition, there is the potential for consumers to participate in media production themselves via
relatively inexpensive video equipment.

Undoubtedly, the technologies introduced by a variety of large corporations in the 1970s and 1980s provided the film industry with some
wonderful new distribution outlets. Despite claims of unfair competition and piracy, the Hollywood majors are indeed benefitting from a
variety of outlets. We have seen how home video has become an enormously profitable market for Hollywood companies, and cable continues
to provide additional revenue for film distributors. In addition, the large
Hollywood companies' involvement in these new technologies via
ownership of cable channels and systems, video companies, etc., has
meant even further profits.

Diversified revenues   For some time now, the Hollywood majors have
not depended solely on revenues from theatrical exhibition. But these
latest distribution outlets have meant that revenues are even further
diversified, which adds even more power to the majors' operations.
Quite simply, there are many more markets for their products. Hollywood executive Frank Rothman observed: "When television started in
the 1950s, there was a strong view that that was the end of Hollywood.
When cable came, we thought that would kill our sales to networks.
None of these things happened. Every time the market expands, the
combination is greater than before."[1]

Realignments in the television industry have meant adjustments in
markets for the majors. Yet these changes, in many instances, have led
to even more business for the majors. Even though the studios have
sold fewer movies to the major networks, independent stations have
been more interested in Hollywood films, as well as syndicated TV
programming.

With so many more markets, it has also been possible for some smaller
companies to survive or find new life, at least for a while. For instance,
Republic Pictures was able to profit in the 1980s from the new outlets
for film release (especially videocassettes), as well as from television
production. Under new ownership in 1987, Republic capitalized on its
library by "squeezing every possible dollar out of its films" and keeping

costs down for production of made-for-TV movies. By the end of the decade, Republic had tripled its sales from these various sources.[2]

Spreading the risks For the film industry, then, more outlets have translated into less risk.

Video and cable release of films have provided extra benefits for films which did well in theaters, and given "legs" to films which did not do well in theatrical release. Furthermore, globalization tendencies have opened new markets, to further reduce the risk of producing big budget films.

As Asu Aksoy and Kevin Robins point out,

> The ability to coordinate and exploit different media outlets means that major production companies can now spread risks over increasingly segmented audiences.
>
> If part of the success of the Hollywood majors can be explained by the rationalization of production costs, we would argue that what has made them the dominant powers in the film business has been the ability to get their films (whatever their production cost) to a worldwide audience. And it was this ability – that is to say, control over the distribution side of the business – that allowed the majors to continue their dominance even after the Paramount Decree.[3]

New trends in film financing As a result of new distribution technologies, there have been some claims that film production is less risky as there is an increased need for product. However, with the average negative cost for a Hollywood film reported to be well over $25 million and advertising costs rising, the majors, at least, argue that there is even more risk.

While many of the majors rely on in-house productions, independents look for financing sources in many locations. And new distribution outlets have led to a wider range of pre-buy or pre-licensing deals. This is not necessarily new, as TV networks, foreign distribution outlets and other sources have been involved in such deals in the past. But important new sources are pay cable and home video companies, and sometimes these new players also become directly involved in production. Examples include HBO's production program, discussed in chapter 5, and Vestron's production activity mentioned in chapter 6. Other income sources are represented by the expanding market for entertainment-related merchandise, as discussed in chapter 8.[4]

New sources of funds have also come from new owners of distribution and production companies. With an increased need for product, the Hollywood companies have become attractive to those wanting to (and now able to) expand their communications empires. Examples include Turner's and Paretti's brief flings with MGM, Murdoch's takeover of Fox, the Sony and Matsushita purchases of Columbia and MCA, and the struggle over Paramount in 1993–4. It is not surprising that these corporations were interested in Hollywood investments. The value of the libraries of the major studios alone represent a sizable asset. For instance, in 1987 MCA's 3,000 films were valued at $1.5 billion.[5]

Meanwhile, Hollywood companies developed their own devices for raising funds. Disney has been quite successful raising production funding through public offerings such as Silver Screen Partners. Meanwhile, Twentieth Century Fox raised $63 million through limited partnership funds called American Entertainment Partners, formed by Shearson Lehman Brothers. Other financial innovations will no doubt follow, as the majors seek others to carry the risk of blockbuster filmmaking.

Hooray for success Hollywood in the 1980s represented more than just a dream factory – it was an industry that brought home the bacon. New distribution outlets (as well as enhanced advertising campaigns) brought a new level of popularity to movies, and Hollywood reaped the benefits.

Aksoy and Robins observe: "With the emergence of competition from television and cable channels, film companies are now extending these cascading strategies and playing on the time of release across different media." Enormous profits were made with wildly successful blockbusters, such as *Batman*, *Terminator 2*, *Jurassic Park*, and countless others. But even further rewards came from distributing American cultural products throughout the world. More than once the US film industry received praise for its success in foreign markets, representing one of the strongest net export industries in the country. More and more global markets provided revenue for the expansion by Hollywood companies abroad, thus representing an enterprise which the USA seemed destined to control through the turn of the century.

Continuity in the 1990s

"The More Things Change, the More They Remain the Same"
Dennis Stanfill, former Fox chairman

But even though there have been these dramatic developments in the production, distribution and exhibition of filmed entertainment, what has actually changed about the film industry? After having looked more closely at Hollywood in the 1970s and 1980s, it is possible to conclude that there is a good deal of continuity as well as change.

More commodities   While there are new means of producing and distributing filmed entertainment, Hollywood's creative efforts are still aimed at creating commodities. In other words, the potential of video, cable and satellite technologies have been developed with profit, rather than expanded communication and/or enlightenment, in mind. In other words, the film industry's primary motivation has to do with profits, not necessarily with film. As a few of the Hollywood executives confessed in the early 1980s, they do not care whether or not their products are exhibited in theaters or in the home, as long as they get paid their "fair share." But it may also be true that the corporations that represent Hollywood may not necessarily be as locked into films as one might think. As Thomas Guback points out, "the ultimate product of the motion picture business is profit; motion pictures are but means to that end."[6]

It is important to note that despite these motivations, the introduction of new technological wonders by corporate innovators does not always succeed. Despite the power of large corporations, there are still examples of failure and misjudgment, sometimes leading to huge losses, as with other commodities. Among the examples covered in this study are the early attempts by Hollywood to enter broadcasting, the introduction of videodiscs, and a pay-per-transaction arrangement for video retailing.

The point, however, is that the development of technologies that have vast potential for enlightenment and understanding has been controlled by the business sector of our society, and by a relatively small set of players within that sector.

More films?   One would think with these new outlets for films on a global scale, more production would follow logically. Well, at least for a while in the mid-1980s, film production blossomed. 1985 was the busiest filming period for Hollywood in 12 years, while film production reportedly was up 50 percent in 1986. Yet the total domestic theatrical releases by all companies increased only 4 percent to 472 titles in 1986. Since then, the number of domestic film releases has varied: 466 in 1988, 472 in 1989, 379 in 1990 and 424 in 1991.[7]

Indeed, at the beginning of the 1990s, the majors even released fewer films than in previous years. The distributors blame the situation on megasalaries for stars and high distribution costs (advertising and prints), which continued to rise during the decade.[8] But these increasing costs can be associated directly with the blockbuster mentality that pervades the industry as well as the inflated costs associated with the major studios' operations.[9]

That's entertainment! As Erik Barnouw suggests in the quotation at the beginning of this chapter, technologies are often envisioned as new possibilities for enlightenment and democracy. However, their actual development may be something else.

Once again, the new technologies discussed in this volume have evolved as forms of entertainment. Yes, there are informational programs on cable and even pay cable. Yes, there are documentary videos and informational programs available on videocassettes. But the *dominant* use of these new media forms is entertainment. No, nothing against a good laugh, a good cry, a mindless romp through outer space. The point, again, is that we were promised so much more.

Many popular writers and social scientists, and more than a few government inquiries, have argued that there may be serious consequences of such a preoccupation with being passively entertained, rather than being creative and informed.[10] It also might be noted that since this phenomenon has occurred with the introduction of most new communication technologies, as Barnouw suggests, we might look to the social setting in which these technological developments occur, rather than the technologies themselves. This view was echoed by an industry visionary, Bob Stein of the Voyager Company, when asked about the future of laser technology:

> Technologies don't grow up in a vacuum, they grow up – in this case – under moribund imperialist life in the late 20th century. . . . The same crap that is coming out of Hollywood is going to come out of these technologies by and large. If things don't change radically socially, then we're going to be using one tiny-tiny bit of the potential of the technology.[11]

Some may hold out for new creative possibilities that may be provided by some new entertainment technologies, promoting alternatives to the passive experiences presented by the culture industry. For instance, after observing his children exploring and playing with computers, James Monaco expressed hope that "there will be millions more like them who will take their rightful place with the priests of sounds and images and experience the joy of creation as often as the dubious pleasure of consumption."[12] Yet, the "joy" of consumption still may be overpowering to many viewers, especially when surrounded by appealing and/or subversive commercial pitches to accept a more passive, pay-per society mentality.

More channels for advertising Many of the discussions of the new communications technologies connected to the information revolution seem to avoid the issue of advertising via these new outlets. While more consumer choice or diversity is praised, the possibilities of new technologies as more exact marketing devices are less often acknowledged.

As we have seen in chapter 8, the latest distribution outlets for Hollywood films have incorporated more deliberate and extensive advertising and marketing campaigns than in the past. While these trends might have intensified without new communication outlets, the new technologies have nevertheless assisted in the further commercialization of our culture.

Property is property Another concept that has changed little throughout these developments is the notion of culture as property. In other words, the introduction of cable, home video, or satellite communication has not altered the accepted perception of cultural or creative expression which is owned rather than shared. The Disney culture may be international, reaching beyond national and cultural boundaries, but it is *owned* by the Disney company.

The notion of culture as property is illustrated quite well with the issue of piracy, a problem which has accelerated with some of the new communication technologies discussed in this book, and especially in relation to video technology. Again, the entertainment industry has turned to the state to protect its interests (i.e. profits) by enforcing the notion of culture as property, a value which automatically accompanies the development of these new technologies in capitalist societies.

We also are reminded from this discussion that technologies may be changing some of the ways in which we experience entertainment and information in the 1990s, but the relations of production remain the same. There has been no revolution in social relations.[13]

Uneven distribution The boom in new distribution outlets and markets has been enormously lucrative for the film industry and its leaders.

During a decade when the gap between the poor and the rich in the USA became even more glaring, many of the Hollywood majors reported record profits and the corporate heads of the largest companies were rewarded for their success, often with profit incentives and stock options.

A survey by the *Los Angeles Times* in 1984 indicated that "more than 100 stars, directors, producers, writers, agents and studio executives have built fortunes of $50 million or more in the last few years."[14] The salaries of Hollywood stars continue to skyrocket,[15] while executive salaries and compensations have reached all-time highs. Steven J. Ross (Time Warner) topped Forbes' list of best paid chief executives, receiving combined compensation of $302 million in 1990. Martin S. Davis of Paramount made the list for the second year, as did Michael D. Eisner of Disney.[16] At the end of 1992, Eisner made an astounding move, cashing in over $90 million in stock options, prompting other executives to do the same in order to avoid potential tax hikes by the Clinton administration during 1993. Again, what has changed about these tales of the wealthy becoming wealthier? Not a lot.

Meanwhile, Hollywood unions were losing members and strength, suffering from the proliferation of non-union films and runaway production, and giving in to concessions demanded by prosperous (and some would argue, greedy) studios.[17]

Another question of distribution relates to how much new technology is really needed, at what cost and to whom. When asked his opinion of HDTV, one might have expected Ted Turner – head of Turner Entertainment, which has benefited from many of the recent technological changes – to wax eloquent on the advantages of this specific technology. His response, however, was surprising (again, typical for Turner):

> Over half the people on earth don't have enough to eat and probably a third of the people don't have any TV at all. It's gonna be mega-billions to convert over to that, and I think there are a lot more things that can be done with that money before the rich world pigs out on high-density color TV. We oughta supply people that don't have electricity with electricity before we do that.[18]

Of course, that would provide a larger audience for Turner's expanding regular-TV audience, but nevertheless, his thoughts remind us that constant technological change is not always automatically necessary for real human progress.

Myth-busting

Having looked more closely at the latest technologies employed by the film industry and some of the other developments over the last few decades, it is possible to examine the promises and myths introduced in chapter 1: (1) more competition, (2) industrial conflict, and (3) more diversity.

Myth 1: competition – concentration versus independence Despite the claim that the new technologies introduced in the 1970s and 1980s would foster competition, this has not been the case, as much of the evidence in this study has indicated.

With the enhanced need for product or software, the Hollywood majors were poised and ready to supply it. While the majors already received income from diverse resources, new distribution outlets meant even further diversification. Despite the initial skirmishes and claims of foul play, the majors were well positioned (or made the necessary adjustments) to maintain their prominence, not only in the traditional film industry, but in the larger culture industry. They were able and willing to build alliances with other companies – outside the traditional film industry or even with new "competitors" – as well as developing interdependencies between old and new technologies. In addition, they have benefitted from relaxed government regulation, thus merging into large synergistic corporations that control huge chunks of popular cultural production, not only in the USA but around the world.

The majors' strength might be contrasted to a typical independent filmmaker who only produces films, and thus is unable to capitalize on or draw strength from these diversified revenues. And, if there was one observation that prevailed in Hollywood at the beginning of the 1990s, it was the difficulties faced by independents. The majors' entry into exhibition further exacerbated the situation. As one independent observed, "You have all these screens, but they're showing the same eight movies over and over again, as opposed to giving (smaller) films a chance to find their audience."[19]

So the majors rule the entertainment roost. If there is any doubt about concentration in the traditional film industry, recall that the top five or six distribution companies regularly receive nearly 90 percent of domestic (North American) theatrical film rentals and still dominate the distribution of motion pictures to home video and cable markets. Indeed, the notion of competition in the traditional film industry is a legendary myth, and remains so as Hollywood looks toward the 21st century.

Myth 2: industrial conflict Throughout this book, there have been references to "the film industry." And in many of the developments during the last decades, "the film industry" has been pitted against other entertainment or communications industries – broadcasting, cable, and home video. This is the rhetoric of the industries themselves and the government representatives who regulate or deregulate them. Yet, there are several reasons why this terminology is misleading, especially for those who seek to understand the impact of these activities on our culture.

Increasingly, the same products are seen in all these supposedly-separate industries. As noted in the first chapter and illustrated in subsequent chapters, popular cultural products are continuously duplicated, reworked and reproduced. Thus to think about the unique contribution of "film" is myopic.

Furthermore, the giant communications corporations are involved in many, if not all, of these activities. As discussed in chapter 4, all of the Hollywood majors have subsidiaries which deal with film, television, music, cable, and home video. Most of the larger companies also are involved in publishing, theme parks, and merchandising. Thus, how is it possible to separate the interests of these corporations into specific "industries"? More often than not, when Jack Valenti represents "the film industry," he must qualify his remarks to account for the various corporations that also are involved heavily in other sectors. (Time Warner and Fox presented these kinds of problem in the late 1980s/early 1990s.) As Aksoy and Robins conclude:

> The major Hollywood companies are being turned into image empires with tentacles reaching down, not only to movies and TV programmes, but also to books, records, and even hardware. The feature film business no longer exists in its own right, but is increasingly becoming part of an integrated, global image business, central to the broader media strategies of entertainment companies and conglomerates. However, the major studios are the fundamental building blocks of the emerging entertainment megacompanies.[20]

Certainly there are differences in the characteristics of various distribution outlets for entertainment, necessitating some differences in industry structures and policies. Indeed, there are differences in the essences of these various media, as Marshall McLuhan and Harold Innis showed us in their work.

Yet these differences are breaking down and it might behoove us to think in terms of *transindustrial* activities, emphasizing the overlapping strategies of a relatively few corporations producing and distributing entertainment and cultural products. Again, we might also revisit the notion of a *culture industry*, as depicted by the Frankfurt School theorists in the 1930s. One need not argue that the effects of the culture industry are uniform or overpowering (as the Frankfurt School assumed) to accept that there are shared interests and activities among these various business sectors, and to resist the notion that there is constant industrial conflict, as many industry and government representatives would contend. Further, it is possible, without sinking to economic reductionism, to accept the terminology popular with the corporations themselves, as they stress the notion of "synergy" between their various operations. But this brings us to the question of diversity, the next myth of the information age.

Myth 3: diversity or more of the same?   A common theme in past discussions of new technologies is the enhanced diversity offered the consumer, with terms such as "television of abundance" and "technologies of freedom."[21] Yet, the more common observation these days is that the range of programming has not been enhanced with new distribution outlets. *Channels* magazine observed in 1987, it is more like "old wine in many new bottles." As British communications scholar, Graham Murdock has argued: "It is possible to greatly increase the number of channels and the number of goods in circulation without significantly extending diversity. More does not necessarily mean different. It can also mean more of the same thing distributed in a variety of ways. ...Diversity is not multiplicity."[22]

After a decade of new cable channels and home video options, it is no longer an academic exercise to predict less true diversity. Articles in the popular press, editorial cartoons, public opinion polls, and even writers of popular songs (e.g. Bruce Springsteen) reflect the disillusionment with the promises of more diversity through new entertainment technologies. For instance, in early 1992 an Associated Press survey reported that 40 percent of people in the USA believed that cable and video rentals made it easier to find programs they wanted to see, while one-third of those polled said that cable and VCRs made no difference and 20 percent claimed that choices had become even worse.[23]

As we have seen in this study, the new distribution outlets which have been introduced over the last few decades have provided us (for a price) with at least the outlets (or conduits) for cultural diversity. We are no longer prisoners of the "tyranny" of watching or listening to the same sources, at the same time. Yet, by looking at the narrow range of producers and the typical duplication of programming, it is possible to argue that similar ideas, values and expressions are reproduced in these different outlets. In other words, a form of *cultural synergy* has coincided with the corporate synergy stressed by the megacorporations which produce and distribute cultural products. The economic logic is compelling, as once a character or story is created and developed (and, of course, owned), there are advantages in moving it into different formats. For instance, it is not unusual to find films made into television programs, because the same companies that often produce and distribute major films also produce prime-time programming. With a popular film, there is no need to make a pilot, which can cost around $2.2 million per hour. And, while some films do not transfer into successful television fare, they still have the advantage of being recognized immediately by audiences.[24] Roger Rabbit, the movie, becomes Roger Rabbit, the cartoon, becomes Roger Rabbit, the video, etc. The production savings and promotional value of different outlets seems obvious. But the result is less diversity from channel to channel (or conduit to conduit).

The notion of cultural synergy implies that characters, stories and ideas are made into products for different outlets. However, what often occurs is that we see the same products on different outlets, or, in other words, we experience *recycled culture*. While cable offers many more channels than previous systems, much of the programming includes recycled TV shows, movies, or documentaries. While videocassette versions of films provide the opportunity to see a movie in the comfort of our homes, the film still is recycled from another outlet, and will be recycled again for network television, again for syndicated television, etc. While many fans enjoy seeing their favorite TV programs, movies, etc. over and over again, and can even "own" their own copies, it seems disturbing that our culture may not be actually evolving, but merely recycling. At the very least, there is much less diversity than promised when new distribution outlets display the same programming as previous outlets.

Moving into the 21st Century

Promises, promises. What purpose do they serve? It might be argued that the public has not cried out for these new technologies, nor for more competition in the culture industry, nor for more diverse, uplifting programming. But if a market is to develop, the public – or consumers – must be convinced of the positive attributes of new technological wonders, whether they be computers, electronic banking machines, videocassette recorders or fiber-optic cable systems.

But it also might be argued that it is not difficult for people to tap into these optimistic visions of the future. After all, a classic American tradition is to link technology with progress. The dawning of a new age (an "information age") also may be a compelling vision, especially when it may be possible to reignite an increasingly fading American economy with more jobs and more prosperity.

Yet given the history of past technologies which have failed to live up to their promises, plus some strong indications that more enlightenment, diversity, and other positive attributes may not automatically accompany new technologies, more active promotion of the notion of "technological progress" may be necessary these days. Thus, these positive projections serve to enhance the acceptability of the continuous introduction of new technologies, new commodities, and new markets. Of course, new markets *must* be promoted as inherently positive and appealing, and consequently glowing forecasts and hopeful promises are inevitably pinned to emerging cultural technologies, as they are to any new technological development with the promise of new profits. Whether or not those technologies are really necessary or beneficial for the betterment of society is rarely part of the discussion, if there is indeed any public discussion at all.

While many of the promises of the latest technologies may indeed be myths, Hollywood has always thrived on myths. That much seems unchanged. Many other characteristics of Hollywood also remain. Despite the revolutionary technological developments of the last few decades, the social relations of corporate Hollywood remain unscathed. But what about changes in the future?

Hollywood seems poised and ready for the next century. Despite the continuing rhetoric of technophobia, the major Hollywood corporations seem more than ever ready for change. That is, ready to capitalize on change and ready to diversify activities wherever profits may lead.

Certainly the megacorporations that dominate the entertainment world are not invincible. There are no guarantees that they will always survive and make the right decisions. As noted at the beginning of this chapter, Hollywood in the 1990s must still depend on unpredictable audiences, inevitable government influences and other political and economic vagaries. Ultimately, their own grand plans and dreams may prove fatal, as some predict when looking at the skyrocketing costs of talent and continually expanding budgets for major Hollywood films.

It remains to be seen if the public will ever be offered anything really new or challenging from future technological developments or other industrial changes. But it also remains to be seen how the public ultimately will respond. How long will audiences – especially with increasing access to the tools and technologies of culture – continue to play the role of consumers of cultural values and products not of their own making?

Meanwhile, the major Hollywood players move on. The Big Boys demonstrated their flexibility in the 1980s by expanding beyond movies in theaters and on television, to concepts and characters on videocassettes and cable channels, and (the same) concepts and characters in theme parks, video games and T-shirts. These same companies are poised and ready to supply similar products to the new electronic highways of the future. Thus, for Hollywood, now more than ever, film is only the starting point in a journey . . . beyond the silver screen.

Notes

Chapter 2 The Way We Were: An Historical Look at Hollywood and Technology

1 George Mair, *Inside HBO: The Billion Dollar War Between HBO, Hollywood and the Home Video Revolution*, New York: Dodd, Mead & Co., 1988, p. 13.
2 Jack Valenti, "Managing Changes in Technology," *Variety*, 14 January 1987, p. 8.
3 Another example: "Hollywood has always been ambivalent about new delivery technologies. In the 1950s, television was thought to be the death knell for the movies. But the networks soon became a significant aftermarket for theatrical films and a substantial revenue source for the studios." In "Simon Says: Foreign Sales will Drive Hollywood in Nineties," *Video Business*, 19 May 1989, p. 36.
4 For instance, see Raymond Fielding, *A Technological History of Motion Pictures and Television*, Berkeley: University of California Press, 1967; James Limbacher, *Four Aspects of Film*, New York: Brussel & Brussel, 1968. Examples of other studies which look at specific technologies include R. T. Ryan, *A History of Motion Picture Color Technology*, New York: Focal Press, 1978; Harry M. Geduld, *The Birth of the Talkies: From Edison to Jolson*, Bloomington: Indiana University Press, 1975; Brian Coe, *The History of Movie Photography*, New York: New York Zoetrope, 1982; and Martin Quigley, *New Screen Techniques*, New York: Quigley, 1953.
5 David Bordwell, Janet Staiger and Kristin Thompson, *The Classical Hollywood Cinema: Film Style and Mode of Production to 1960*, New York: Columbia University Press, 1985, p. 251.
6 For a more detailed history of the introduction of sound, see Douglas Gomery's work, including "The Coming of Sound to American Cinema,"

Ph.D. dissertation, University of Wisconsin-Madison, 1975; "Problems in Film History: How Fox Innovated Sound," *Quarterly Review of Film Studies* 1, no. 3, August 1976.

7   Robert C. Allen and Douglas Gomery, *Film History: Theory and Practice*, New York: Alfred A. Knopf, 1985, p. 123. Also see Bordwell et al., *The Classical Hollywood Cinema*, chapter 23, for a discussion of the transition to sound.

8   See N. R. Danelian, *AT&T: The Story of Industrial Conquest*, New York: Vanguard, 1939; Janet Wasko, *Movies and Money: Financing the American Film Industry*, Norwood, N.J.: Ablex, 1982, pp. 60–9.

9   Wasko, *Movies and Money*, pp. 77–97.

10   Erik Barnouw, *The Golden Web*, New York: Oxford Press, 1968, p. 103.

11   Michelle Hilmes, *Hollywood and Broadcasting: From Radio to Cable*, Urbana, Ill.: University of Illinois Press, 1990, p. 7.

12   Ibid., pp. 33–5; Gomery, "The Coming of Sound," p. 130.

13   Hilmes, *Hollywood and Broadcasting*, p. 36.

14   Jonathan Buchsbaum, "Zukor Buys Protection: The Paramount Stock Purchase of 1929," *Cine-Tracts*, no. 8, Summer–Fall 1979.

15   Hilmes, *Hollywood and Broadcasting*, pp. 55–70.

16   See Arthur Knight, *The Liveliest Art*, New York: Macmillan, 1957, p. 292; Garth Jowett, *Film: The Democratic Art*, Boston: Little Brown, 1975, p. 349.

17   Hilmes, *Hollywood and Broadcasting*, p. 72.

18   Douglas Gomery, "Failed Opportunities: The Integration of the US Motion Picture and Television Industries," *Quarterly Review of Film Studies*, Summer 1984, p. 224; Douglas Gomery, "Theater Television: The Missing Link on Technological Change in the US Motion Picture Industry," *Velvet Light Trap* 21, Summer 1985, pp. 54–61.

19   See Gary N. Hess, *An Historical Study of the DuMont Television Network*, New York: Arno Press, 1979.

20   Hilmes, *Hollywood and Broadcasting*, pp. 118–119; Gomery, "Failed Opportunities," pp. 219–27.

21   Hilmes, *Hollywood and Broadcasting*, pp. 120–5; Gomery, "Failed Opportunities," p. 223.

22   Hilmes, *Hollywood and Broadcasting*, p. 126.

23   Ibid., pp. 127–8.

24   See Mark Freed, "An Analysis of the Failure of Subscription Television in California in 1964," unpublished master's thesis, University of Oregon, December 1969.

25   Hilmes, *Hollywood and Broadcasting*, pp. 133–7. The Paramount decrees refer to the antitrust suit against the five fully integrated Hollywood majors and three other distributors in the 1940s, which was settled through a series of consent decrees beginning in 1948. The majors were required to divorce their production and distribution activities from exhibition, to refrain from price setting and other anti-competitive agreements, and to distribute their films "theater by theater, picture by picture". For more details, see Michael

Conant, *Antitrust in the Motion Picture Industry*, Berkeley, Calif.: University of California Press, 1960.

26 Ibid., pp. 117–18. For more on interaction between film and television, see Thomas H. Guback and Dennis J. Dombkowski, "Television and Hollywood: Economic Relations in the 1970s," *Journal of Broadcasting* 20, Fall 1976; Frederic Stuart, "The Effects of Television on the Motion Picture Industry: 1948–1960," and Barry R. Litman, "The Economics of the Television Market for Theatrical Movies," in Robert Allen, ed., *The American Motion Picture Industry*, Carbondale, Ill.: Southern Illinois University Press, 1982.

27 Another technological development that Hollywood took advantage of was phonograph records and music products, which have not been dealt with here. For further discussion, see Roland Gelatt, *The Fabulous Phonograph 1877–1977*, New York: Collier Books, 1977, especially pp. 250–5, 325–32; Steve Chapple and Reebee Garofalo, *Rock 'n' Roll is Here to Pay: The History and Politics of the Music Industry*, Chicago: Nelson-Hall, 1977.

28 Morris Ernst, *The First Freedom*, New York: The Macmillan Co., 1946, p. 197.

29 Edward Branigan, "Color and Cinema: Problems in the Writing of History", in Paul Kerr, ed., *The Hollywood Film Industry*, Routledge & Kegan Paul, 1986, pp. 122–5; Allen and Gomery, *Film History*, pp. 109–13.

30 Eileen Meehan, "Critical Theorizing on Broadcast History," *Journal of Broadcasting and Electronic Media* 30, no. 4, Fall 1986, pp. 393–411.

31 Branigan, "Color and Cinema," pp. 125–8; Allen and Gomery, *Film History*, pp. 112–13; Stephen Heath, "The Cinematic Apparatus: Technology as Historical and Cultural Form," in Teresa de Lauretis and Stephen Heath, *The Cinematic Apparatus*, New York: St Martin's Press, 1980, p. 5.

32 Stephen Neale, *Cinema and Technology: Image, Sound, Colour*, Bloomington, Ind.: Indiana University Press, 1985, p. 159.

33 For example, Richard Emil Hincha, "Twentieth Century Fox's Cinemascope: An Industrial Organization Analysis of its Development, Marketing and Adoption," Ph.D. dissertation, University of Wisconsin-Madison, 1989.

34 Geoff Hodgson, *Economics and Institutions*, Cambridge: Polity Press, 1988.

35 Michael Storper and Susan Christopherson, "Flexible Specialisation and Regional Industrial Agglomerations: The Case of the U.S. Motion Picture Industry," *Cambridge Journal of Economics* 13, no. 2, 1987, pp. 104–17.

36 Asu Aksoy and Kevin Robins, "Hollywood for the 21st Century: Global Competition for Critical Mass in Image Markets," *Cambridge Journal of Economics* 16, no. 1, 1992, pp. 1–22.

37 Jean-Louis Comolli, "Technique et idéologie: Caméra, perspective, profondeur de champ," *Cahiers du Cinéma*, May–June 1971. For translations of Comolli's key articles, see Nick Browne, ed., *Cahiers du Cinéma: 1969–1972: The Politics of Representation*, Cambridge, Mass.: Harvard University Press, 1990.

38 See de Lauretis and Heath, *The Cinematic Apparatus*; Branigan, "Color and Cinema"; Allen and Gomery, *Film History*.

39 See Russell Jacoby's *The Last Intellectual: American Culture in the Age of Academe*, New York: Basic Books, 1987, for an excellent discussion of the use of academic jargon and ivory-tower intellectualization by leftist scholars.
40 Branigan, "Color and Cinema."
41 Bordwell et al., *The Classical Hollywood Cinema*.
42 Ibid., p. 243.
43 Andrew Britton, "The Philosophy of the Pigeonhole: Wisconsin Formalism and 'The Classical Style,'" *CineAction!*, Winter 1988–9, p. 48.
44 See Thomas H. Guback, "Are We Looking at the Right Things in Films?" Paper from Society for Cinema Studies conference, Philadelphia, Penn., 1978.
45 Hilmes, *Hollywood and Broadcasting*, p. 4.
46 MARHO, *Visions of History*, New York: Pantheon Books, 1983, p. ix.
47 For more discussion of the approach used in this volume, see Eileen R. Meehan, Vincent Mosco, and Janet Wasko, "Rethinking Political Economy: Change and Continuity," *Journal of Communications* 43(4), Autumn 1993.

Chapter 3 Film Production in the Information Age

1 Frank Dutro, lecture at the American Film Institute, Los Angeles, Calif., 5 August 1991. See Andy Marx, "Screenwriters Getting Computer-Age Assist," *Variety*, 20 September 1993, pp. 7–8.
2 See Harvey Berger, "The PC Goes to Hollywood," *PC*, 16 October 1984.
3 Jim Nash, "IS: The Hottest Thing to Hit Hollywood Since the Phone," *Computerworld*, 24 December 1990, p. 45.
4 James Daly, "Scripting Hollywood Success with IS," *Computerworld*, 20 November 1989, pp. 7, 82.
5 Presentation by Randy Blim, Sr Vice President, Pacific Video, at Laser Pacific, Los Angeles, Calif., 9 August 1991.
6 Charles Eidsvik, "Machines of the Invisible: Changes in Film Technology in the Age of Video," *Film Quarterly*, Winter 1988/89, pp. 18–23.
7 See James Monaco, "Into the 90's," *American Film*, January/February 1989, pp. 24–7.
8 William A. Koch, "Eastman Video Tape & Future Imaging Technologies," *American Cinematographer*, March 1984.
9 Quoted in Blim's 1991 presentation; also, see Koch, "Eastman Video Tape"; Don Sutherland, "Film's Comeback," *Audio Visual Communications*, December 1989.
10 See Lee Gregory, 'Imagevision Meets Monty Python," *American Cinematographer*, January 1983; R. Glickman, "Tech Talk: An Available High Resolution Video System," *The Hollywood Reporter*, 3 August 1981.
11 John Francis Lane, "The Coppola Connection," *Sight & Sound*, Autumn 1989, pp. 219–20; John Skow, "Going for the Cheeky Gamble," *Time*, 25 January 1982; Thomas M. Pryor, "Cost Aside, Coppola's 'Heart' Reflects

Top Technical Research," *Variety*, 17 January 1982, p. 3; Judy E. Klein, "Coppola Makes 'Rumble Fish' – The Coppola Way," *Boxoffice*, November 1983, pp. 10–11.

12 See Brian Winston, "HDTV in Hollywood: Lights, Cameras, Inaction," in John V. Pavlik and Everette E. Dennis, eds, *Demystifying Media Technology*, London: Mayfield Publishing Co., 1993, pp. 109–17; Raymond Fielding, "Recent Electronic Innovations in Professional Motion Picture Production," *Journal of Film and Video* 36, Spring, 1984; Richard W. Stevenson, "Pushing Video in the Film Capitol," *New York Times*, 6 November 1991, p. D1:3.

13 Ken Jurek, "HDTV Stakes," *Audio Visual Communications*, December 1989. See also Norm Alster, "TV's High-Stakes, High-Tech Battle," *Fortune*, 24 October 1988, p. 161–70.

14 Peter Newcomb, "Cutting Edge," *Forbes*, 29 April 1991.

15 Broadcasters were told by FCC officials at a conference in January 1993 that a "winning HDTV system" would be named by the end of February, followed by field tests and an ultimate FCC decision by 1994: "Can You Profit from the Digital Revolution?," Association of Independent Television Stations (INTV) conference panel, San Francisco, Calif., 25 January 1993. See "HDTV Decision Likely to be Delayed One More Time for Retesting," *Communications Daily*, January 26, 1993; Edmund Andrews, "Foes Hook Up for HDTV," *Register Guard*, 25 May 1993.

16 See Susan Levin, "High Definition Transfers to 35 mm," *American Cinematographer*, May 1986. *The 1991 International Television & Video Almanac*, New York: Quigley Publishing, 1991, p. 603, reported that three feature films were shot in high definition video in 1988, including *Julia and Julia*, *Crack in the Mirror*, and *Do It Up*, as well as the TV movie, *Innocent Victims*.

17 Presentation by J. Richard West, Director, Technical Services, Sony High Definition Facilities Inc., Culver City, California, 9 August 1991.

18 Winston, "HDTV in Hollywood," p. 117. Also see David E. Sanger, "Stalking the Next Walkman," *New York Times*, 23 February 1992.

19 "Hollywood's Brave New World," *Los Angeles Times*, 23 December 1990.

20 Ibid.

21 Susan Borden, "The New Business of High Definition," *Audio Visual Communications*, December 1989; Rupert Stow, "Twist & Shout in High-Definition Effects," *Audio Visual Communications*, December 1989.

22 Rebo's *Performance Pieces* became the first high definition originated feature to win an award at a major film festival (Cannes) in 1989. It is interesting to note that one of Rebo's founders is a member of the Japanese Ministry of Trade and Industry. See Borden, "The New Business of High Definition," p. 32; Stow, "Twist & Shout in High-Definition Effects"; Newcomb, "Cutting Edge." For a list of HDTV productions worldwide in 1990, see Joseph Flaherty, "High-Definition Television: Technical and Political Issues," in Pavlik and Dennis, *Demystifying Media Technology*, pp. 99–109.

23 Ron Sherriffs, informal conversation, Eugene, Oregon, 9 March 1992.

24 Mario Orazio, "In Search of 'The Film Look,'" *TV Technology*, November 1990; "Video Technology in Film Making," *New York Times*, 12 March 1985.

25 "Hollywood's Brave New World."

26 Blim presentation, 1991. This sentiment was echoed by Alex Ben-Block, Executive Editor, *Hollywood Reporter*, in a lecture at Directors Guild of America, Los Angeles, Calif., 2 August 1991.

27 Eidsvik, "Machines of the Invisible."

28 Winston, "HDTV in Hollywood," p. 114.

29 See Stewart Brand, *The Media Lab: Inventing the Future at MIT*, New York: Viking Press, 1987, pp. 72–6; Joseph Turow, *Media Systems in Society*, New York: Longman, 1992, p. 7.

30 Also called a video record operator, and organized by the soundmen's local affiliated with the technicians' union which dominates the industry, the International Association of Theatrical and Stage Employees (IATSE).

31 James B. Brandt, "Video Assist: Past, Present and Future," *American Cinematographer*, June 1991.

32 Commercial directors have found the video assist process problematic, as their "creative power is diverted to the client." See Kirk Paulsen, "Video Assist Matte System," *American Cinematographer*, November 1985, p. 105.

33 Brandt, "Video Assist."

34 Paul Hirsch and David Rosenblum, film editors, lecture at the Directors Guild of America, Los Angeles, Calif., 8 August 1991.

35 Michael Nielsen, "Labor's Stake in the Electronic Revolution," *Jump Cut*, no. 35, April 1990, p. 80; Koch, "Eastman Video Tape"; Skip Ferderber, "Sting's Concert Film," *American Cinematographer*, February 1986.

36 Bob Lasiewicz, "Computers in the Editing Room," *American Cinematographer*, June 1985.

37 See "Time Code Basics," *American Cinematographer*, March 1983; Gary H. Anderson, "Understanding Video Edit Systems," *American Cinematographer*, January 1984; "Montage and Editorial Editing Systems...," *Television/Radio Age*, 1 October 1984.

38 Richard Nisbet, "Post-Production of *Opportunity Knocks*," *American Cinematographer*, November 1985, pp. 100, 103. Also see Michael Stanton, "*Mussolini* – Electronic Editing," *American Cinematographer*, June 1986, p. 85.

39 Emory M. Cohen, "The Electronic Laboratory – A Working Reality," *SMPTE Journal*, November 1988, p. 915.

40 However, there are some exceptions. For instance, *The Godfather III* was cut on a Montage editing system.

41 Hirsch and Rosenblum, lecture, 1991.

42 Sean Mitchell, "Editing: The Kindest Cut," *Los Angeles Times*, 23 March 1990.

43 Nielsen, "Labor's Stake," pp. 78–84.

44 Emory M. Cohen, "Volatile Video Transfer Scene," *American Cinematographer*, February 1989, p. 82.

45 Hirsch and Rosenblum, lecture, 1991. Also see Hans Fantel, "New Tech-
    nology Moving Into Films," *New York Times*, 12 March 1985.
46 See Winston, "HDTV in Hollywood," p. 114.
47 Harlan Kennedy, "Radical Sheik," *American Film*, December 1990, p. 32.
    For more on electronic editing, see Anderson, "Understanding Video Edit
    Systems"; Richard Patterson, "Film Style Video Editing Systems," *American
    Cinematographer*, January 1985; Stanton, "*Mussolini* – Electronic Editing."
48 Kirk Honeycutt, "Pushing the Envelope with Visual Effects," *Los Angeles
    Times*, 19 March 1990, p. F1.
49 See "2001 Entertainment: Personal FX," *Discover*, November 1988; Richard
    Wolkimir, "High Tech Hokum is Changing the Way Movies are Made,"
    The Smithsonian, October 1990; Richard Zoglin, "Lights! Camera! Special
    Effects!" *Time*, 16 June 1986, pp. 92–3.
50 Similar computer graphic techniques were used by Industrial Light & Magic
    for the film *Willow*. See Ron Magid, "ILM Gets a Piece of the Action,"
    American Cinematographer, January 1992; "Make Sticky, Morph!", *Time*,
    8 July 1991, p. 56. Morphing also was used in *The Abyss* to create the
    undulating sea creature called the Pseudopod. See "Lights! Action! Disk
    Drives!," *Newsweek*, 22 July 1991, p. 54; Bob Fisher, "The Dawning of the
    Digital Age," *American Cinematographer*, April 1992, pp. 71–2; Janet Maslin,
    "Movie Wizards Tell Cyborgs' Secrets," *New York Times*, 21 February 1992;
    David Hutchinson, "Digital Dawn," *SFX* 3, pp. 48–58; "Technology in the
    Movie Industry: Special Report," *Wall Street Journal*, 16 September 1985.
51 See David A. Kaplan, "Believe in Magic," *Newsweek*, 14 June 1993, pp.
    60–1.
52 Bob Fisher, "The Dawning of the Digital Age"; see also Alfred D. Harrell,
    "AFI/Apple Alliance Bears Fruit," *American Cinematographer*, April 1992.
53 "Lights! Action! Disk Drives!."
54 "2001 Entertainment."
55 Honeycutt, "Pushing the Envelope."
56 Harrell, "AFI/Apple Alliance," p. 92.
57 One film during the late eighties entitled *Lookers* dealt with the idea of
    computerized actors. Also see Kathleen K. Wiegner and Julie Schlax, "But
    Can She Act?," *Forbes*, 10 December 1990; Edith Myers, "Behind the
    Scenes," *Datamation*, March 1982, pp. 36–42, Harrell, "AFI/Apple Alli-
    ance," p. 92.
58 Mimeographed material from Apogee Productions.
59 Wolkomir, "High Tech Hokum." Also, see Magid, "ICM Gets a Piece of
    the Action."
60 "Lights! Action! Disk Drives!"; Kaplan, "Believe." See Thomas G. Smith,
    Industrial Light and Magic: The Art of Special Effects, New York: Ballantine
    Books, 1986 (excerpt in "Reel Illusions," *Omni*, June 1987, pp. 71–6). For
    more on Lucasfilm, see Dale Pollock, *Skywalking: The Life and Films of
    George Lucas*, New York: Harmony Books, 1983; Charles Champlin, *George
    Lucas: The Creative Impulse*, New York: Harry N. Abrams, 1992.
61 Chris Willman "'Dick Tracy' Brings in Arresting New Cinema Sound

System," *Los Angeles Times*, 30 May 1990. Also see Martha Groves, "'Star Wars' Scores Go Digital at Lucas' Skywalker Ranch," *Los Angeles Times*, 24 March 1990, p. F10.

62 Several special sections of trade magazines have focused on the animation revival: *Variety*, March 1992; *The Hollywood Reporter*, 26 January 1993, pp. S1–S76; Ray Bennett, "Animation Draws Winning Hand," *Daily Variety*, 5 February 1993. Also see Aljean Harmetz, "Video Alters Economics of Movie Animation," *New York Times*, 1 May 1985; Charles Solomon, "That Won't Be All, Folks, as Cartoons Make a Comeback," *Los Angeles Times*, 25 March 1990, p. F1.

63 Larry Rohter, "The Feature-Length Cartoon Returns," *New York Times*, 16 May 1991, p. c17.

64 Solomon, "That Won't Be All."

65 David Wilson, "Colour Box: New Films for Old," *Sight & Sound*, Summer 1985, p. 147.

66 Susan Linfield, "The Color of Money," *American Film*, January/February, 1987.

67 Wilson, "Colour Box."

68 Linfield, "The Color of Money," p. 30.

69 See Jack Mathews, "Colorization Debate Takes on a New Hue," *Los Angeles Times*, 16 March 1989; Don Shannon, "Panel Weighs 'Moral Rights' of Film Alteration," *Los Angeles Times*, 25 October 1989.

70 Robert S. Birchard, "My Hair is Red, My Eyes are Blue," *American Cinematographer*, October 1985, p. 76; Linfield, "The Color of Money," p. 30.

71 Wilson, "Colour Box."

72 Birchard, "My Hair is Red," pp. 75–7.

73 Linfield, "The Color of Money," p. 30.

74 Wilson, "Colour Box."

75 Greg Dawson, "Into the 90s: Ted Turner," *American Film*, January/February 1989, p. 39.

76 See Nielsen, "Labor's Stake."

77 Ibid., p. 83.

78 *Spaceballs* is an example of a film which satirizes the sci-fi genre which is rich in special effects, yet the film still had to incorporate some of the same special effects techniques in the process.

79 This sentiment is repeated consistently in discussions with Hollywood "insiders," and is a common theme of those interviewed by Tom Brokaw for NBC's documentary on "The New Hollywood," aired in March 1990.

80 Wolkomir, "High Tech Hokum," p. 124.

81 Frank Thompson, "The Big Squeeze," *American Film*, February 1990, pp. 40–3.

82 Ibid.

83 Nick Burns, "Big Screen to Small: Film Style and Television," unpublished paper, University of Oregon, 1990.

84 Eidsvik, "Machines of the Invisible."

85   See David Bordwell, Janet Staiger and Kristin Thompson, *The Classical Hollywood Cinema: Film Style and Mode of Production to 1960*, New York: Columbia University Press, 1985.

86   Presentation by Karl Malden, President, Academy of Motion Picture Arts and Sciences, Los Angeles, Calif., 7 August 1991.

87   Presentation by James Hineman, Deputy Director, American Film Institute, Los Angeles, Calif., 5 August 1991; Harrell, "AFI/Apple Alliance Bears Fruit."

Chapter 4 The Big Boys: The Hollywood Majors

1   "Is Tinseltown about to Meet its Terminator," *The Economist*, 25 May 1991, pp. 71–2.

2   John Micklethwait, "The Entertainment Industry: Raising the Stakes," *The Economist*, 4 January 1990, pp. S3–S18.

3   Neal Koch, "The Paramount Challenge: Make Hits New Ways," *Channels*, February 1989, pp. 44–5.

4   Unless otherwise noted, the material in this section is from Paramount's Annual Reports and Form 10Ks, 1991–2.

5   Other Paramount first-run syndicated programming includes *Entertainment Tonight, The Arsenio Hall Show, Hard Copy*, and *Maury Povich*.

6   Joe Mandese, "Hollywood's Top Gun," *Marketing and Media Decisions*, March 1988, pp. 109–14.

7   Skip Wollenberg, "2 Media Giants Ally with QVC Bid," *San Francisco Chronicle*, 18 October 1993, p. B1; "Street Talk," *USA Today*, 14 September 1992, p. 3B; Paul Wiseman, "Paramount Leaves QVC Bid on Hold," *USA Today*, 28 September 1993, p. B1.

8   Unless otherwise noted, the material in this section is from Time Warner Annual Reports and Form 10Ks, 1989–92.

9   This amount does not include first-run or repeat network revenues for network series, pilots, mini-series or made-for-television movies, but includes "revenues relating to Home Box Office of $155 million."

10   "Time Warner," *Business Week*, 22 July 1991.

11   See John Taylor, *Storming the Magic Kingdom*, New York: Knopf, 1987; Ron Grover, *The Disney Touch*, Homewood, Ill.: Business One Irwin, 1991.

12   Grover, *The Disney Touch*, pp. 137–9.

13   In their Form 10K for 1990, the company reported that their film library included 194 full-length live action features, 29 full-length animated color features and 529 cartoon shorts. Unless otherwise stated, material in this section was taken from the Walt Disney Company Annual Reports and Form 10Ks, 1990–3.

14   Touchstone Pictures was formed in 1984 (before the management/ownership shuffle) with the release of *Splash*.

15   Grover, *The Disney Touch*, p. 231.

16 Ibid., chapter 15.

17 See Laura Landro, "Cablevision to Pay $75 Million for Rights to Offer Disney Channel to Its Subscribers," *Wall Street Journal*, 10 October 1984.

18 Grover, *The Disney Touch*, pp. 149–50.

19 Ibid., p. 150.

20 The Phoenix/Scottsdale area of Arizona was the first. Michael Adams, "Hooked on Disney," *Successful Meetings*, September 1990, pp. 48–55.

21 Grover, *The Disney Touch*, pp. 186, 190.

22 S. G. Warburg Securities and Co. Inc., International Offering of Shares for Euro Disneyland. SCA, 5 October 1989, cited in Grover, *The Disney Touch*, p. 187.

23 Grover, *The Disney Touch*, p. 188.

24 Ibid., pp. 192–4; Terry Ilott and Michael Williams, "MCA Plays Catch-Up in Global Parks," *Variety*, 18 March 1991, p. 1, 110.

25 Brian Coleman and Thomas R. King, "Euro Disney Rescue Package Wins Approval," *Wall Street Journal*, 15 March 1994.

26 Ibid., p. 174. MGM filed a suit against Disney in May 1988, challenging the agreement. See MGM/UA Communications Co. and MGM Grand Inc. v. The Walt Disney Co., California Superior Court, Case No. C686329.

27 Ibid., pp. 176–80.

28 Ibid., p. 181.

29 For a detailed description of the Fox takeover, see Alex Ben Block, *Outfoxed: Marvin Davis, Barry Diller, Joan Rivers, and the Inside Story of America's Fourth Television Network*, New York: St Martin's Press, 1990. Unless otherwise noted, the information presented in this section is from the The News Corporation Limited's Annual Reports 1990–2.

30 For more on Murdoch and his company, see William Shawcross, *Murdoch*, New York: Simon & Schuster, 1992.

31 Some pruning of the Murdoch empire was done between 1991 and 1992, as several magazines, a half interest in Sky Television, and other enterprises were sold. The company still had substantial debt problems in early 1993, as it sought to restructure its balance sheet through various bond offerings. See Linda Keslar, "News Maps out $2 Bil Trip to Bond Markets," *Daily Variety*, 25 January 1993, p. 6; Deirdre Camoly, "Murdoch Keeps Ties to Eight Magazines," *New York Times*, 17 May 1991.

32 See "Giant Pay Giants," *Television Business International*, December/January 1993, p. 38.

33 The News Corporation's 1992 Annual Report states: "Twentieth Century Fox Film is one of only seven major film studios in the world."

34 This represented Fox's affiliate station count as of January 1993. The Fox programs offered included "The Simpsons", "America's Most Wanted", "Married . . . with Children".

35 The News Corporation Limited, Annual Report, 1987, p. 54.

36 Ibid.

37 Ronald Grover, Mark Landler, and Richard A. Melcher, "Is Tinseltown Too Tough for Rupert Murdoch?" *Business Week*, 1 February 1993, p. 56.

38 Ronald Grover, "When Columbia Met Sony . . . A Love Story," *Business*

Week, 9 October 1989. Unless otherwise noted, the material in this section is from Sony's Annual Reports and Form 10Ks, 1991–3.

39 To get Peters and Guber out of their five-year contract with Warner, Sony also gave Warner a 50 percent interest in CBS Record Club, the right to distribute Columbia films on cable, the stock that Columbia owned in Jerry Weintraub Entertainment, and exchanged its 35 percent interest in Burbank Studio for the Lorimar studio lot in Culver City (formerly MGM). *1991 International Motion Picture Almanac*, New York: Quigley Publishing, 1991.

40 Grover, "When Columbia Met Sony," p. 44.

41 Sony Corp. Annual Report, 1990, p. 1.

42 Ted Elrick, "The Occidental Tourist," *DGA News*, March–April 1990, p. 9; this point was also confirmed by Henry Ishil, Largo Entertainment, in a presentation at the Directors Guild of America, Los Angeles, 2 August 1991.

43 Ronald Grover, "Invasion of the Studio Snatchers," *Business Week*, 16 October 1990, pp. 52–4.

44 David Williams, "Sony's Hollywood Gambit," *Tokyo Business Today*, December 1989, pp. 14–19.

45 Sony Corp. Annual Report, 1991.

46 Bill Inman, "Big Mat Goes to Hollywood," *Business*, December 1990, pp. 86–90.

47 Marc Beauchamp, "Doing the Hollywood Shuffle," *Forbes*, 19 October 1987, pp. 35–6.

48 Anthony Michael Sabino, "Buon Giorno, Hollywood: Pathe Communications Leads the European Invasion in its Takeover of MGM Studios," *Journal of European Business*, March/April 1991, pp. 26–8.

49 Linda Rapattoni, "Judge says Parretti Must Give Up MGM," *Variety*, 8 January 1992, pp. 5, 14.

50 Peter Bart, "Ciao, Giancarlo," *Variety*, 8 January 1992, p. 14.

51 Among Orion's critically acclaimed films have been *Platoon*, *Dancing with Wolves*, and *Silence of the Lambs*. See Ron Grover, "Orion is still Starcrossed," *Business Week*, 4 May 1992.

52 By mid-1991, the box office take from *Dances with Wolves*, was $183 million, and from *The Silence of the Lambs* $130 million. See *1992 International Motion Picture Almanac*, p. 19A.

53 Orion Pictures Corporation, Form 10K, 1992.

54 See Robert Marich and Kirk Honeycutt, "Revived Orion Taking Business 'Step by Step,'" *The Hollywood Reporter*, 26 January 1993, pp. 1, 14.

55 Orion Pictures Corporation, Form 10K, op. cit.

56 Alan Citron, "Bill Seeks to Protect Culture from Overseas," *Los Angeles Times*, 11 October 1991, p. D2:3. HR 3533 was considered by the House Subcommittee on Commerce, Consumer Protection and Competitiveness. The bill was primarily written to block control of US national landmarks and parks, but would limit foreign ownership of domestic "cultural business enterprises" to 50 percent. The aim was to block further foreign ownership of the major Hollywood studios, but still allow for foreign investments. Interestingly, the Motion Picture Association of America

opposed the legislation on the ground that it represented a trade barrier. See Stan Soocher, "Legislators Review Show Bills; Congressional Update," *Entertainment Law & Finance*, December 1991, p. 1.

57 "Japan Goes to Hollywood," *Newsweek*, 9 October 1989.

58 Bill Nothstine, "Matsushita Mangles 'Mr Baseball'?" *Oregon Sports News*, Spring 1993, p. 73.

59 Maggie Mahar, "Adventures in Wonderland: Sony's Fling in Show Biz," *Barron's*, 7 October 1991, p. 9; "Hooked by Hollywood," *The Economist*, 21 September 1991, pp. 79–80; Alan Citron and Leslie Helm, "Matsushita Plays a Low-Key Profile at MCA for Now," *Los Angeles Times*, 17 November 1991, p. D1:5.

60 David E. Sanger, "Stalking the Next Walkman," *New York Times*, 23 February 1992; Victor F. Zonana, "Global Media," *Los Angeles Times*, 5 January 1992, p. D1:2.

61 For recent discussions of the Fin-Syn debate, see John Lippman, "FCC Reopens the Debate on Syndication," *Los Angeles Times*, 1 January 1993, D2:3; John Lippman, "Fight over Lucrative TV Reruns to Resume," *Los Angeles Times*, 6 November 1992, p. D1:5; Edmund L. Andrews, "Rerun Rights Proposal Angers Hollywood Studios," *New York Times*, 7 April 1991, Sec. 1, p. 22; Ronald Grover, "Shootout on Hollywood and Vine," *Business Week*, 8 January 1990.

62 Andrews, "Rerun Rights."

63 New Line Cinema is one example. Founded in 1967, the company has shown a profit every year. Committed to "strategic diversification" and an explicit policy of not "emulating old-line major studios," New Line targets movies to specific audience segments and specific distribution channels, building profitable "franchises" (see chapter 8) with the *Nightmare on Elm Street* and *Teenage Mutant Ninja Turtles*. For "upscale audiences," New Line added its Fine Line division in 1990, which released *The Player* in 1992. See New Line Cinema Annual Report, 1991.

64 A. D. Murphy, "North American Theatrical Film Rentals Market Shares, 1970–1992," *Daily Variety*, 13 January 1993. See also A. D. Murphy, "WB Takes Lethal Share," *Variety*, 25 January 1993, p. 18.

65 See Alan Citron, "The Hollywood that Can't Say No," *Los Angeles Times*, 13 December 1992, p. D1:4.

66 See especially Ronald Brownstein, *The Power and the Glitter: The Hollywood–Washington Connection*, New York: Vintage Books, 1992.

Chapter 5 The Wired Nation and the Electronic Superhighway: Cable Television, Pay Cable, Pay-Per-View and Beyond

1 See Federal Communications Commission, "New Television Networks: Entry, Jurisdiction, Ownership and Regulation," Final Report, Network

Inquiry Special Staff, Washington, D.C.: Government Printing Office, 1980; K. Gordon, J. D. Levy and R. S. Preece, "FCC Policy on Cable Ownership," Staff Report, Office of Plans and Policy, Federal Communications Commission, Washington, D.C.: Government Printing Office, 1981; J. D. Levy and F. O. Setzer, "Measurement of Concentration in Home Video Markets," Staff Report, Office of Plans and Policy, Federal Communications Commission, Washington, D.C.: Government Printing Office, 1982; US House of Representatives, "Telecommunications in Transition: The Status of Competition of Telecommunications Industry," Report by the Majority Staff of the Subcommittee on Telecommunications, Consumer Protection, and Finance, Committee on Energy and Commerce, 97th Cong., 1st Sess., Washington, D.C.: Government Printing Office, 1981; and US House of Representatives, "Media Concentration, Parts 1 and 2," Hearings before the Subcommittee on General Oversight and Minority Enterprise, Committee on Small Business, 96th Cong., 1st Sess., Washington, D.C.: Government Printing Office, 1981.

2　Steven S. Wildman and Bruce M. Owen, *Video Economics*, Cambridge: Harvard University Press, 1992. Also see J. R. Meyer, R. W. Wilson, M. A. Baughcum, F. Burton, and L. Caouette, *The Economics of Competition in the Telecommunications Industry*, Cambridge, Mass: Oelgeschlager, Gunn & Hain, 1980.

3　Cited in Christopher Sterling, "Cable and Pay Television," in Benjamin M. Compaine, ed., *Who Owns the Media?*, White Plains, NY: Knowledge Industry Publications, 1982, p. 308.

4　Pamela G. Hollie, "Hollywood Offers Pay-TV Challenge," *New York Times*, 28 April 1980.

5　Ibid.

6　George Mair, *Inside HBO: The Billion Dollar War Between HBO, Hollywood and the Home Video Revolution*, New York: Dodd, Mead & Co., 1988, p. 19.

7　For regulation pertaining to pay cable, see Cable Television Report and Order, 36 FCC2d 143, 190 (1972), aff'd sub nom.; Home Box Office v. FCC, 567 F.2d 9, 13 (DC Cir.), cert. denied, <=85> 434 US 829 (1977); Cable Television Syndicated Program Exclusivity Rules, 79 FCC2d 652 (1980) (repealing rules on distant signal carriage and syndicated program exclusivity), aff'd sub nom.

8　Mair, *Inside HBO*, p. 43.

9　Don Garbera, "At Home with Home Box Office," *Video Systems*, February 1990.

10　Mair, *Inside HBO*, p. 25.

11　Sterling, "Cable and Pay Television."

12　Mair, *Inside HBO*, p. 42.

13　Stratford P. Sherman, "Coming Soon: Hollywood's Epic Shakeout," *Fortune*, 30 April 1984, p. 208.

14　Mair, *Inside HBO*, pp. 44, 72.

15　Ibid., p. 78.

16 Ibid., p. 73. HBO has continued its production activities, also moving into television. During 1991, the company created two production divisions (HBO Independent Productions and HBO Worldwide Pictures), bought out Citadel Productions, and made deals with other television production companies. See "Companies on the Move," *Variety*, 6 January 1992, p. 80.

17 Thomas J. Murray, "Hollywood Battles for New Markets," *Duns Review*, June 1980; *Cable Marketing*, May 1982, p. 65.

18 Mair, *Inside HBO*, pp. 42–3, 63.

19 Ibid., p. 13.

20 For more background, see Michelle Hilmes, *Hollywood and Broadcasting: From Radio to Cable*, Urbana, Ill.: University of Illinois Press, 1990, p. 174.

21 Mair, *Inside HBO*, p. 64.

22 Jack Banks, "The Institutional Analysis of the Pay Cable Market," *Studies in Communication & Culture*, Spring 1988, p. 3.

23 See Paul Blustein, "Hollywood Challenges HBO Clout in Lucrative Cable-Movie Business," *Wall Street Journal*, 11 August 1980; also see Thomas H. Guback, "Motion Pictures," in Compaine, *Who Owns the Media?*

24 Blustein, "Hollywood Challenges HBO Clout"; Murray, "Hollywood Battles for New Markets."

25 "Getty's Pay-TV Venture is Sued by Justice Unit," *Wall Street Journal*, 5 August 1980.

26 See United States of America, Plaintiff, v. Columbia Picture Industries, Inc.; Getty Oil Company; MCA, Inc.; Paramount Pictures Corporation; and Twentieth Century Fox Film Corporation, Defendants, and Premiere, Intervenor-Defendant, 80 Civ. 4438 (GLG), United States District Court, Southern District of New York, 507 F. Supp. 412; 6 Media L. Rep. 2336; 1980–81 Trade Cas. (CCH) P63,698, 31 December 1980.

27 Lawrence J. White, "Antitrust and Video Market: The Merger of Showtime and The Movie Channel as a Case Study," in Eli M. Noam, ed., *Video Media Competition: Regulation, Economics, and Technology*, New York: Columbia University Press, 1985, pp. 338–63.

28 See Banks, "The Institutional Analysis," p. 135.

29 See Ann Crittenden, "Coke's Entertainment Formula," *Channels of Communication,* September 1986.

30 Mair, *Inside HBO,* p. 76.

31 "A New Shooter in Tinseltown," *Newsweek*, 13 December 1982, p. 106.

32 "TriStar Spells Out Finance Plans," *Broadcasting*, 29 October 1984, p. 56; "NATD withdraws Opposition to TriStar," *Variety*, 21 September 1983, p. 38.

33 "TriStar Gets Go-Ahead from Justice," *Broadcasting*, 19 September 1983, p. 35; Tom Girard, "Justice Dept. Greenlights TriStar," *Variety*, 21 September 1983, pp. 3, 29.

34 "TriStar Spells Out."

35 "TriStar Executives' Salaries Revealed," *Variety*, 14 November 1984, p. 3.

36 "CBS Mulling Sale of Its Equity in TriStar Pictures Partnership," *Variety*, 25 September 1985, p. 5.

37 Mark Lewyn, "Why Cable Companies are Playing So Rough, *Business Week*, 12 August 1991, p. 67.

38 *Broadcast & Cable Market Place 1992*, New Providence, New Jersey: R. R. Bowker, 1993, p. xxiii.

39 John MacManus, "Will Marketing Stop the Regulators?" *Advertising Age*, 10 December 1990, p. S1.

40 *Broadcasting & Cable Market Place 1992*, p. F100.

41 Standard & Poor's Industry Surveys, "Leisure," 4 July 1991, p. L40.

42 Standard & Poor's Industry Surveys, "Media," 7 February 1991, p. M29.

43 Wayne Walley, "Local Ad Sales Surging in Cable," *Advertising Age*, 15 April 1991, p. 20; MacManus, "Will Marketing Stop the Regulators?."

44 Janet Stilson, "Cable Ad Sales Dent Broadcast Revenues," *Electronic Media* 20, April 1987, p. 3.

45 *Broadcasting Yearbook 1991*, Washington, DC: Broadcasting Publications, 1991, p. D-3.

46 "Cable Changes the Systems from Within," *Channels/Field Guide 1990*, p. 90; *Broadcasting Yearbook 1991*.

47 Standard & Poor's, "Media."

48 Susan Hornik, "Basically, Cable Hits a Hot Spot," *Advertising Age*, 8 April 1991, p. 41.

49 *Broadcasting & Cable Market Place 1992*, p. xxiii.

50 Mark Lewyn, "Why Cable Companies are Playing so Rough," *Business Week*, 12 August 1991, p. 67.

51 Mike Evans, "The Inflation Bite is Back," *Industry Week*, 15 April 1991, p. 82. For the 1991 General Accounting Office Survey of Cable Rates, see 102nd Cong. 1st Sess., 137 Cong Rec S 11091, Vol. 137 No. 116.

52 Standard & Poor's, "Media," 6 June 1991, p. M4.

53 "Keeping the Lions at Bay," *Channels/Field Guide 1991*, p. 56.

54 See David Waterman, "The Failure of Cultural Programming on Cable TV: An Economic Interpretation," *Journal of Communication*, Summer 1986.

55 John Dempsey, "Is USA Net a Web Wannabe?" *Variety*, 1 July 1991, p. 57.

56 Kathryn Harris, "Mind over Rock Videos," *Forbes*, 21 January 1991, pp. 49–51.

57 Robert Sobel, "Carving Out an Audience: How Three Top Cable Networks are Building on Their Loyal Base," *Advertising Age*, 8 April 1991, pp. 43–4.

58 Jane Weaver, "The World is Flat: Cable Networks Brace for their First-Ever Soft Upfront," *Mediaweek*, 3 June 1991.

59 See John Eckhouse, "Interactive Ads will Home in on Consumers," *San Francisco Chronicle*, 1 October 1993, p. B2; "Big-name Players Fill Home Shopping Roster," *The Oregonian*, 29 June 1993; Steven W. Colford, "Infomercial Intros," *Advertising Age*, 8 April 1991.

60 John Dempsey, "Court TV Net's in Session," *Variety*, 1 July 1991.

61 Standard & Poor's, "Leisure."

62 Elizabeth Kolbert, "New Cable Channels Fight for Room," *Register-Guard*, 10 January 1993, p. 10B.

63 John Dempsey, "Cablers Cautiously Await Rereg," *Daily Variety*, 5 January 1993.

64 Standard & Poor's, "Media," 7 February 1991, p. M30.

65 See research by Paul Kagan Associates, reported in Sterling, "Cable and Pay Television," p. 434.

66 *Broadcasting Yearbook 1991.*

67 "VCR and Paycable Penetration," *Variety*, 13 September 1989.

68 Standard & Poor's, "Leisure," p. L4.

69 Dean M. Krugman and D. Eckrich, "Differences in Cable and Pay-cable Audiences," *Journal of Advertising Research* 22, no. 4, 1982, pp. 23–9; J. T. Rothe, M. G. Harvey, and G. C. Michael, "The Impact of Cable Television on Subscriber and Nonsubscriber Behavior," *Journal of Advertising Research* 23, no. 4, 1983, pp. 15–23.

70 John Motavalli, "Pay Cable Markets: In Search of a Strategy," *Channels Field Guide '87.*

71 See Richard Katz, "Preview Review," *Channels*, February 1990.

72 John Dempsey, "MCA & Cable Nets in Four-Way Foreplay," *Variety*, 22 October 1990

73 Sherman, "Coming Soon."

74 Michael Cieply, "MCA Sells Film Rights to CBS . . ." *Los Angeles Times*, 9 April 1990.

75 Sherman, "Coming Soon."

76 Tom Girard, "Candid Col Gives Details of HBO Pact," *Variety*, 7 November 1984.

77 Sherman, "Coming Soon."

78 "Showtime/Movie Channel and Paramount: Power through Partnership," *Broadcasting*, 2 January 1984.

79 John Motavalli, "Pay Cable Markets: In Search of a Strategy," *Channels Field Guide '87.*

80 Tom Girard, "HBO, 20th-Fox See Accord on Non-Exclusive Pic Deal Running Through Eighties," *Variety*, 14 March 1984.

81 See "Cable Report: HBO's 'Could Be' Exclusive," *Television Radio Age*, 23 June 1986; "HBO & Orion Still Going Steady as Paycabler Picks Up 14 Films," *Variety*, 27 February 1985; Kathryn Harris, "HBO Signs Deal for Exclusive Pay-TV Rights to Warner Movies," *Los Angeles Times*, 5 June 1986.

82 Alex Ben Block, "Shoot-out in Pay TV," *Forbes*, 22 September 1986. Also, see Tom Bierbaum, "Showtime, HBO Want Exclusives on Cable Pics," *Variety*, 16 April 1986; Motavalli, "Pay Cable Markets"; "Cable Report."

83 Richard W. Stevenson, "Carolco Flexes its Muscle Overseas," *New York Times*, 26 June 1991.

84 Banks, "The Institutional Analysis," p. 45.

85 Ronald Bettig, "The Impact of New Communications Technology on Filmed-Entertainment Copyrights," unpublished Ph.D. dissertation, University of Illinois, 1989.

86 See US House Judiciary Committee, Subcommittee No. 3, *Copyright Law Revision – Part 2* and *Part 3*, Hearings on H. R. 4347, 5680, 6831, 89th Cong., 1st Sess. (1965); and US Senate Judiciary Committee, Subcommittee on Patents, Trademarks, and Copyrights, *Copyright Law Revision – CATV*, Hearings on S. 1006, 89th Cong., 2nd Sess. (1966).

87 United Artists Television Inc. v. Fortnightly Corp., 255F. Supp. 177 (SDNY 1966), aff'd 377 F.2d 872 (2d Cct. 1967).

88 Bettig, "The Impact of New Communications," pp. 220–1.

89 Ibid., p. 226.

90 Ibid., p. 229.

91 Title 17 USC Section 111: Limitations on Exclusive Rights: Secondary Transmissions, d) Compulsory Licensing for Secondary Transmissions by Cable Systems.

92 For further discussion of cable compulsory licensing issues, see US Department of Commerce, National Telecommunications and Information Administration, *Video Program Distribution and Cable Television: Current Policy Issues and Recommendations*, June 1988.

93 *Broadcasting Yearbook 1991*, p. A-7; Stan Soocher, "Sorting Out New Cable Rereg Law," *Entertainment Law and Finance*, September 1992.

94 Richard W. Stevenson, "A Push for Pay-Per-View TV," *New York Times*, 11 June 1985, p. D-1.

95 Twentieth Century Fox, Form 10K, 1985, p. 8.

96 Mair, *Inside HBO*, p. 57.

97 David Waterman, "Pre-recorded Home Video and the Distribution of Theatrical Feature Films," in Noam, *Video Media Competition*, pp. 221–243.

98 Lewyn, "Why Cable Companies."

99 Public Law 102–385, Cable Television Consumer Protection and Competition Act of 1992, 102nd Congress, 2d Session, 5 October 1992.

100 See 138 Congressional Record S 712, Vol. 138 No. 10, Cable Television Consumer Protection Act.

101 Soocher, "Sorting Out."

102 Ibid.

103 See CFR Sections 76.57–76.61 (1984); Quincy Cable TV, Inc. v. FCC, 768 F.2d 1434, 1463 (DC Circuit 1985), cert. denied sub nom; National Association of Broadcasters v. Quincy Cable TV, Inc., 476 US 1169 (1986).

104 Anthony Ramirez, "High-Tech TV: So Near, Yet so Far Away," *New York Times*, 30 March 1992, D8:4.

105 Fairfax County's Media General system had held the record for the most channels, with a 120-channel capacity with programming offered on 96.

106 Rich Brown, "Time Warner Pay Takes Quantum Leap," *Broadcasting*, 26 October 1992, p. 53.

107 Peter M. Nichols, "Videotape's Growing Rival: Pay-Per-View TV," *New*

York Times, 30 March 1992, p. D8:3. Also see Barry Layne, "Time Warner Box $27 mil, 150-Channel N.Y. Cable System," *The Hollywood Reporter*, 8 March 1991.

108   James Barron, "150 Remedies to the Wail, 'There's Nothing on TV,'" *New York Times*, 19 December 1991, p. B3:3; Paula Span, "Quantity Time on Cable," *Washington Post*, 12 February 1992, p. C1.

109   Span "Quantity Time on Cable."

110   Brandon Tartikoff, Keynote address, National Association for Television Programming Executives (NATPE), 24 January 1993, San Francisco, Calif. See also "500 Channels and Nothing to Watch," *Time*, 14 December 1992, p. 22.

111   Viacom had earlier announced that it would be using Scientific Atlanta's digital compression system on a limited basis. See Paula Parisi, "TCI Putting Compression into Action Next Summer," *The Hollywood Reporter*, 3 December 1992. Around the same time, Zenith announced a method "to increase cable capacity sharply, using a new transmission method for digitally compressed standard TV and HDTV, sending 16 streams of digital data along a single cable channel. Cable operators will be able to cram in up to 23 movie channels, 9 live video channels, or 2 HDTV channels – vs. 1 show per channel today. System will be ready in about two years." See William D. Marbach, "Zenith's Digital Scheme for Cable TV," *Business Week*, 14 December 1992, p. 97.

112   Parisi, "TCI Putting Compression into Action."

113   Span, "Quantity Time on Cable."

114   Federal Communications Commission, Telephone Company–Cable Television Cross Ownership Rules, Sections 63.54–63.58, Further Notice of Proposed Rulemaking, First Report and Order and Second Further Notice of Inquiry, 7 FCC Rcd 300 (1991).

115   See Richard Karpinski, "After FCC Decision . . . Industry Faces a Host of Video Dial Tone Scenarios," *Telephony*, 27 July 1992; David Kelly, "FCC Gives Telcos Access to Cable," *Hollywood Reporter*, 25 October 1991; Anne Rackham, "Teamwork Looks Likely in New Cable Service Ventures," *The Los Angeles Business Journal*, 9 December 1991, p. 34.

116   Kelly, "FCC Gives Telcos Access."

117   Federal Communications Commission, Telephone Company-Cable Television Cross-Ownership Rules, Sections 63.54–63.58, CC Docket no. 87–266; 7 FCC Rcd 5781 (adopted July 16, 1992).

118   Cheryl A. Tritt, Chief, FCC Common Carrier Bureau, "Communacopia: The Evolution of Communications," Goldman Sachs & Company Telecommunications Conference, New York City, 13 November 1992.

119   Jeff Bater, "FCC Approves TV-on-Phone-Line Rule," United Press International Report, 16 July 1992.

120   Ibid.

121   Edmund L. Andrews, "Telephone Companies to Get Right to Transmit Television," *New York Times*, 16 July 1992, p. A1:1.

122   The prohibition applies to cities of 5,000 or more, unless the telephone

company receives a waiver from the FCC. Some 250 cable systems in rural areas are owned by small, independent phone companies. Cable Communication Policy Act of 1984, Public Law No. 987–549 @ 601 (3) 1984 US Code Cong. and Ad News (98 Stat.) 2779, 2781.

123 Bills dealing with telephone entry into cable included HR 2437 (1989), HR 2546 (1991), S. 1068 (1989), S. 2800 (1990), and S. 1200 (1991).

124 Also see Thomas McCarroll, "A Giant Tug-of-Wire," *Time*, 24 February 1992, p. 36.

125 See Dennis Wharton, "Bell Rings in with TV Telco Suit, " *Daily Variety*, 18 December 1992, p. 1.

126 McCarroll, "A Giant Tug-of-Wire."

127 Ibid.

128 Susan Kinsman "Telephone and Cable Industry Battle for Billions," *The Hartford Courant*, 23 November 1992, p. A1.

129 McCarroll, "A Giant Tug-of-Wire."

130 American Interests, "Wired for Failure? With the Global Telecommunications Revolution Leave the US Behind?" *Federal News Service*, 24 January 1992, transcript.

131 For instance, NYNEX was indicted in 1990 on criminal-contempt charges for providing computerized information in 1986 in violation of a federal court order. See McCarroll, "A Giant Tug-of-Wire."

132 Ibid.

133 Ibid.

134 See Andrew Calabrese and Janet Wasko, "All Wired Up and No Place to Go: The Search for Public Space in US Cable Development," *Gazette* 49, 1992, pp. 136–148; American Interests, "Wired for Failure?" A commentary piece in *Business Week* argued in late 1991 that the phone company should be able to compete with cable, as well as own some programming interests, and that cable should be able to enter the phone business. See Peter Coy, "Cable TV: For a Better Picture, Try Competition," *Business Week*, 23 December 1991, p. 58.

135 "A.T.&T. to Play a Role in Delivering Cable TV Programs," *New York Times*, 5 May 1992, D4:3; Doris Toumarkine, "AT&T Providing Digital Compression Technology," *Hollywood Reporter*, 5 May 1992.

136 "IBM nears Cable TV Agreement," *Register Guard*, 25 August 1992, p. 6C.

137 Andrew Kupper, "Any Movie, Anytime," *Fortune*, 25 January 1993, p. 83.

138 Joseph Weber and Peter Coy, "Look Ma – No Cable: It's Video-by-Phone," *Business Week*, 16 November 1992, p. 86.

139 Kupper, "Any Movie, Anytime."

140 Weber and Coy, "Look Ma–No Cable."

141 Ibid.; Tritt, "Communacopia."

142 Geraldine Fabrikant, "A Phone Company Buys Entry Into Cable Television Business," *New York Times,* 10 February 1993, p. A1:1.

143 Ken Terry, "Time Warner Breaks New Cable Ground," *Billboard,* 6 February 1993; Matt Rothman, "Time Warner Readying Florida

'Superhighway,'" *Daily Variety*, 27 January 1993, p. 1; Diane Mermigas, "Time Warner Steps into the Future," *Electronic Media*, 1 February 1993.

144 Rothman, "Time Warner Readying Florida 'Superhighway.'"
145 Parisi, "TCI Putting Compression into Action."
146 McCarroll, "A Giant Tug-of-Wire."
147 See FCC, Telephone Company–Cable Television–Cross Ownership Rules, MPAA comments, especially Note 291 and 293; 324–6. Also, John Lippman, "Diller Seeks to Form New Cable Venture," *Los Angeles Times*, 10 December 1992, p. D1:5.
148 Mermigas, "Time Warner Steps into the Future."
149 See Karpinski, "After FCC Decision"; Rothman "Time Warner Reading Florida 'Superhighway' "; Wharton, "Bell Rings in"; Toumarkine, "AT&T Providing Digital Compression"; Cindy Skrycki and Paul Farhi, "Hollywood on the Phone," *Washington Post*, 22 October 1992, p. A1; Seth Goldstein, "Blockbuster Sizes Up PPV Potential," *Billboard*, 30 January 1993, p. 11.
150 Mary E. Thyfault, "Promise to Keep: Telecom Development is a Clinton Principle, if not a Principal Concern," *Information Week*, 30 November 1992.
151 According to Rep. Boucher (D-Va.) (member of both House Commerce and House Judiciary Committees), the House could combine three bills into one package. Currently separate bills include one allowing telcos to enter cable business (Boucher and Rep. Oxley (R-O.) introduced in 1992), a bill to codify court rulings allowing the regional telephone companies into the information services line of business, while imposing rules against cross-subsidy (to be proposed by House Telecom Subcommittee Chmn. Markey (D-Mass.), and ex-Sen., now VP, Gore's bill allowing telephone companies to share facilities and networks. See "Boucher Considers 3-Part Legislative Strategy for Telco Issues," *Communications Daily*, 22 January 1993, p. 1.
152 Randy Sukow, "Congress: The Telco-Cable Battleground," *Broadcasting*, 4 January 1993, p. 51.
153 See Ellen Messmer, "Fighting for Justice on the New Frontier: The Electronic Frontier Foundation's Cofounder Explores the Rights of the Citizens of Cyberspace," *Network World*, 11 January 1993, p. S19. See also Jeffrey Chester and Kathryn Montgomery, "Media in Transition: Independents and the Future of Television," *NVR Reports* #10, November 1992.
154 Sloan Commission on Cable Communications, *On the Cable: The Television of Abundance*, New York: McGraw Hill, 1970.
155 See Doug Kellner, "Public Access Television and the Struggle for Democracy," in Janet Wasko and Vincent Mosco, eds., *Democratic Communication in the Information Age*, Toronto: Garamond Press, 1992; Douglas Kellner, *Television and the Crisis of Democracy*, Boulder, Colorado: Westview Press, 1990.
156 Peter Marks, "Cable Television Experiments with 150 Channels," *Register-Guard*, 7 July 1992, p. 5B.

157 Elizabeth Kolbert, "With 500 Channels, How Could Anyone Learn What's On?" *New York Times*, 4 January 1993.

158 Vincent Mosco, *The Pay-Per Society*, Norwood, N.J.: Ablex Publications, 1988.

Chapter 6 Talkin' 'Bout a Revolution: Home Video

1 "Homevideo Track," *Variety*, 13 July 1988, p. 40.

2 A. M. Rubin and C. R. Bantz, "Utility of Videocassette Recorders," *American Behavioral Scientist*, May/June, 1987, p. 472.

3 *1991 International Motion Picture Almanac*, New York: Quigley Publishing, 1991, p. 603.

4 *Standard & Poor's Industry Surveys*, 11 March 1993, p. L21–2.

5 "President of MPAA Describes Film Industry's Biggest Threat . . . including Home Video Recorders," *New York Times*, 5 May 1985, Sec, II, p. 1.

6 "MPAA's Valenti Offers Truce in CES Keynote Speech," *Video Business*, 20 January 1989, p. 6, cited in Daniel Moret, "The New Nickelodeons: A Political Economy of the Home Video Industry with Particular Emphasis on Video Software Retailers," unpublished MA thesis, University of Oregon, March 1991, pp. 85–6.

7 Albert Abramson, "A Short History of Television Recording," *Journal of the SMPTE*, February 1955, reprinted in Raymond Fielding, *A Technological History of Motion Pictures and Television*, Berkeley, Calif: University of California Press, 1967, p. 250; Aaron Foisi Nmungwun, *Video Recording Technology: Its Impact on Media and Home Entertainment*, Hillsdale, N.J.: Lawrence Erlbaum Publishers, 1989, pp. 1–2.

8 Nmungwun, *Video Recording Technology*, pp. 38–48, 100–1; Abramson, "A Short History," p. 250.

9 Nmungwun, *Video Recording Technology*, p. 101; Abramson "A Short History," (p. 250) reports that Hartley and Ives also were in England.

10 See Albert Abramson, *Electronic Motion Pictures*, Berkeley, Calif.: University of California Press, 1955.

11 Abramson, "A Short History," p. 251; Nmungwun, *Video Recording Technology*, p. 2.

12 See Mike Nielsen, "Hollywood High Frontier: The Emergence of Electronic Cinema," *Journal of Film and Video* XXXVI, Spring 1984, pp. 34–5; Eric Smoodin, "Motion Pictures and Television, 1930–1945: A Pre-history of the Relations Between the Two Media," *Journal of Film and Video* 34, no. 3, Summer 1982; Edward Buscombe, "Thinking it Differently: Television and the Film Industry," *Quarterly Review of Film Studies*, Summer 1984; Douglas Gomery, "Failed Opportunities: The Integration of the U.S. Motion Picture and Television Industries," *Quarterly Review of Film Studies*, Summer 1984; Douglas Gomery, "Theatre Television: The Missing

Link of Technological Change in the U.S. Motion Picture Industry," *The Velvet Light Trap*, no. 21, Summer 1985; and "Theatre Television: A History," *SMPTE Journal* 98, no. 2, February 1989.

13 Nmungwun, *Video Recording Technology*, p. 109. For a discussion of live versus recorded network programming, see Robert Vianello, "The Rise of the Telefilm," *Quarterly Review of Film Studies*, Summer 1984.

14 See Nmungwun, *Video Recording Technology*, pp. 109–11.

15 Peter Hammar, "The Birth of the VTR," *Broadcast Engineering*, June 1986, p. 158; Abramson, "A Short History," p. 250.

16 Crosby's company was eventually acquired by the 3M Company in 1956, after producing several high-frequency data recorders based on the longitudinal VTR for the US Army Signal Corps. Nmungwun, *Video Recording Technology,* p. 118.

17 *1991 International Motion Picture Almanac*, p. 343.

18 Nmungwun, *Video Recording Technology*, p. 137; *1991 International Motion Picture Almanac*, p. 343.

19 An often-reported speech by Sarnoff in 1951 included three wishes for his 50th anniversary in radio in 1956 – one of his requests was for a video recording device to be created by RCA engineers. Nmungwun, *Video Recording Technology*, p. 120.

20 Hammar, "The Birth of the VTR," p. 160; Abramson, "A Short History," p. 253; James Lardner, *Fast Forward: Hollywood, the Japanese and the Onslaught of the VCR*, New York: W. W. Norton, 1987, pp. 56–8.

21 *1991 International Motion Picture Almanac*, p. 343; Lardner, *Fast Forward*, p. 59; Nmungwun, *Video Recording Technology*, p. 112. An interesting historical note: Ray Dolby, the creator of Dolby sound, was involved with the development of Ampex's video recording systems from August 1952, and then worked on similar technology for the military. See Lardner, *Fast Forward*, p. 58; Nmungwun, *Video Recording Technology*, pp. 125–8; and Dick Roraback, "The Man Behind Silence: Dolby," *The Oregonian*, 29 May 1988, pp. D1, D4.

22 Unless otherwise noted, the following sections rely on Lardner, *Fast Forward*, and Nmungwun, *Video Recording Technology*.

23 See Nick Lyons, *The Sony Vision*, New York: Crown Publishers, 1976.

24 Ampex also worked with the Japanese company Toshiba, and actually produced a consumer-oriented cartridge system in the early 1970s called Instavision.

25 Lardner, *Fast Forward*, p. 81.

26 Sony also decided to share the U-Matic technology with other companies, leading to the first inter-manufacturer agreement between Matsushita and JVC. U-Matics are still used worldwide, with 31 different models available in 1983. See Nmungwun, *Video Recording Technology*, pp. 148–9; and Lardner, *Fast Forward*, pp. 71–73.

27 These companies included Sony, Ampex, CBS, Toshiba, Matsushita, North American NV Philips, Telefunken, RCA, Avco, American Photocopy

Equipment, Arvin, Technical Operations Inc., and Japan Electron Laboratory Co. Nmungwun, *Video Recording Technology*, pp. 149–53.

28 Michael Wiese, *Home Video: Producing for the Home Market*, Westport, CT: M.Wiese, 1986, p. 3; *1991 International Motion Picture Almanac*, pp. 343–4.

29 In his book, *RCA* (New York: Stein and Day, 1986), Robert Sobel reports $400 million (p. 255); Nmungwun (*Video Recording Technology*, p. 182) cites $580 million. Also see Margaret B. W. Graham, *RCA and the VideoDisc: The Business of Research*, New York: Cambridge University Press, 1986.

30 Sobel, *RCA*, p. 254–5.

31 US Department of Commerce, "1988 U.S. Industrial Outlook – Household Durables," January 1988, p. 47:7. At the beginning of the nineties, Beta still maintained its strength in a few markets: 90 percent in Mexico and 70 percent in Indonesia. Nmungwun, *Video Recording Technology*, pp. 153–6.

32 Susan Chira, "Sony to Make VHS Recorders," *The Oregonian*, 12 January 1988, pp. A1, A10; David Lachenbruch, "Here, Buy Another," *Channels/ Field Guide 1989*, p. 126.

33 David E. Whiteside, Otis Port and Larry Armstrong, "Sony Isn't Mourning the 'Death' of Betamax," *Business Week*, 25 January 1988, p. 37.

34 Lardner, *Fast Forward*, pp. 305–6.

35 Although several US firms marketed 8 mm format video equipment in the early nineties, it was still produced by Japanese companies. See *Channels*, January 1987, p. 88; Lardner, *Fast Forward*, pp. 307–11.

36 Ellen Schmid, "Compact Disc Video," *Electronic Media*, 27 July 1987, pp. 18, 22.

37 "Order Sought Against 'TV Genie'," *Register Guard*, 14 March 1987.

38 Lardner, *Fast Forward*, p. 302.

39 "What's Next!" *Video Review*, December 1986, p. 63.

40 Steven Schwartz, "The Strange Tale of the Dual-Deck VCR," *Video Review*, March 1989, pp. 25–6; "Go, Toshiba Settle Suit," *Variety*, 20 July 1988, p. 71; "Two VCR Makers Settle 2-Deck Suit," *Variety*, 10 August 1988, p. 34.

41 Lardner, *Fast Forward*, p. 302; Schwartz, "The Strange Tale"; "Pres. MPAA Opposes Sharp Co. . . . ," *New York Times*, 6 March 1985; "Movie Industry is Worried about a Videocassette Recorder," *Wall Street Journal*, 30 January 1985, p. 29.

42 Schwartz, "The Strange Tale."

43 Ibid. "Go-Video Accord Set with Samsung," *New York Times*, 3 March 1989. See also Gene G. Marcial, "Sneak Preview: The Next VCRs," *Business Week*, 11 July 1988, p. 88; "Go Video Adds Sony," *Variety*, 4 May 1988, p. 519.

44 Hans Fantel, "New VCR Allows Instant Tape-to-Tape Copying," *Register-Guard*, 2 November 1990.

45 Dennis Hunt, "The Format Battle Rages On," *Los Angeles Times*, 6 June 1986.
46 US Department of Commerce, "1988 U.S. Industrial Outlook," p. 47.7; Nmungwun, *Video Recording Technology*, p. 164; Electrical Industry Association, "Consumer Electronics U.S. Sales," January 1992.
47 Lardner, *Fast Forward*, p. 313.
48 Electrical Industry Association documentation in *1989 International Television and Video Almanac*, New York: Quigley Publishing, 1989, p. 399.
49 Lachenbruch, "Here, Buy Another," p. 126.
50 Electrical Industry Association, "Consumer Electronics U.S. Sales."
51 Doyle Dane Bernbach Inc., *The Media Scene: What Will It Look Like?*, 1982.
52 Tom Bierbaum, "Electronics Group Paint a Rosy Pic for H'wood," *Variety*, 14 January 1987, p. 13.
53 "Home Video Track," *Variety*, 27 July 1988, p. 37.
54 "Sales of VCRs are Slowing Down," *Register Guard*, 15 January 1989.
55 Wiese, *Home Video*, p. 23.
56 Wayne Thompson, "Advice to Help in Buying VCR," *The Oregonian*, 17 May 1988.
57 US Department of Commerce, "1988 U.S. Industrial Outlook," p. 47.7.
58 See Mark R. Levy, "Program Playback Preferences in VCR Households," *Journal of Broadcasting* 24, no. 3, Summer 1980; Mark R. Levy, "The Time-Shifting Use of Home Video Recorders," *Journal of Broadcasting* 27, no. 3, Summer 1983; Donald E. Agostino, Herbert A. Terry, and Rolland C. Johnson, *Home Video: A Report on the Status, Projected Development and Consumer Use of Videocassette Recorders and Videodisc Players in the United States*, FCC Network Inquiry Special Staff, November 1979.
59 The Betamax cases include: Universal City Studios, Inc., et al. v. Sony Corp. of America Inc., et al., 480 F. Supp. 429 (C.D. Cal 1979); Sony Corp. of America, Inc. et al. v. Universal City Studios, Inc., et al., 659 F. 2d 963 (9th Oct. 1981); and Sony Corp. of America, Inc., et al. v. Universal City Studios, Inc., et al., 464 U.S. 417, 104 S. Ct. 774 (1984).
60 Lardner, *Fast Forward*, p. 34.
61 Ibid., p. 36.
62 See Title 17 U.S.C. Section 106.
63 See 480 F. Supp. 429.
64 Lardner, *Fast Forward*, p. 204.
65 See US House, H.R. 4783, 97th Cong., 1 Sess., 20 October 1981; US House, H.R. 5705, 97th Cong., lst Sess., 3 March 1982; US Senate, S. 31, S. 32, S. 33, 98th Cong., 1st Sess, 26 January 1981.
66 US House, Committee on the Judiciary, Subcommittee on Courts, Civil Liberties, and the Administration of Justice, *Home Recording of Copyrighted Works, Part 1 and Part 2*, Hearings on H.R. 4783, H.R. 4794, H.R. 4808, H.R. 5250, H.R. 5488, and H.R. 5705, 97th Cong., 1st Sess and 2nd Sess, 12–14 April, 24 June, 11 August, 22–23 Sept. 1982. Hearings also

took place in the Senate: US Senate, Committee on the Judiciary, *Copyright Infringements (Audio and Video Recorders)*, Hearings on S. 1758, 30 November 1981, and 21 April 1982. Also see "Home Truths for Hollywood," *The Economist*, 30 July 1983.

67　Lardner, *Fast Forward*, p. 250–1.

68　Ibid., p. 253.

69　464 US 417, 104 S. Ct. 774.

70　Lardner, *Fast Forward*, pp. 274–5.

71　Mark R. Levy, "Program Playback Preferences," p. 335.

72　Mark R. Levy, "The Time-Shifting Use," pp. 267–8.

73　See Bruce A. Austin, "The Film Industry, Its Audience and New Communications Technologies," in Austin, ed., *Current Research in Film*, vol. II, Norwood, N.J.: Ablex Publications, 1985.

74　Nmungwun, *Video Recording Technology*, p. 161; statistics also cited by the International Federation of Phonogram and Videogram Producers, London, reported in *Variety*, 14 January 1987.

75　William A. Koch, "Eastman Video Tape and Future Imaging Technologies," *American Cinematographer*, March 1984, p. 83.

76　Study cited in Terry L. Childers and Dean M. Krugman, "The Competitive Environment of Pay-Per-View," *Journal of Broadcasting and Electronic Media* 31, no. 3, Summer 1987, pp. 335–42.

77　"Sales of VCRs are Slowing Down," *Register Guard*, 15 January 1989.

78　Lachenbruch, "Here, Buy Another," p. 126.

79　Terry Atkinson, "VCR Programming: Making Life Easier Using Bar Codes," *Los Angeles Times*, 17 July 1989, VI, p. 1.9.

80　Lardner, *Fast Forward*, p. 184.

81　Ibid., p. 174.

82　Blay's enterprise was so successful that in 1978 Fox bought Magnetic for $7.8 million. Ibid., pp. 172–3; George Rush, "Home Video Wars," *American Film*, April 1985, pp. 61–3.

83　Lardner, *Fast Forward*, p. 176.

84　Title 17 U.S.C. Section 109: Limitations on Exclusive Rights: Effect of Transfer of Particular Copy or Phonorecord, reads: "the owner of a particular copy or phonorecord lawfully made under this title, or any person authorized by the owner, is entitled, without the authority of the copyright owner, to sell or otherwise dispose of the possession of that copy or phonorecord."

85　Lardner, *Fast Forward*, p. 180.

86　Rush, "Home Video Wars."

87　Lardner, *Fast Forward*, pp. 188–9.

88　Ibid., p. 197.

89　Ibid., p. 201.

90　Ibid., p. 202.

91　See US House, Committee on the Judiciary, House Report 98–987, 31 August 1983; and US Senate, Committee on the Judiciary, Senate Report 98–162, 23 June 1983.

92 US Senate, Committee on the Judiciary, *Home Video Recording*, Hearing on Providing Information on the Issue of Home Video Recording, 99th Cong., 2d Sess., 23 September 1986. Also see Robyn Norwood, "VCR Anti-Copying Device Urged," *Los Angeles Times*, 24 September 1986.

93 "Rentrak Tests P-P-T Outside," *Variety*, 10 August 1988, p. 33.

94 The system known as Playcount was tested in Australia, but was partially owned by Capital Cities/ABC Video Enterprises. Al Stewart, "Depth Deals Get Shallow Start," *Billboard*, 13 August 1988, p. 89.

95 Jennifer Stern, "The Case of the Missing Movies," *Video Review*, October 1988, pp. 23, 26; "Pay-per-view Tapes Expected on Market," *Register-Guard*, 5 May 1991.

96 Wiese, *Home Video*, p. 23; Miriam Furman, "VCR Prices Decline," *Leisure Time Electronics*, January 1986, p. 46.

97 Wiese, *Home Video*, p. 25.

98 Tom Bierbaum, "Distrib Upheavals Cloud Industry," *Variety*, 20 July 1988, p. 71.

99 Wiese and others have relied on data from the Fairfield Group for these revenue estimates.

100 *Top Gun* cost around $17.5 million to produce, but brought in $270 million in ticket sales and another $50 million in video sales by 1988. See "Home Video Had a Spotty 1987," *Variety*, p. 96; Joe Handese, "Hollywood's Top Gun," *Marketing and Media Decisions*, March 1988, pp. 109–14.

101 "Home Video Had a Spotty 1987," *Variety*, p. 89.

102 Dennis Hunt, "Gods Must Be Crazy Tops the Foreign-Film Survey . . .," *Los Angeles Times*, 28 November 1986.

103 Mark Christiansen, Vice-President, Western Division Manager, MGM/UA Distribution Co., lecture at the University of Oregon, November 1990; Moret, "The New Nickelodeons," p. 86.

104 Jim McCullaugh, "A Title Business is A-1 for Sales," *Billboard*, 20 August 1988, p. 5.

105 As one industry executive explains, "A lot of those are great movies that many fans would love. But we have to do what's dictated by the economics of the market. It's a shame that people are waiting for certain movies that may never come out." See Dennis Hunt, "Looking for a Beloved Film? Good Luck," *Los Angeles Times*, 8 December 1989, p. F26.

106 *Video Marketing Newsletter*, 10 August 1986, p. 3.

107 Peter McAlevy, "Studio Commandos," *Newsweek*, 12 May 1986.

108 Ed Hulse, "Hollywood's Video Invasion," *Video Review*, February 1989, p. 84.

109 Peter Bart, "Stars to Studios: Pass the Bucks," *Variety*, 24 September 1990, p. 108.

110 Ibid., pp. 1, 108.

111 Ron Grover, *The Disney Touch*, Homewood, Ill.: Business One Irwin, 1991, p. 138.

112 See Tom Bierbaum, "RCA/Colpix Home Video Dumps Seven of its Distribs Overboard," *Variety*, 27 April 1988, p. 32.

113 David Waterman, "Pre-recorded Home Video and the Distribution of Theatrical Feature Films," in Eli Noam, ed., *Video Media Competition: Regulation, Economics and Technology*, New York: Colombia University Press, 1985, p. 228.

114 Tom Bierbaum, "Focus on Service Campaign Spotlighted at NAVD Meet," *Variety*, 10 May 1989.

115 An advance is money given to a rights holder by a rights purchaser in expectation of sales. Sometimes, it is refundable. Also, guarantees are sometimes used as bargaining chips in competitive bidding for a product. A guarantee is a one-shot, up-front payment from a distributor, manufacturer or retailer to a rights holder to secure various rights to a property. The amount is based on expectation of earnings, and is normally not refundable if earnings fall short of amount. Other terms relating to the home video industry are explained in "Glossary of Home Video Terms," *Variety*, 28 September 1983, pp. 42, 133.

116 "Near Record Fee for 'Prizzi' Rights," *Variety*, 19 June 1985.

117 "Home Video Had a Spotty 1987," p. 96.

118 Geraldine Fabrikant, "As Video Soars, Vestron Slips," *New York Times*, 23 May 1987, p. 33.

119 Waterman, "Pre-recorded Home Video", p. 228.

120 M. J. Alvarez, "Lessons in Vertical Integration in Film and Video," *Video Software Dealer*, December 1988, pp. 36–40, in Moret, "The New Nickelodeons," p. 86.

121 See Al Stewart, "Warner HV Joins Rental Price Increase," *Variety*, 25 April 1990.

122 Max Alexander, "Actors Wake Up to the Small Screen," *Variety*, May 1990, pp. 39–40.

123 Lardner, *Fast Forward*, p. 316.

124 "Home Video Had a Spotty 1987," p. 89.

125 Goldman Sachs investment report, cited in Grover, *The Disney Touch*, p. 137.

126 Marc Berman, "Rentals Reap Bulk of 1991 Vid Harvest," *Variety*, 6 January 1991, p. 22; B. Apar, "Vegas Vid Summit," *Video Business*, 26 January 1990, pp. 1, 12; Standard & Poor's Industry Surveys, p. L25. For figures from 1984–7, see "The Competition Looks On: Hollywood, The Nets and Cable Try to Gauge VCR's Impact," *Time*, 24 December 1984.

127 See the annual *International Television and Video Almanac* for lists of video distributors, producers, and other video companies.

128 Lawrence Cohn, "New Economy of Scale in Hollywood," *Variety*, 14 January 1987, p. 64.

129 See Fabrikant, "As Video Soars. . . ."

130 "Commtron Drops Half of Lines," *Variety*, 4 May 1988, p. 520.

131 "WHV Reassigns 2 Top Managers," *Variety*, 27 July 1988, p. 36.

132 Berman, "Rentals Reap Bulk."

133 Standard & Poor's Industry Surveys, p. L25.

134 Tom Bierbaum, "Nelson Ent. Deals with Orion," *Variety*, 10 August 1988, p. 35.

135 *Video Marketing Newsletter* 8, no. 1, 5 January 1986, p. 1.

136 Fabrikant, "As Video Soars . . .", p. 18.

137 "Home Video Had a Spotty 1987," p. 89; Lisa Gubernick, "Where's the Payoff?" *Forbes*, 25 July 1988, p. 69; Joshua Hammer, "The Crash of a Moviemaker," *Newsweek*, 4 September 1989, p. 46; Karry Hannon, "A Sad Story," *Forbes*, 14 May 1990, p. 10.

138 Max Alexander, "MHE Banks on Feature Plans," *Variety*, 1 October 1990.

139 Hulse, "Hollywood's Video Invasion," p. 29; "Action Intl. Mulls Studio Courtship," *Variety*, 1 October 1990.

140 James B. Meigs, "E.T. Comes Home," *Video Review*, September 1988, p. 32.

141 Ibid., p. 34.

142 "Batman Lacks Anti-Copying Device," *The Oregonian*, 28 November 1989; see also "The Macrovision Mess," *Video Review*, December 1986.

143 "Technicolor Buyout Accelerates Consolidation," *Video Business*, 30 September 1988, p. 6; "Estimated Market Share of Selected Video Duplicators," *Video Business*, 25 May 1990, p. 38.

144 Andy Wickstrom, "Video Duplicators see Plenty of Room to Grow," *Video Business*, 10 April 1992, p. 6; "To EP or not EP," *Video Business*, 22 January 1993, p. 38.

145 "Commtron Drops Half of Lines."

146 Berman, "Rentals Reap Bulk."

147 Bierbaum, "Focus on Service Campaign."

148 "BVHV . . ." *Variety*, 24 September 1990, p. 22.

149 Bierbaum, "Focus on Service Campaign."

150 Waterman, "Pre-recorded Home Video," p. 226.

151 J. Peters, "Racking up Business," *Video Business*, 7 July 1989, p. 18.

152 Tom Bierbaum, "Home Video Suppliers and Distribs Go Head to Head," *Variety*, 13 July 1988, p. 39.

153 Al Stewart, "Major Suppliers Have it All from A to B Video Titles," *Billboard*, 28 May 1988.

154 "Convention Capsules," *Billboard*, 20 August 1988.

155 "Dealers Ponder Downside of Vid Distrib Cutbacks," *Billboard*, 15 August 1988, pp. 1, 89.

156 See Moret, "The New Nickelodeons," p. 89.

157 See Bierbaum, "RCA/Colpix"; "Commtron Drops Half of Lines."

158 "Dealers Ponder," *Billboard*; also see Paul Sweeting and Ira Mayer, "Without a Studio Partner, A Hit is Hard to Find," *Channels/Field Guide 1988*, p. 127.

159 Moret, "The New Nickelodeons," p. 98. Several sources indicated a sharp decline in dealer purchases of B films during 1988. See Dennis Hunt, "Why B-Movies are Harder to Find at Your Video Store," *Los Angeles Times*, 17 March 1989.

160   Stewart, "Major Suppliers Have it All."
161   Wiese, *Home Video*, 267; Waterman, "Pre-recorded Home Video," p. 226.
162   "Home Video Track," *Variety*, 10 May 1989.
163   "Home Video Track," *Variety*, 20 July 1988.
164   See Moret, "The New Nickelodeons," pp. 87–9.
165   "VSDA Reports Sales Up 4.3 percent," *Variety*, 10 August 1988, p. 33.
166   Ira Mayer, "Good-bye, Easy Growth," *Channels/Field Guide 1989*, p. 106; Moret, "The New Nickelodeons," p. 56.
167   Moret, "The New Nickelodeons," p. 56; Berman, "Rentals Reap Bulk."
168   Moret, "The New Nickelodeons," p. 58.
169   "Disney's 'Limited Gold II' Targets Sales Record," *Variety*, 27 March 1985, p. 36. Gross margin is the difference between the price a retailer buys a product for and the price he sells it at; the margin before expenses. "Glossary of Home Video Terms."
170   Moret, "The New Nickelodeons," pp. 37–8. Modderno estimated that X-rated films accounted for 50–70 percent of revenues for the first video stores. See C. Modderno, "Videos' Success Means the End of Boob Tube," *USA Today*, p. 9A.
171   Wiese, *Home Video*, p. 247; Moret ("The New Nickelodeons," pp. 43–4) cites *Video Business* estimates of between 25,000 and 29,000 stores.
172   "52 percent of Vidstores Report Increased Rentals," *Variety*, 10 May 1989; *1993 Video Store Retailer Survey*, pp. 5–6.
173   "Study Reinforces Depth-of-Copy Gripes," *Variety*, 10 August 1988, p. 33; "52 percent of Vidstores Report," *Variety*; Furman, "VCR Prices"; *1993 Video Store Retailer Survey*, p. 10.
174   See Stern, "The Case of the Missing Movies."
175   Moret, "The New Nickelodeons," p. 39; also see Wiese, *Home Video*, p. 29.
176   Moret, "The New Nickelodeons," pp. 72–3.
177   B. Story, "The Video Store Top 100: Video Retailing Muscles Up," *Video Store*, December 1989, pp. 44–6; *1993 Video Store Retailer Survey*, pp. 14–16.
178   "52 percent of Vidstores Report," *Variety*.
179   Paul Dunwiddie, "Blockbuster Video Keeps 'em Reeling," *Register-Guard*, 19 December 1989.
180   See *Video Store Magazine's* annual retailer survey for more details.
181   See Ira Mayer and Paul Sweeting, "There's Many a Way to Get That $2.25 a Night," *Channels/Field Guide* 1988, p. 128.
182   See Furman, "VCR Prices."
183   Mayer and Sweeting, "There's Many a Way."
184   David Rowe, "Speaking Out," *Video Software Dealer*, May, 1988, p. 4, cited in Moret, "The New Nickelodeons," p. 40.
185   Story, "The Video Store Top 100"; "The Top 100: An Annual Ranking of the Largest Video Retail Chains," *Video Store Magazine*, December 1992.
186   Bruce Haring, "1988 Annual: New Vid Franchises Take Big Bucks," *Billboard*, 13 August, 1988, p. 58.

187 Standard & Poor's Industry Surueys, 'Leisure Time," 11 March 1993; p. L26; "Companies on the Move," *Variety*, 6 January 1992, p. 76.
188 Moret, "The New Nickelodeons," p. 67.
189 "Blockbuster Gains During Recession," *Register-Guard*, 21 January 1992.
190 Dunwiddie, "Blockbuster Video Keeps 'em Reeling."
191 R. Gunnerson, "U.S. Home Video Report," *Billboard*, 5 January 1991, pp. V15, V21–2; "The Top 100," p. 15.
192 Moret, "The New Nickelodeons," p. 69.
193 Nancy Rivera Brooks, "Fast-Forward Market," *Los Angeles Times*, 30 June 1986.
194 Moret, "The New Nickelodeons," p. 75.
195 Lardner, *Fast Forward*, p. 313.
196 Wiese, *Home Video*, p. 261.
197 Moret, "The New Nickelodeons," pp. 75, 77.
198 Mayer and Sweeting, "There's Many a Way"; Moret, "The New Nickelodeons," pp. 75–6.
199 Tom Bierbaum, " 'Focus on Service' Campaign," *Variety*, 10 May 1989; Moret, "The New Nickelodeons," p. 94.
200 Moret, "The New Nickelodeons," p. 95; also see R. Lee Sullivan, "A Feature Role for Video Sell-Through," *Discount Merchandiser*, November 1990, pp. 52, 64–7.
201 Mike Duff, "Video II: The Rebirth," *Supermarket Business*, November 1990, pp. 45–8, 55.
202 Moret, "The New Nickelodeons," p. 75.
203 National Association of Record Merchandisers survey, 1985, in Wiese, *Home Video*, p. 248.
204 Cited in Wiese, *Home Video*, p. 249.
205 Mayer and Sweeting, "There's Many a Way."
206 *Standard & Poor's Industry Surveys*, p. L26.
207 Wiese, *Home Video*, p. 265; Moret, "The New Nickelodeons," pp. 45, 52, 55.
208 M. Hendrickson, "Competition Pressures," *Video Business*, 19 May 1989, p. 40, cited in Moret, "The New Nickelodeons," p. 40; "Survey Says: B Films Lag," *Video Business*, November 1987, p. 55, cited in Moret, p. 52.
209 See *1991 International Television and Video Almanac*, p. 605.
210 "Erol's Plans Promo," *Variety*, 27 April 1988, p. 32; "Commtron Drops Half of Lines."
211 *1991 International Television and Video Almanac*, p. 604.
212 Dennis Hunt "Videolog: Adult Films Go After a Different Market," *Los Angeles Times*, 18 October 1985, Calendar section, p. 17.
213 Hunt, "Why, B-Movies are Harder to Find"; Moret, "The New Nickelodeons," p. 54; see Wiese, *Home Video*, p. 266.
214 Berman, "Rentals Reap Bulk."
215 *1991 International Motion Picture Almanac*, p. 605.
216 Wiese, *Home Video*, p. 25.
217 Ibid., p. 267.

218 Mayer, "Good-bye, Easy Growth," p. 106.
219 Lardner, *Fast Forward*, p. 323.
220 "Home Truths for Hollywood."
221 Peter M. Nichols, "Home Video," *New York Times*, 16 May 1991, p. C22.
222 See Ronald Bettig, "The Impact of New Communications Technology on Filmed-Entertainment Copyrights," unpublished Ph.D. dissertation, University of Illinois, 1989.
223 *1991 International Television and Video Almanac*, p. 604.
224 See Baharuddin Aziz, "ASEAN Copyright Law: U.S. Intellectual Property Interests in the Information Age – Political Economic Analysis," unpublished Ph.D. dissertation, University of Oregon, August 1990.
225 Waterman, "Pre-recorded Home Video," p. 8.
226 See "Orion Chief Predicts Tape 'Ice Age'," *Billboard*, 23 April 1988; Lardner, op. cit., pp. 313–15.
227 See Austin, "The Film Industry."
228 "Do Videocassette Rentals Pose Threat to Film Industry?," *New York Times*, 24 November 1985.
229 T. Thompson, "The Twilight of the Drive-In," *American Film*, July/August 1983, pp. 44–9. For an irreverant and controversial look at what remains of drive-in culture, see Joe Bob Briggs, *Joe Bob Goes to the Drive-In*, New York: Delacorte Press, 1987.
230 Deirdre Fanning, "The Best of the Show is Over," *Forbes*, 19 October 1988, pp. 101–5.
231 *1991 International Motion Picture Almanac*, p. 604.
232 Richard Mahler, "VCRs vs. TV Stations," *Electronic Media*, 17 August 1987, p. 30.
233 Cited in Terry L. Childers and Dean M. Krugman, "The Competitive Environment of Pay-Per-View," *Journal of Broadcasting and Electronic Media* 31, no. 3, Summer 1987, p. 336.
234 Video release of a film also has been timed with Academy Award promotions, and there are many examples of boosted video revenues from Oscar-winning or nominated films in video release. See Nancy Spiller and Dennis Hunt, "Does Oscar Mean More in Video Dollars?," *Los Angeles Times*, 26 March 1989; Al Stewart, "Oscar Gives Homevids a New Lease on Life," *Variety*, 21 March 1990.
235 Jack Mathews, "Summer Hits: The Seeds of Video's Spring," *Los Angeles Times Magazine*, 28 May 1989, pp. 31–2.
236 I. Slifkin, "King's Sematary Inspires More Hollywood Plots," *Video Business*, 6 October 1989, in Moret, "The New Nickelodeons," p. 110; Hulse, "Hollywood's Video Invasion," p. 28.
237 Jack Mathews, "Summer Hits: The Seeds of Video's Spring," *Los Angeles Times Magazine*, 28 May 1989, pp. 31–2.
238 Hulse, "Hollywood's Video Invasion," p. 85.
239 Vincent Canby, "VCRs are Calling the Shots in the Movie Business," *Register-Guard*, 5 January 1990, p. 10D.

240 Anton Wilson, *Cinema Workshop*, ASC Holding Corp., 1983, pp. 82–3.
241 Wilson, *Cinema Workshop*, pp. 64, 83.
242 Ibid., p. 253.
243 Nick Burns, "Big Screen to Small: Film Style and Television," unpublished manuscript, University of Oregon, December 1991.
244 Hulse, "Hollywood's Video Invasion," p. 84.
245 Frank Spotnitz, "What's Next?" *American Film*, January/February 1989, p. 32.
246 Meigs, "E.T. Comes Home."
247 "Sales of VCRs are Slowing Down," *Washington Post*, 15 January 1989.
248 Frank Beerman, "Madison Square Garden to Start HV Label," *Variety*, 13 July 1988, p. 39.
249 G. Ptacek, "Making it into the Minors," *Video Business*, 3 November 1989, pp. 26–7, cited in Moret, "The New Nickelodeons," p. 98.

Chapter 7 The Silver Screen: Theatrical Exhibition in the Information Age

1 Aljean Harmetz, "Hollywood's Video Gamble," *New York Times Magazine*, 28 March 1982, p. 42.
2 Ibid.
3 Michael Schwartz, "Turning Movie Houses into Video Houses," *Channels*, April/May 1982.
4 Will Tusher, "Forget the Obit, Theaters Won't Die," *Variety*, 1 January 1986.
5 "Gen Cinema Says VCRs are a Help to Exhibition Biz," *Variety*, 14 January 1987, p. 7.
6 Tusher, "Forget the Obit."
7 Lloyd Paseman, "Movie Theaters Flourish in Video Era," *Register-Guard*, 21 July 1987.
8 Alexander Auerbach, "Big Screen + Little Screen = Big Money," *Boxoffice*, May 1984.
9 Ruth Ryon, "Theater Firms Think Big to Bring Back 'Lost' Movie Patrons," *Los Angeles Times*, 29 June 1986.
10 The *1993 International Motion Picture Almanac* (New York: Quigley Publishing, 1993, p. 23A) reported that there were 24,570 screens at the end of 1991, an increase of 3.7 percent from 1990. While there was a slump in the number of drive-in screens (908), the number of indoor screens was on the rise again. Also see Thomas H. Guback, "The Evolution of the Motion Picture Theater Business in the 1980s," *Journal of Communications*, Spring 1987, pp. 60–77.
11 Cameron Stauth, "The Cineplex Complex," *American Film*, December 1990, pp. 16–17.

12 See Kathryn Harris, "Squeezing the Customers," *Forbes*, 23 July 1990, pp. 39–40.

13 Bill Barol, "The Last Picture Shows," *Newsweek*, 8 June 1987.

14 Karen Stabiner, "The Shape of Theaters to Come," *American Film*, September 1982.

15 Dan Cray, "Movies Begin Moving Toward Upfront Deals," *Mediaweek*, 3 June 1991.

16 Harmetz, "Hollywood's Video Gamble," p. 43.

17 For more on splitting agreements, see Guback, "The Evolution of the Motion Picture Theater Business"; Dan Morain, "Probe Continues into Movie Theater 'Split' Agreements," *Los Angeles Times*, 27 June 1986.

18 A. D. Murphy, "Cinemas to Survive Hi-Tech Era," *Variety*, 4 August 1982.

19 In 1990, there were 31 US circuits with 100 screens or more. *1991 International Motion Picture Almanac*, p. 23A.

20 Will Tusher, "Distribution's Theater Boys Near Peak," *Variety*, 7 January 1987.

21 Harris, "Squeezing the Customers."

22 Richard Trainor, "Major Powers," *Sight and Sound*, Winter 1987/88, pp. 26–30.

23 Gerald F. Phillips, "The Recent Acquisition of Theater Circuits by Major Distributors," *The Entertainment and Sports Lawyer*, Winter 1987, pp. 1–23; "The Return of Hollywood: Fun and Profit," *The Economist*, 29 October 1988, pp. 21–4.

24 Harris, "Squeezing the Customers"; Trainor, "Major Powers."

25 Lawrence Cohn, "New Economy of Scale in Hollywood," *Variety*, 14 January 1987, p. 44.

26 Trainor, "Major Powers."

27 Mark Ivey, "The Show-Biz Giant that has Hollywood Spooked," *Business Week*, 28 November 1988, pp. 174–8.

28 See Diane Mermigas, "Viacom Sale Stuns Firm's Top Brass," *Electronic Media*, 9 March 1988, p. 3.

29 "The Return of Hollywood," *The Economist*.

30 Trainor, "Major Powers."

31 See Doris Tovmarkine, "MovieFone, Pacer/CATS Tie Knot," *The Hollywood Reporter*, 23 February 1992.

32 Ryon, "Theater Firms Think Big."

33 Michael Nielsen, "Labor's Stake in the Electronic Cinema Revolution," *Jump Cut*, no. 35, p. 82.

34 See Chris Willman, " 'Dick Tracy' Brings in Arresting New Cinema Sound System," *Los Angeles Times*, 30 May 1990, p. F2.

35 Charles Champlin, "The Home Audience is Listening," *Los Angeles Times*, 30 May 1990, p. F1.

36 Allan Stegeman, "The Large-Screen Film: A Viable Entertainment Alternative to High Definition Television," *Journal of Film and Video*, Spring 1984; Jim Stokes, "IMAX and OMNIMAX: The Biggest Screens," *Back Stage*, 5 July 1984; Francis Boyes, "Voyage of Discovery: Imax Systems

Corp. Takes Space Fans to the Movies," *Canadian Business*, October 1984; Stabiner, "The Shape of Theaters to Come."

37 George Englund produced a short fictional film in 1981, featuring his wife, Cloris Leachman, and Imax technology. By the end of 1991, a later Imax film, *The Dream is Alive*, had grossed $70 million worldwide since its opening in 1985. "Top 100 All-Time Film Rental Champs," *Variety*, 6 January 1992, p. 86.

38 Bill Krohn and Harley W. Lond, "Showscan: A New Type of Exhibition for a Revolutionary Film Process," *Boxoffice*, February 1984.

39 Pat Dowell and Ray Heinrich, "Bigger than Life," *American Film*, May 1984.

40 Stabiner, "The Shape of Theaters to Come," p. 53.

41 Frank Spotnitz, "What Next?," *American Film*, January/February 1989, p. 35.

42 Gregory Solman, "Through the Looking Glass," *American Film*, September 1990, p. 50.

43 Spotnitz, "What Next?," p. 35.

44 Steve Ditlea, "Data Suit: Artificial Intelligence," *Omni*, September 1988, p. 22.

45 Spotnitz, "What Next?," p. 35.

46 Simon Perry, "Film Trade Ponders Video Projection," *Variety*, 9 January 1989.

47 Jack Valenti, "Managing Changes in Technology," *Variety*, 14 January 1987, p. 8. See also Schwartz, "Turning Movie Houses into Video Houses."

48 See Stegeman, "The Large-Screen Film."

49 Edmund Andrews, "Foes Hook Up for HDTV," *Register-Guard*, 25 May 1993, p. 1A.

50 A group of cable operators announced the formation of Cable Television Laboratories, Inc. as a research and development consortium which would offer HDTV programming. See Peter Newcomb, "Cutting Edge," *Forbes*, 29 April 1991.

51 For instance, HDTV sets for the home retailed for around $35,000 in 1991. See Newcomb, "Cutting Edge"; Stephen Kindel, "Pictures at an Exhibition," *Forbes*, 1 August 1983.

52 Krista Van Lewen, "Will Consumers Buy HDTV?," *Satellite Communications*, January 1989, pp. 23–4.

53 Nielsen, "Labor's Stake," p. 84.

Chapter 8 Hollywood Meets Madison Ave.: The Commercialization of US Films

1 M. B. Haralovich, "Film Advertising, the Film Industry, and the Pin-up: The Industry's Accommodations to Social Forces in the 1940s," in Bruce A. Austin, ed., *Current Research in Film: Audiences, Economics, and Law*,

Vol. 1, Norwood, NJ: Ablex Publishing, 1985; Janet Staiger, "Announcing Wares, Winning Patrons, Voicing Ideals: Thinking about the History and Theory of Film Advertising," *Cinema Journal* 29, no. 3, Spring 1990; Jane Gaines and Charlotte Herzog, eds, *Fabrications: Costume and the Female Body*, New York American Film Institute Readers/Routledge, 1990.

2 See Thomas H. Guback, "Hollywood's International Market," in Tino Balio, *The American Film Industry*, Madison, Wisc.: University of Wisconsin Press, 1976.

3 Staiger, "Announcing Wares."

4 S. Spillman, "Marketers Race to Leave Their Brand on Films," *Advertising Age*, 1 July 1985.

5 D. Kalish, "Now Showing: Products!" *Marketing and Media*, 23 August 1988.

6 Spillman, "Marketers Race"; N. A. Lang, "You Oughta Be in Pictures," *Beverage World*, April 1990.

7 Lang, "You Oughta Be in Pictures"; Lois P. Sheinfeld, "Dangerous Liaisons," *Film Comment*, September/October 1989, p. 70.

8 D. Hajdu, "Commercials on Cassette," *Video Review*, December 1988.

9 Lang, "You Oughta Be in Pictures"; Michael Fleming, "Product Pluggola Padding Pic Producers' Budgets," *Variety*, 9 May 1990.

10 Sheinfeld, "Dangerous Liaisons," p. 71.

11 Hajdu, "Commercials on Cassette."

12 Ibid.

13 Kalish, "Now Showing: Products!"

14 Lang, "You Oughta Be in Pictures."

15 "The Ad Line is Increasingly Becoming the Thing for Costly Features," *Variety*, 4 April 1990.

16 Marcy Magiera, "Coming Attractions: Movie Tie-Ins Galore," *Advertising Age*, 28 May 1990.

17 Michael Fleming, "Turtles, Toons and Toys 'R' In," *Variety*, 18 April 1990.

18 Ibid.

19 Kalish, "Now Showing: Products!"

20 Sheinfeld, "Dangerous Liaisons," p. 71.

21 Spillman, "Marketers Race."

22 L. Loro and Marcy Magiera, "Philly Products Angle for Ringside in 'Rocky V'," *Advertising Age*, 5 February 1990.

23 Spillman, "Marketers Race."

24 "The Ad Line is Increasingly Becoming the Thing," *Variety*.

25 Hajdu, "Commercials on Cassette."

26 Ibid.

27 Sheinfeld, "Dangerous Liaisons," pp. 70–2.

28 Fleming, "Turtles, Toons and Toys."

29 Jon Silbert, "When Screens Become Billboards," *American Film*, May 1989.

30 "Simpsons' Suit Cites Oregonians," *Register-Guard*, 14 June 1990.

31 S. W. Colford, "Tobacco Critic Opens New Front," *Advertising Age*, 27 March 1989; A. Lallande, "The Capital Cutting Room, *Marketing and Media Decisions*, 23 August 1989.

32 "CSPI Calls for Movie Subtitles Identifying Paid Products," *Broadcasting*, 3 April 1989.

33 R. Rothenberg, "Movies Become Another Vehicle for Advertisers," *Register-Guard*, 23 June 1991.

34 Lang, "You Oughta Be in Pictures."

35 Lallande, "The Capital Cutting Room."

36 Marcy Magiera, "Madison Avenue Hits Hollywood," *Advertising Age*, 10 December 1990.

37 Marcy Magiera, "Disney Move May Slow Theater Ads," *Advertising Age*, 12 February 1990; "Theaters Go Commercial," *Register-Guard*, 25 January 1987.

38 Marcy Magiera, "Studio Ad Bans Aid In-Theater Media," *Advertising Age*, 6 October 1990.

39 "Selling Goes to the Movies," *Sales and Marketing Management*, February 1990; "Theaters Go Commercial," *Register-Guard*.

40 Magiera, "Studio Ad Bans."

41 S. Hume and Marcy Magiera, "What Do Moviegoers Think of Ads?," *Advertising Age*, 23 April 1990.

42 Ibid.

43 Ibid.

44 Marcy Magiera, "A Real Movie Treat," *Advertising Age*, 10 December 1990.

45 Janet Stilson, "Programmers Struggle for Fewer New Dollars," *Electronic Media*, 17 August 1987, p. 32; "Vid Blurbs Shoot to Match Success of 'Top Gun' Ad," *Variety*, 13 July 1988, pp. 39–40.

46 Hajdu, "Commercials on Cassette."

47 Ibid.

48 M. Walley, "Nielsen Ratings: Video's Savior?," *Advertising Age*, 22 August 1988.

49 Ibid.

50 Marcy Magiera, "Pizza Hut Ties In with Turtles Video," *Advertising Age*, 30 July 1990.

51 J. Peters, "Studios Split on Videos as Premiums," *Variety*, 13 June 1990.

52 K. Fitzgerald and J. Leisse-Erickson, "'Willow' Stirs Promo Frenzy," *Advertising Age*, 16 May 1988.

53 Pamela Ellis-Simons, "Screen Gems?," *Marketing and Media Decisions*, 23 November 1988.

54 Ronald Grover, "Hitching a Ride on Hollywood's Hot Streak," *Business Week*, 11 July 1988.

55 Ellis-Simons, "Screen Gems?."

56 B. Hulin-Salkin, "Movie Tie-ins," *Incentive*, June 1989.

57 Ellis-Simons, "Screen Gems?."

58 Marcy Magiera, "Hollywood Cools Off Summer Film Tie-ins," *Advertising Age*, 15 April 1991.

59   I. Mayer, "Good-bye, Easy Growth," *Channels/Field Guide 1989*.

60   Magiera, "Hollywood Cools Off."

61   Marcy Magiera, "Videos Aim $85M at Kids," *Advertising Age*, 17 June 1991, p. 16.

62   Lester J. Borden, "Merchandising and Distribution Techniques of Programmes," paper presented at New Dimensions in Television meeting Venice, Italy, March 1981.

63   G. Cebrzynski, " 'I Didn't See the Movie, But I Drank the Wine'," *Marketing News*, 16 April 1990, p. 4.

64   Jay L. Johnson, "Licensing: A $66.5 Billion Industry," *Discount Merchandiser*, June 1991, pp. 36–41, 76–8.

65   For example, the National Basketball Association reported receiving over $1 billion from licensing activities in 1991, while just one player – Michael Jordan – was to receive $21.2 million from his product endorsements during 1992. "Morning Briefings," *Register-Guard*, 30 January 1992. See also Janet Wasko and Mark Phillips, "Teal's the Deal in Sports Merchandising," *Oregon Sports News*, Spring 1993, pp. 48–51.

66   Pete Williams, "Recession Hits Foundation of House of Cards," *USA Today Baseball Weekly*, 2 January 1992, p. 24.

67   Ellis-Simons, "Screen Gems'?."

68   Fleming, "Product Pluggola."

69   Jay Blickstein, "Trek Merchandise Sales Beaming Up," *Variety*, 2 December 1991, p. 54.

70   "Nightmare Called Freddy Becomes Toymaker Dream," *Register-Guard*, 7 September 1989.

71   David Fox, " 'Jurassic' Stomps Record," *Los Angeles Times*, 15 June 1993.

72   See Richard Schickel, *The Disney Version*, New York: Avon Books, 1968.

73   Charles Solomon, *Enchanted Drawings*, New York: Alfred A. Knopf, 1989.

74   Ibid.

75   Larry Carlat, "Bombs Away," *Variety*, 30 May 1990.

76   See " 'Dick Tracy' Seen as Risky Business," *Variety*, 30 May 1990.

77   Larry Carlat, "How It Really Works," *Variety*, 30 May 1990; The Walt Disney Company, Form 10K, 1990.

78   Ellis-Simons, "Screen Gems?."

79   Johnson, "Licensing."

80   See Fleming, "Product Pluggola."

81   Borden, "Merchandisng and Distribution Techniques."

82   Garth Alexander, "No Toys in Tokyo Puts 'Turtles' in the Soup," *Variety*, 15 April 1991.

83   Grover, "Hitching a Ride."

84   Fleming, "Product Pluggola."

85   See James P. Forkan, "Licensees Hope for Movie Magic," *Advertising Age*, 22 February, 1988.

86   " 'Dick Tracy'," *Variety*.

87   Ibid.

88   Kathleen Day, "Being Famous Pays in Licensing Game," *Los Angeles Times*, 6 October 1985.

89   Ellis-Simons, "Screen Gems?."

90   Carlat, "How It Really Works."

91   Borden, "Merchandising and Distribution Techniques."

92   Grover, "Hitching a Ride."

93   Carlat, "Bombs Away."

94   "Will the Summer Stifle 'Simpsons' Sizzle?" *Variety*, 30 May 1990.

95   Ellis-Simons, "Screen Gems?."

96   See "'Simpsons' Suit Cites Oregonians," *Register-Guard*, 14 June 1991; and the following discussion of Disney.

97   Along with the growth of video game popularity has been a growing concern over the number of hours spent by young game players, as well as the violent and militaristic content that characterizes many of the games. For more discussion, see Terri Toles, "Video Games and American Military Ideology," in Vincent Mosco and Janet Wasko, eds., *Critical Communications Review, Volume 3: Popular Culture and Media Events*, Norwood, N.J.: Ablex Publications, 1985; Marsha Kinder, *Playing with Power in Movies, Television and Video Games*, Berkeley, Calif.: University of California Press, 1991; Patricia Marks Greenfield, *Mind and Media: The Effects of Television, Video Games and Computers*. Cambridge, Mass: Harvard University Press, 1984; Geoffrey R. Loftus, *Mind at Play: The Psychology of Video Games*. New York: Basic Books, 1983.

98   Philip Elmer-Dewitt, "The Amazing Video Game Boom," *Time*, 27 September 1993, p. 68. Also see Standard & Poor's Industry Surveys, "Leisure Time," pp. L51–3, for more recent data on the video game industry.

99   See Geoffrey Deitz, "Studios Play Along with Video Games," *Variety*, 18 November 1991, for more details on deals involving video game versions of feature films.

100 The Walt Disney Company, Form 10K, 1990.

101 Greg Evans, "Marketing 'Dick Tracy': A Breathless Success," *Variety*, 15 August 1990.

102 Hulin-Salkin, "Movie Tie-ins."

103 The Walt Disney Company, Form 10K, 1990.

104 Stephew Koepp, "Do You Believe in Magic?" *Time*, 25 April 1988.

105 Another estimate was that Disney's share of the licensed goods market in the USA was over $2 billion at retail in 1990. Johnson, "Licensing."

106 The Walt Disney Company, Form 10K, 1990.

107 Ronald Grover, *The Disney Touch*, Homewood, Illinois: Business One, 1991.

108 The Walt Disney Company, Form 10K, 1990.

109 Grover, *The Disney Touch*.

110 The Walt Disney Company, Form 10K, 1990.

111 Penny Gill, "The Disney Stores Blend Retailing and Entertainment," *Stores*, June 1991, pp. 20–4.

112 The Walt Disney Company, Form 10K, 1990.

113 See Grover, *The Disney Touch*.

114 Borden, "Merchandising and Distribution Techniques," p. 5.

115 Carlat, "How It Really Works."
116 "The Ad Line is Increasingly Becoming the Thing," *Variety*.
117 See Day, "Being Famous Pays."
118 Cyndee Miller, "Disney Plans Global Expansion of its Stores," *Marketing News*, 13 May 1991, pp. 1, 22.
119 Sheinfield, "Dangerous Liaisons," p. 72.
120 C. Bernstein "The Leisure Empire," *Time*, 24 December 1990.
121 Fleming, "Turtles, Toons and Toys."
122 Thorstein Veblen, "The Theory of the Leisure Class: An Economic Study of Institutions," (1899) published in Max Lerner, ed., *The Portable Veblen*, New York: The Viking Press, 1948.
123 R. K. L. Collins, "Sneakers that Kill: Kids and Conspicuous Consumption," *Media and Values*, Fall/Winter 1990.
124 Eileen Meehan, "Conceptualizing Culture as Commodity: The Problem of Television," *Critical Studies in Mass Communication* 3, 1986, pp. 448–57.

Chapter 9 Around the World in Nanoseconds: International Markets for Filmed Entertainment

1 David Hancock and André Lange, *IDATE Industrial Analyses*, Vol. 1: *The World Film and Television Market*, Institut de L'audiovisuel et des Télécommunications en Europe, Montpellier, France, October 1992, p. 103. Hancock and Lange, like many others, bemoan the lack of accurate statistics for world audiovisual markets, especially from the American majors. The IDATE data utilizes information from investment banks, such as Goldman Sachs, as well as from the MPAA and the AFMA. However, the MPAA still does not issue statistics on video and television markets, and as *Variety* noted recently, "guards the all-media feature revenue grand total with impressive efficiency." *Variety*'s estimate for "all-media feature revenue" – "feature film revenues from video, pay TV, free TV, cable TV and other post-theatrical markets" was $14–15 billion for 1992. See A. D. Murphy, "Int'l Rentals for '92 Total $1.44 Billion," *Daily Variety*, 16 June 1993.
2 *The 1991 International Motion Picture Almanac* (New York: Quigley Publishing, 1991, p. 19A) reports that US distributors operate in more than 80 markets around the world; however, the top 15 represent 75 percent of their business.
3 For a more complete discussion of these activities, see André Lange and Anthony Renaud, "The Future of the European Audiovisual Industry," The European Institute for the Media, Media Monograph No. 10, Manchester, England, pp. 24–6.
4 Thomas Joseph Cryan, David W. Johnson, James S. Crane, and Anthony Cammarata, "Strategies for the International Production and Distribution

of Feature Films in the 1990s," *Loyola Entertainment Law Journal* 8, 1988, p. 6.

5 MPAA Document, "Worldwide Estimates of Population, Television Households/Sets, and VCRs, 1989."

6 Jeremy Coopman, "Report: Grim '90s for Euro TV Biz," *Variety*, 9 May 1990.

7 "B'casters, Production Honchos Promote Eurowide Program Market at Confab," *Variety*, 4 October, 1989.

8 Frank Segers, "As DBS Services Surge, H'wood Girds for Birds," *Variety*, 11 July 1990; MPAA, "Worldwide Estimates."

9 "ITA Sees Vid Boom Behind Euro Unity," *Variety*, 21 March 1990.

10 Hancock and Lange, IDATE, pp. 135–7; also see Don Groves, "That's Entertainment? Path to Unified Europe in 1992 is Rocky, says British Study," *Variety*, 13 December 1989; Howard G. Chua-Eoan, "Movie Muscle," *Time*, 28 May 1990.

11 Hancock and Lange, IDATE, p. 137; also see Bruce Alderman, "Yank Majors Cleaning Up at French Wickets . . . ," *Variety*, 21 March 1990.

12 Henry Sutton, "The $64,000 Question in Cannes," *The European*, 11 May, 1990.

13 Tapio Varis, "International Flow of Television Programmes," Reports and Papers on Mass Communication, No. 100, Unesco, Paris.

14 Preben Sepstrup, "Transnationalization of Television in Western Europe," in Christian W. Thomsen, ed., *Cultural Transfer or Electronic Imperialism?* Heidelberg: Carl Winter Universitätsverlag, 1989, pp. 110–11; Anthony Pragnell, "Television in Europe: Quality and Values in a Time of Change," Manchester, England: The European Institute for the Media, Media Monograph No. 5.

15 "We may not be able to export our automobiles, but we are exporting our culture in the form of movies," notes an MCA executive in Chua-Eoan, "Movie Muscle," p. 42.

16 Hancock and Lange, IDATE, p. 103; also see John Micklethwait, "A Survey of the Entertainment Industry," *The Economist*, 23 December 1989, p. 4; George Lucas, "World Market is Last Crusade," *Wall Street Journal*, 13 July 1989; A. D. Murphy, "Globe Gobbling Up US Pix in Record Doses," *Variety*, 13 June 1990.

17 Murphy, "Globe Gobbling."

18 Geraldine Fabrikant, "When World Raves, Studios Jump," *New York Times*, 7 March 1990.

19 Hancock and Lange, IDATE, p. 107; also see "Movie Moguls Watch How They Play in Pisa," *Register-Guard*, 25 June 1990.

20 Richard Gold, "Take Heart, Orion Pix Tells Shareholders," *Variety*, 4 July 1990.

21 Chua-Eoan, "Movie Muscle," p. 42.

22 "American TV Loses its Visa," *Channels/Field Guide 1990*, pp. 46–7.

23 Hancock and Lange, IDATE, p. 107.

24 Ibid., p. 113.

25 Gladys D. and Oswald H. Ganley, *Global Political Fallout: The VCR's First Decade, 1976–1985*, Norwood, N.J.: Ablex Publishing, 1987, p. 1.
26 Paul Harris, "Quotas are Inevitable, Maxwell Warns Solons: US Urged to Make Concessions, Not War," *Variety*, 25 October 1989.
27 "AFMA Sales by Country and Media," *Variety*, 22 February 1990.
28 Murphy, "Globe Gobbling"; Chua-Eoan, "Movie Muscle."
29 "ITA Sees Vid Boom," *Variety*.
30 See Segers, "As DBS Services Surge."
31 Don Groves, "Who Will Rule Britannia's Skies?" *Variety*, 21 March 1990.
32 Don Groves, "MPEA Prez Karlin Slams French, Spanish Trade Restrictions," *Variety*, 20 June 1990.
33 Jeremy Coopman, "CIT Sez Satellite's Days are Numbered . . .," *Variety*, 20 June 1990.
34 Jeremy Coopman, "Euro Entertainment Revenues to Double in Next Decade, Sez Analyst," *Variety*, 7 March 1990.
35 Aljean Harmetz, "Hollywood Starts an Invasion of Europe's Booming Market," *New York Times*, 11 January 1990.
36 For the history of the US film industry's global activities see Thomas H. Guback, *The International Film Industry: Western Europe and America since 1945*, Bloomington, Indiana: Indiana University Press, 1969; Manjunath Pendakur, *Canadian Dreams and American Control: The Political Economy of the Canadian Film Industry*, Detroit, Michigan: Wayne State University Press, 1990; and Kristin Thompson, *Exporting Entertainment: America in the World Film Market, 1907–34*, London: BFI Pub., 1985. More recent analysis of international film markets is presented by Thomas H. Guback in "Non Market Factors in the International Distribution of American Films," in Bruce A. Austin, ed., *Current Research in Film*, Vol. 1, Norwood, N.J.: Ablex Publishing, 1985; "Government Financial Support to the Film Industry in the U.S.," in Bruce A. Austin, ed., *Current Research in Film*, Vol. 3, Norwood, N.J.: Ablex Publishing, 1987; and "Capital, Labor Power and the Identity of Film," in Bruce A. Austin, ed., *Current Research in Film*, Vol. 5, Norwood, N.J.: Ablex Publishing, 1989.
37 "Fighting for Hollywood's Fair Share," *Channels*, November 1989, p. 98.
38 Ernest Gill, "Old Worldsters Unite to Fight Yanks," *Variety*, 8 June 1988.
39 Alderman, "Yank Majors Cleaning Up."
40 Sutton, "The $64,000 Question in Cannes"; for a discussion of the disadvantages for nations that rely on imported films, see Thomas H. Guback, "Should a Nation Have its Own Film Industry?," *Directions* 3, no. 1, 1989, Program on Communication and Development Studies, Northwestern University.
41 Groves, "That's Entertainment?."
42 Pragnell has observed other advantages of the US market: "The existence of a television-oriented single-language audience of more than 200 million people, with competitive and well-funded networks serving a largely homogeneous advertising market and the 24-hour broadcasting day." "Television in Europe," p. 13.

43 See Lange and Renaud, "The Future of the European Audiovisual Industry," pp. 297–9.
44 "Canada's Market Position Come '92 Debated at Toronto Trade Forum," *Variety*, 20 September 1989.
45 There are numerous references to recent difficulties of independent companies. See, for instance, Thomas Garvin, "Independents' Day," *Screen International*, 12 May 1990.
46 Lucas, "World Market is Last Crusade."
47 Merrill Brown, "Hollywood Wins Again," *Channels*, September 1988, p. 34.
48 Council of Europe, "European Convention on Transfrontier Television," European Treaty Series No. 132, 1989. For background on the directive and other European regulatory activities, see Lange and Renaud, "The Future of the European Audiovisual Industry," pp. 65–77; also, Robert Villeneuve, "Europe in the Audiovisual Age," in Thomsen, *Cultural Transfer or Electronic Imperialism?*
49 Chua-Eoan, "Movie Muscle."
50 Groves, "That's Entertainment?"; "Boxoffice Rise Inspires Hope among Italo Industryites," *Variety*, 20 June 1990.
51 Chua-Eoan, "Movie Muscle."
52 Gill, "Old Worldsters Unite to Fight Yanks."
53 "Labor Party in Britain Pushing for Filming Boost," *Variety*, 6 June 1990. Also see Jean-Noël Dibie, *Aid for Cinematographic and Audio-Visual Production in Europe*, London: John Libbey, 1993, a study commissioned by the Council of Europe reviewing subsidy plans for European and non-European countries.
54 Don Groves, "Invasion of the Talent Snatchers," *Variety*, 4 April 1990, p. 13.
55 Farah Nayeri, "Film vs. Homevideo: It's a Gallic War," *Variety*, 21 March 1990.
56 Groves, "MPEA Prez Karlin."
57 Micklethwait, "A Survey of the Entertainment Industry," p. 17, *New York Times*, 24 October 1989.
58 Groves, "MPEA Prez Karlin."
59 See Simon Morgan, "European Television: Broadcasting in the 1990s," *International Media Law*, November 1989, p. 90; Thomas H. Guback, "What the Quota Means," *Television Quarterly* 24:3, 1990, p. B1.
60 Bruce Alderman, "EC's Bangemann: Nations Unlikely to Bolster Quotas by Making Them National Law," *Variety*, 8 November 1989.
61 "MPEA to Change Guard Overseas," *Variety*, 23 May 1990; "The International Movie Marketplace: Mother Lode, or Just Fool's Gold?," *Variety*, 22 February 1989.
62 "Fighting for Hollywood's Fair Share," *Channels*.
63 "House Resolution Blasts EC TV Quotas," *Daily Variety*, 24 October 1989; also see "Aggressive US Stance on Quotas May Have Hurt More than Helped," *Variety*, 4 October 1989.
64 "The International Movie Marketplace," *Variety*.

65 "Film Industry Urges Congress to Revise Propaganda Labeling," *Variety*, 4 April 1990.
66 "The International Movie Marketplace," *Variety*.
67 See CBS Inc., "Trade Barriers to US Motion Picture and Television, Pre-recorded Entertainment, Publishing and Advertising Industries," September 1984 (reprinted in *International Satellite and Cable Television: Resource Manual for the Fourth Biennial Communications Law Symposium*, University of California, 1985, pp. 238–59); US Congress, Joint Economic Committee, Subcommittee on Trade, Productivity, and Economic Growth, *International Piracy Involving Intellectual Property*, Hearings, 99th Cong., 2d. Sess., 31 March 1985; and Motion Picture Export Association, "Trade Barriers to Exports of U.S. Filmed Entertainment: A Report of the United States Trade Representative," February 1991.
68 See Baharuddin Aziz, "ASEAN Copyright Law: US Intellectual Property Interests in the Information Age – Political Economic Analysis," unpublished Ph. D. dissertation, University of Oregon, August 1990. For more on the proliferation of video technology internationally, see Douglas A. Boyd, Joseph D. Straubhaar, and John A. Lent, *Videocassette Recorders in the Third World*, New York: Longman, 1989.
69 See Jong-Hyun Lee, "A Political Economic Study of the Korean Film Industry," unpublished Master's thesis, University of Oregon, June 1989.
70 Bruce Alderman, "NBC Seeking Global Partners," *Variety*, 13 September 1990.
71 Philip Schlesinger, "Trading in Fictions: What Do We Know about British Television Imports and Exports?," *European Journal of Communication* 1, 1986, pp. 282–5.
72 Pragnell, "Television in Europe," pp. 13–14; Harris, "Quotas are Inevitable."
73 There are over 500 film festivals around the world, although many of the most important ones, such as Cannes and Monte Carlo, are as much film markets as competitive festivals. See "In Quest of a Filmfest," and International Film Festival Guide, *Variety*, 24 January 1990.
74 The AFMA reported in their "World Sales" survey for 1988, the following sales by film market: AFM: $308 million; Cannes: $235 million; MIFED: $193 million; compared to $193 million for non-market sales.
75 John Lippman, "No-frills NATPE Cuts the Glitz and Gets Down to Business," *Variety*, 10 January 1990.
76 Alderman, "NBC Seeking Global Partners."
77 Chua-Eoan, "Movie Muscle"; Amy Dawes, "Global Batmania Lifts Warner to Foreign Mark," *Variety*, 28 February 1990, p. 7.
78 Fabrikant, "When World Raves."
79 Dawes, "Global Batmania."
80 Todd McCarthy, "Warner Bros. Intl. Chalks Up 4th Record Year for Rentals," *Variety*, 18 January 1989, p. 13.
81 Don Groves, "Vigorous Rentals Push UIP to $380 Million," *Variety*, 31 August 1988, pp. 5, 37.

82 Alderman, "NBC Seeking Global Partners."

83 Kruger, "Europe 1992 Brims with Possibilities."

84 "Video Flash Covers Homevideo Market as 'Decade of Home Entertainment' Opens," *Variety*, 13 June 1990.

85 Jack Kindred, "West German Distributors Join in Prepping for Unification," *Variety*, 20 June 1990.

86 "The International Movie Marketplace," *Variety*.

87 Deborah Young, "The Big Thaw: It's Started an Avalanche of Deals," *Variety*, 27 June 1990.

88 Coopman, "Euro Entertainment."

89 Lange and Renaud, "The Future of the European Audiovisual Industry," p. 63; Denis McQuail and Karen Siune, *New Media Politics: Comparative Perspectives in Western Europe*, Beverly Hills, Calif.: Sage Publications, 1986, p. 39.

90 "American TV Loses its Visa," *Channels/Field Guide 1990*, p. 47.

91 Helen Guider, "Strange Bedfellows Make Good Biz Sense in TV Coprods," *Variety*, 9 May 1990; Bruce Alderman, "ABC Spells Out Euro Strategy," *Variety*, 4 Oct. 1990.

92 Lange and Renaud, "The Future of the European Audiovisual Industry," p. 64; "Yank-Brit $50 Mil Cable Project," *Variety*, 21 March 1990.

93 Chua-Eoan, "Movie Muscle"; Fabrikant, "When World Raves"; "Time Warner to Help Build Theaters in Soviet Union," *New York Times*, 7 March 1990.

94 Groves, "That's Entertainment?."

95 Dawes, "Global Batmania"; also, see "It's New; It's Colossal; It Even Has Free Parking," *Business Week*, 4 July 1988.

96 Aljean Harmetz, "Hollywood Starts an Invasion of Europe's Booming Market," *New York Times*, 11 January 1990, p. C19.

97 "Disney Announces Expansion Plans," *New York Times*, 17 March 1990; Mike Williams, "French Count Eggs Before MCA/U Hatches Theme Park," *Variety*, 13 June 1990.

98 "20th Fox Forms British Unit to Develop Film Comedies," *Variety*, 9 May 1990.

99 Young, "The Big Thaw"; Kathleen A. Hughes, "Hollywood Turns to Russia with Love," *Wall Street Journal*, 4 June 1990.

100 Harmetz, "Hollywood Starts an Invasion."

101 Garvin, "Independents' Day."

102 Ibid.

103 Alderman, "NBC Seeking Global Partners."

104 Alderman, "ABC Spells Out Euro Strategy."

105 Guider, "Strange Bedfellows"; Deborah Young, "East Europe's Star Rises at Cannes," *Variety*, 23 May 1990.

106 Garvin, "Independents' Day."

107 Don Groves, "Snugly Americans Cozy up to Europe," *Variety*, 24 January 1990.

108   "Movie Moguls Watch How They Play in Pisa," *Register-Guard*, 25 June 1990.

109   Ibid.

110   Joseph D. Phillips, "Film Conglomerate Blockbusters: International Appeal and Product Homogenization," in Robert Allen, ed., *The American Motion Picture Industry*, Carbondale, Ill.: Southern Illinois University Press, 1982.

111   Fabrikant, "When World Raves."

112   Ibid.

113   Chua-Eoan, "Movie Muscle." *Variety* estimated that crime or police thrillers would represent over 35 percent of the box office in 1990. See Lawrence Cohn, "Cop Pix Collar Summer Lineup," *Variety*, 13 June 1990.

114   "It's Back to the Drawing Board as Animation Market Heats Up," *Variety*, 10 January 1990, p. 102.

115   Fall releases included *The Godfather III*, *Rocky V*, *Young Guns 2*, *A Nightmare on Elm Street 6*, *The Exorcist 3* and a sequel to *Chinatown*, entitled *The Two Jakes*.

116   Chua-Eoan, "Movie Muscle"; Anne Thompson, "They're Back!," *Variety*, 13 June 1990, p. 42.

117   "American TV Loses its Visa," *Channels/Field Guide 1990*, p. 48.

118   See Janet Wasko, "Hollywood, New Technologies and International Banking: A Formula for Financial Success," in Bruce A. Austin, ed., *Current Research in Film: Audiences, Economics, and Law,* Vol. 1, Norwood, N.J.: Ablex Publishing, 1985.

119   Don Groves, "There's No Business like Show Business, More Banks Say; Investments Lucrative," *Variety*, 14 June 1989.

120   Chua-Eoan, "Movie Muscle."

121   Kip Meek and Sarah Wilton, "Banking on the British," *Screen International*, 12 May 1990, p. 30.

122   Cryan, Johnson, and Cammarata, "Strategies," p. 3.

123   Kruger, "Europe 1992 Brims with Possibilities"; Elizabeth Guider, "Lawfirm Seeks Niche in Europe '92," *Variety*, 10 January 1990, p. 7.

124   Groves, "Invasion of the Talent Snatchers."

125   A more thorough discussion of the attack on the cultural imperialism thesis can be found in Colleen Roach, "The Movement for a New World Information and Communication Order: A Second Wave?," *Media, Culture and Society*, July 1990.

126   For a scathing critique of the classic studies, see Michael Tracey, "The Poisoned Chalice? International Television and the Idea of Dominance," *Daedalus* 114, no. 4, Fall 1985.

127   Sepstrup, "Transnationalization of Television."

128   Graham Murdock, "Critical Inquiry and Audience Activity," in Brenda Dervin, Lawrence Grossberg, Barbara J. O'Keefe, and Ellen Wartella, eds., *Rethinking Communication, Volume 2: Paradigm Exemplars*, Newbury Park, Calif.: Sage Publications, 1989, pp. 229–30.

Chapter 10 Hooray for Hollywood:
Moving into the 21st Century

1 John Micklethwait, "The Entertainment Industry: Raising the Stakes," *The Economist*, July 1983.

2 Michael Barrier, "The Republic for Which He Stands," *Nation's Business*, May 1991, pp. 54–7; Robert Wrubel, "The Ghost of Glitz Past," *Financial World*, 9 January 1990, pp. 56–7.

3 Asu Aksoy and Kevin Robins, "Hollywood for the 21st Century: Global Competition for Critical Mass in Image Markets," *Cambridge Journal of Economics* 16, no. 1, 1992, pp. 1–22.

4 A recent example of the value of these new income sources was the film *Terminator 2*, which sold rights to video, cable, and television to raise production funds, as well as expecting $20 million in licensed merchandise. See "Conan, the Humanitarian," *Time*, 6 July 1991, p. 57.

5 Lawrence Cohn, "New Economy of Scale in Hollywood," *Variety*, 14 January 1987.

6 Thomas H. Guback, "The Structure and Policies of the Theatrical Exhibition Business in the United States," paper presented at the Conference on Culture and Communication, Philadelphia, Penn., 1986.

7 Tom Bierbaum, "Don't Scrap Breadth for Depth . . . ," *Variety*, 16 March 1988, p. 93; *1991 International Motion Picture Almanac*, New York: Quigley Publishing, 1991, p. 26A; "Production Update," *Variety*, 6 January 1992, p. 10; *1993 International Motion Picture Almanac*, New York: Quigley Publishing, 1993, p. 19A.

8 Average US marketing costs (prints and advertising) for new features was over $12 million, as reported in *1993 International Motion Picture Almanac*, p. 19A.

9 See, for instance, Steven Bach, *Final Cut: Dreams and Disaster in the Making of Heaven's Gate*, New York: New American Library, 1985. Also, interesting insights into the majors' typical distribution of film revenues was revealed in the suit filed by Art Buchwald against Paramount Pictures in 1992.

10 For instance, see Neil Postman, *Amusing Ourselves to Death*, New York: Viking Press, 1985; Herbert I. Schiller, *Culture, Inc.*, New York: Oxford University Press, 1990.

11 Frank Spotnitz, "What's Next?" *American Film*, January/February 1989, p. 33.

12 James Monaco, "Into the 90s," *American Film*, January/February, 1989, pp. 24–7.

13 A point emphasized by Sarah Douglas and Thomas H. Guback in "Production and Technology in the Communication/Information Revolution," *Media, Culture and Society* 6, no. 3, July 1984, pp. 233–45.

14 Cited in Marc Cooper, "Concession Stand," *American Film*, December 1987, p. 37.

15 Examples are the salaries for *A Few Good Men*: Jack Nicholson received $500,000 for his relatively small role, while Tom Cruise got $12.5 million for the film. Meanwhile, Arnold Schwarzenegger was reported to have received a $15 million jet, in addition to his salary, for appearing in *Terminator 2*. See Alan Citron, "The Hollywood that Can't Say No," *Los Angeles Times*, 13 December 1992, p. D1:4.

16 Steve Kichen, et al., "Corporate America's Most Powerful People," *Forbes*, 27 May 1991, pp. 214–89.

17 See Cooper, "Concession Stand."

18 Greg Dawson, "Ted Turner," *American Film*, January/February 1989, pp. 38–9.

19 Spotnitz, "What's Next?," p. 30.

20 Aksoy and Robins, "Hollywood for the 21st Century."

21 Sloan Commission on Cable Communication, *On the Cable: The Television of Abundance*, New York: McGraw Hill, 1971; Ithiel de sola Pool, *Technologies of Freedom*, Cambridge, Mass.: Belknap Press, 1983.

22 Graham Murdock, "Programming: Needs and Answers," paper presented at New Dimensions in Television meeting, Venice, Italy, 15 March 1981.

23 "Watering TV's Soup," *Register-Guard*, 23 February 1992.

24 Leo Bogart suggested the notion of cultural synergy in "The American Media System and Its Commercial Culture," Occasional Paper No. 8, Gannett Foundation Media Center, March 1991, p. 5: "The underlying principle is that the transfer of symbolic messages across media boundaries permits a 'synergy' that makes the whole larger and more profitable than the sum of its separate parts." Also see Richard Mahler, "Movie Spinoffs on TV," *American Film*, June 1990, p. 13, and Schiller, *Culture, Inc.*

Index